Reflux Nephropathy Update: 1983

Contributions to Nephrology

Vol. 39

KARGER

S. Karger · Basel · München · Paris · London · New York · Tokyo · Sydney

Reflux Nephropathy Update: 1983

Volume Editors

C.J. Hodson, New Haven, Conn.
R.H. Heptinstall, Baltimore, Md.
J. Winberg, Stockholm

124 figures and 85 tables, 1984

KARGER

S. Karger · Basel · München · Paris · London · New York · Tokyo · Sydney

Contributions to Nephrology

National Library of Medicine, Cataloging in Publication
Reflux nephropathy update, 1983/
volume editors, C.J. Hodson, R.H. Heptinstall, J. Winberg -- Basel; New York: Karger, 1984
(Contributions to nephrology; v. 39)
Proceedings of a workshop sponsored by the Kroc Foundation, and held near Santa Barbara, Calif., Oct. 1982.
Includes index.
1. Pyelonephritis – congresses 2. Vesico-Ureteral Reflux – congresses 3. Pyelonephritis – in infancy & childhood – congresses 4. Vesico-Ureteral Reflux – in infancy & childhood – congresses I. Hodson, C. John (Cecil John) II. Heptinstall, Robert H., 1920– III. Winberg, Jan IV. Kroc Foundation V. Series
W1 C0778UN v. 39 [WJ 351 R3325 1982]
ISBN 3-8055-3807-3

Drug Dosage

The authors and the publisher have exerted every effort to ensure that drug selection and dosage set forth in this text are in accord with current recommendations and practice at the time of publication. However, in view of ongoing research, changes in government regulations, and the constant flow of information relating to drug therapy and drug reactions, the reader is urged to check the package insert for each drug for any change in indications and dosage and for added warnings and precautions. This is particularly important when the recommended agent is a new and/or infrequently employed drug.

Satz: Satzstudio Frohberg, D-6463 Freigericht
Printed in Switzerland by Thür AG Offsetdruck, Pratteln
ISBN 3-8055-3807-3

Contents

Section III: Long-Term Follow-Up

Section IV: Prospective Trial of Surgery versus Conservative Treatment

Section V: Pressure, Voiding Dysfunction and Treatment

Section VI: Bacterial Infection

Section VII: Tamm-Horsfall Protein: An Unsettled Riddle

Section VIII: Sterile Reflux Nephropathy in the Pig

Closing Remarks

Appendix

Preface

The response to the publication of the proceedings of our last Workshop on Reflux Nephropathy held in 1978 led to the attempt to hold a second one in Athens following the International Congress of Nephrology in 1981. This fell through because of a change in policy of our chief sponsor which occurred too late to be remedied. The decision of Dr. *Robert Kroc* and the Kroc Foundation to sponsor a second Workshop in October 1982 at the Foundation's Headquarters near Santa Barbara, California, was thus doubly welcome. This edition of Contributions comprises the proceedings of that Workshop.

The limitation of the number of discussants inherent in this type of intercourse carries with it the impossibility of overall representation, and selection of new work in this field was inevitable. We followed the same principle as before, deliberately downplaying the important aspect of microbiology, for the expression of which there are many available forums, and concentrating on two main themes. First the factors relating directly to vesico-ureteric reflux itself and the changes that may result in kidney and ureter, with or without associated infection. There are at least 3 large ongoing long-term prospective studies in which the decision as to treatment is being based mainly on radiographic evidence of these changes. And it seems imperative to know the relative importance of the pure hydrodynamic effect of forceful reflux, with or without background Obstruction on the one hand and, of Infection on the other. And secondly on the manifold clinical facets; from diagnosis, through course and complications to the end stages. These facets both transmigrate across the traditional medical age groups, i.e. infancy, childhood, adolescence and adulthood, and also involve several of the separate medical disciplines; general medicine pathology, surgery, paediatrics, preventative medicine, and so on. There is thus no ready-made forum in the national or international scenes in which the many aspects of this disease may conveniently be brought together.

There is no doubt that today in those nations where public health and medical standards are high, reflux-associated kidney disease and its complications have greatly altered in the last 30 years, just as has childhood bronchiectasis, and possibly for the same reasons, namely early diagnosis of fever and the free use of antibiotics. What it used to be like and the effects on it of good medical care are vividly portrayed by the experience in South Brazil described in chapter 5.

There is also no doubt that a small percentage of our own population – mainly girls – still acquire renal scarring of this type, and that some end up with renal failure at an early age, though many fewer than heretofore. Their problems are outlined in chapter 14, and are seen to involve the wider issues of society today. The further story of the famous series of infants identified years ago in Christchurch, New Zealand, is told in chapter 13.

What may be called overt and covert disease in adults are addressed in chapters 8 and 10, and the still ugly incidence of end-stage disease in this age group in chapter 9.

Last time the question of bladder dysfunction in children was raised and is again brought forward in chapters 17–19. The astonishingly high bladder pressures being recorded in infants and neonates suggest that this may be an immensely important area for further research. The simplification of classification of bladder dysfunction proposed in chapters 16 and 18 by *van Gool* et al., if generally adopted, will clarify thinking, diagnosis, and perhaps treatment too, of this problem. So far, their results appear to justify this approach. These infants have so far presented with symptomatic urinary tract infection and can so be detected. Are there yet others which do not and are not? Of this there can be no doubt. Some are unearthed in family searches (chapter 4) and others by a simple questionnaire (chapter 18). But, as so many people confess, a simple means of detecting uninfected reflux is still a major requirement. In this context the discussions on chapters 4–12 mention the identification by ultrasonography of foetal urinary abnormalities early-on in pregnancy. This is at least a practical issue for high-risk families.

New to many will be the enormous diagnostic and follow-up potential offered by radionuclides (chapters 1–3) which may in the future replace many present well-established methods. Assuming increasing importance are plasma renin assays both in detecting the child at risk of hypertension (chapter 11) and in the decision to carry out partial or total nephrectomy in those where it is already established (chapters 2 and 6).

The Tamm-Horsfall protein issue is again discussed in considerable detail in chapters 22–24 and emphasis laid on the technical problems of differentiating between it and antibodies to it. Its pathogenetic significance is still unsettled but its value as a marker in disease processes is becoming increasingly appreciated.

Finally, the controversy of high-pressure sterile reflux and kidney damage in the experimental pig is now decided (chapters 25–27), and the question of a cell-mediated autoimmune reaction to sterile kidney damage once again raised (chapter 27). Whether the requisite bladder pressures to give rise to the autoimmune process are reached in the critical period of the first few months of life in man is still to be decided, but chapter 17 certainly suggests they may be.

There is no doubt that the critical period of the generation of this disease *is* the first few months of life for the majority of children. Renal damage is mostly present by the age of 3 years, and the emphasis of the diagnostic search must now shift again and pass into yet another stage of life and even begin in the neonatal ward, or the home crib or cradle, or even the uterus in antenatal clinics.

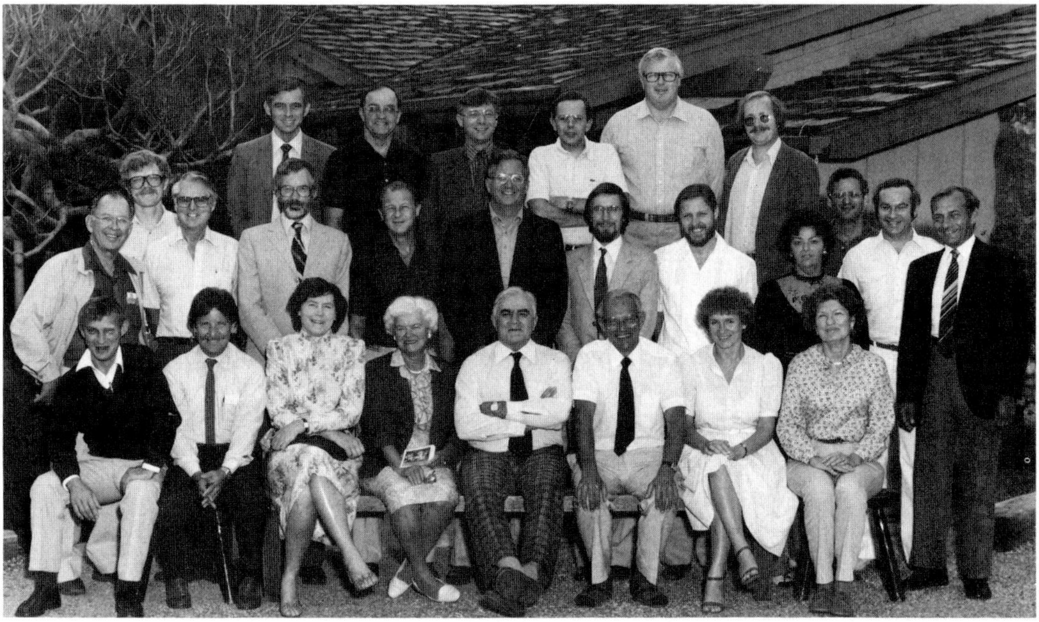

Organizing Chairmen:

Robert H. Heptinstall, M.D.
The Johns Hopkins University
Department of Pathology
600 North Wolfe Street
Baltimore, Md., USA

C. John Hodson, F.R.C.P., F.R.C.R.
Professor of Diagnostic Radiology
Yale University School of Medicine
333 Cedar Street
New Haven, Conn., USA

Professor Jan Winberg
Department of Pediatrics
Karolinska Hospital
Box 60500
S-104 01 Stockholm
Sweden

Contributors

Professor A. William Asscher, K.R.U.F., Institute of Renal Disease, Royal Infirmary, Cardiff CF2 1SZ, Wales, United Kingdom

Peter Avis, Ph.D., Department of Immunology, Health Sciences Center, Memorial University of Newfoundland, St. John's Newfoundland, Canada A1B 3V6

Ross Bailey, M.D., F.R.A.C.P., M.R.C.P., Head of Department of Nephrology, Private Bag, Christchurch Hospital, Christchurch, New Zealand

James J. Conway, M.D., Chairman, Department of Radiology, Division of Nuclear Medicine, Chicago Children's Memorial Hospital,2300 Children's Plaza, Chicago, Ill., USA

Michael Dillon, M.B., F.R.C.P., D.C.H., Consultant Physician, The Hospital for Sick Children, Great Ormond Street, London SC1N 3JH, England

John W. Duckett, Jr., M.D., Director, Department of Urology, Children's Hospital of Pennsylvania, 34th and Civic Center Boulevard, Philadelphia, Pa., USA

Anders Fasth, M.D., Ph.D., Department of Pediatrics II, University of Göteborg, East Hospital, S-416 85 Göteborg, Sweden

Isodore H. & Noemia P. Goldraich, M.D., Centro de Nephrologia Infantil, Rua Marques de Pomtral, 783 Conj. 208, 90000 Porto Alegre RS, Brazil

Jan van Gool, M.D., Department of Pediatric Nephrology, University Children's Hospital, 137 Niewe Gracht, Utrecht 1, The Netherlands

Priscilla Kincaid-Smith, C.B.E., F.R.C.P., Physician in Charge, Director of Nephrology, Royal Melbourne Hospital, Melbourne 3050, Australia

George T. Klauber, M.D., Professor of Urology and Pediatrics, Tufts New England School of Medicine, Boston, Mass., USA

Stephen A. Koff, M.D., Director of Pediatric Urology, University of Ohio State, Children's Hospital, 700 Children's Drive, Columbus, Ohio, USA

Philip G. Ransley, F.R.C.S., Department of Pediatric Nephrology, Institute of Child Health, 30 Guilford Street, London WC1N 1EH, England

Rupert A. Risdon, M.D., Department of Morbid Anatomy, The London Hospital Medical College, The London Hospital, Whitechapel, London E1, England

Stefan B. Svenson, Associate Professor, Department of Bacteriology, National Bacteriologic Laboratory, S-105 21 Stockholm, Sweden

Dr. C. Mark Taylor, The Children's Hospital, Department of Urology, Ladywood Middleway, Birmingham B16 8ET, England

Dr. Kate Verrier-Jones, Senior Pediatric Registrar, K.R.U.F. Institute of Renal Disease, Royal Infirmary, Cardiff CF2 1SZ, Wales, United Kingdom

Richard H.R. White, E.S.Q., F.R.C.P., D.C.H., Consultant Paediatrician and Nephrologist, Department of Nephrology, The Children's Hospital, Ladywood Middleway, Birmingham B15 8ET, England

Acknowledgements

We wish primarily to thank the Kroc Foundation for its decision to fund the Workshop, and Dr. and Mrs. *Robert Kroc* and their Staff at the Foundation for their superb hospitality, personal kindness, and obvious interest throughout the meeting. As Dr. *Donald Whedon* had only been appointed Conference Program Director as of October 1, 1982 an unusual burden fell on both Dr. *Kroc* and Ms. *Bette Heffner* during the formative stages of the meeting, one they bore without sign of stress and with courtesy throughout.

We would extend this thanks for the further promotion of this book which has enabled the Publishers to keep it at a reasonable price.

Particularly also we would like to acknowledge and express gratitude to the projectionist, Mr. *Charles Lawrence*, and to Mr. *Thomas Parker* who so ably taped and subsequently transcribed the discussions. The gastronomists among us extend special appreciation and thanks to Chef *George Greyson* and his staff for their many delicious menus. Rarely can a scientific group have fed so well!

Finally, to our Secretary, Ms. *Donna Lockery*, who has been to endless pains to commit the whole book, manuscripts, and discussions to a word processor, our congratulations and thanks.

Section I: Diagnosis

Contr. Nephrol., vol. 39, pp. 1–19 (Karger, Basel 1984)

1. Radionuclide Cystography

James J. Conway

Department of Radiology, Division of Nuclear Medicine, Chicago Children's Memorial Hospital, Chicago, Ill., USA

Introduction

If one wishes to detect vesicoureteral reflux (VUR) and study the parameters which affect it, then the best method is radionuclide cystography. Radionuclide techniques are more effective than X-ray techniques for detecting VUR but, more importantly, they provide quantitative data relating to the functional parameters which affect it.

X-ray cystography (VCU) has been the traditional method for the detection of VUR. Yet, X-ray techniques are at a major disadvantage since they do not allow the quantitation of parameters affecting bladder function (fig. 1). They are at a further disadvantage since X-ray imaging is primarily a static modality attempting to evaluate a highly dynamic activity of the urinary tract, i.e. the filling and emptying of the bladder.

This presentation is based upon a 12-year experience involving over 3,500 radionuclide examinations. The techniques of direct and indirect radionuclide cystography are contrasted with the traditional X-ray method to point out the major advantages of radionuclide over X-ray methods which mandate its routine use in the initial and follow-up management of the patient with a urinary tract disorder. The aspects of radionuclide cystography which are discussed include the efficacy of radionuclide techniques, the measurement of residual volume, the determination of bladder capacity, the bladder volume at which VUR occurs, the relationship of bladder reflux volume to cessation of VUR and the ability to measure the actual volume of urine which is refluxed.

Direct and Indirect Radionuclide Cystography

Since radionuclide cystography was introduced in 1959 [1], it has evolved into a practical technique for the comprehensive evaluation of

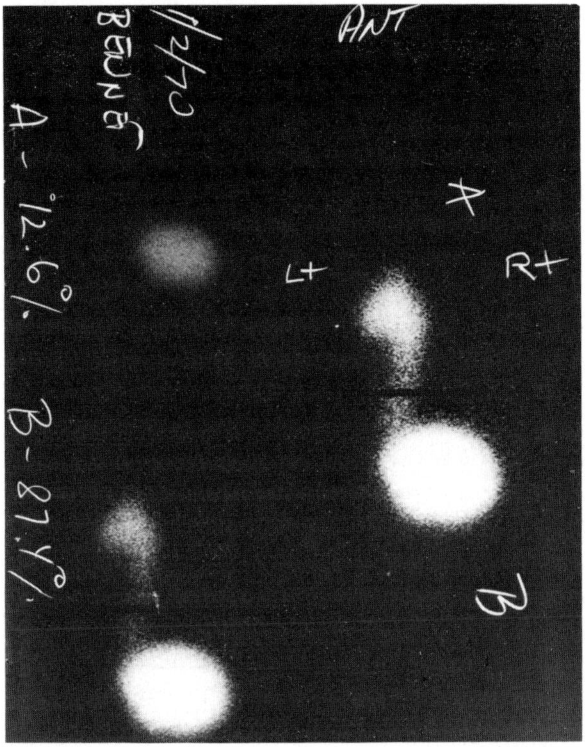

Fig. 1. An early radionuclide cystogram (January, 1970) illustrates splitting the crystal to quantitate the amount of VUR into the upper urinary tracts. Radionuclide cystography lends itself to the quantitation of various parameters of bladder function.

bladder function [2, 5–11, 14, 15, 19, 23]. Radionuclide studies are used for the follow-up management of patients with known VUR and also as an initial means of evaluation in those patients who have a predisposition toward it. Examples are young females with urinary tract infection (UTI) and infants and children with meningomyelocele. More importantly, radionuclide cystography data are accurate prognostic indicators which enable the clinician to predict which patients will resolve their VUR spontaneously [19, 22].

A simple modification of the radionuclide cystography technique also allows one to record bladder pressures during cystography which adds another dimension to the evaluation of bladder dynamics [20, 23]. The radionuclide cystogram, thus, has assumed a significant role in the management of the patient with urodynamic malfunction.

There are basically two radionuclide methods currently in vogue for the evaluation of bladder function. These are the indirect and direct methods of radionuclide cystography.

Indirect Radionuclide Cystography

The concept of indirect radionuclide cystography was introduced by *Dodge* [2] in 1963 and popularized by Handmaker et al. [9] in 1973. Indirect radionuclide cystography is based upon the IV injection of a radionuclide which theoretically is cleared completely through the kidneys within a short interval. Any significant increase of radioactivity in the upper urinary tracts both during or after voiding is due to VUR [2, 9]. The major advantage of the indirect technique is its physiologic method which does not require catheterization [2, 9, 18, 24, 28]. This is a benefit in those patients susceptible to recurrent UTI. Of importance, it has been reported to be as effective as [18, 21, 25, 26], if not more effective, than X-ray cystography in detecting VUR [12, 24, 28].

The disadvantages, when compared with the direct method which requires the instillation of the radionuclide directly into the bladder via a catheter [10, 14, 15], are as follows:

(1) No radionuclides clear completely through the kidneys within a short interval. The rate of clearance is variable from patient to patient due to differing renal function and states of hydration. Patients undergoing radionuclide cystography often have poor renal function, and therefore high levels of background activity potentially can obscure the recognition of small amounts of VUR [10, 18].

(2) The indirect technique evaluates VUR primarily during and after voiding; thus only VUR which occurs with the higher pressures of voiding is recognized. Most VUR, however, occurs at low bladder volumes and low bladder pressures and thus is not recognized with the indirect technique. It is estimated that the indirect radionuclide technique misses approximately 25% of all VUR [15].

(3) Although the indirect method delivers a lower radiation dose to the patient than X-ray cystography, it still is higher than that received with the direct technique [9, 10, 24]. Such radiation dosages are not known to be associated with any significant risk in man; however, a conservative attitude toward the use of radiation would prefer that technique which provides the same or more information for the least radiation dose.

(4) A catheter urine specimen for culture is not obtained with the indirect technique as it is with the direct technique. Repeated catheter cultures of the urine provide a management record of patients undergoing therapy for their urinary tract disorder. There is a significant incidence of unsuspected occult UTI in children who are either on inappropriate antibiotics or do not adhere to their treatment regimen.

(5) Most importantly, the indirect technique does not allow quantitation of data parameters which correlate with the spontaneous cessation of VUR and thus have prognostic management value for the clinician [19, 22].

Thus, the indirect method is more physiologic but is also at a significant disadvantage from a number of parameters.

Direct Radionuclide Cystography

The direct technique has also been described before [13]. A successful study is dependent upon patient cooperation. Critical to this accomplishment is a discussion of the procedure in layman's terms with the child and with the parents. Emphasis is placed upon the simplicity of the study, that there is no pain associated with the catheterization and that any uncomfortable feeling primarily occurs with the complete filling of the bladder. The parent is permitted to remain in the room during the study as long as the child is cooperative. There is no need for consent forms other than the routine hospital consent for diagnostic procedures, since the procedure has been approved for routine use by the Food and Drug Administration.

A Foley catheter is preferred since there is less tendency for the catheter to slip out during filling of the bladder and/or movement of the patient. In general, one uses a number 8 Foley catheter for female infants up to 1 year of age, a number 10 Foley catheter between 1 and 3 years of age, and a number 12 Foley catheter for 3 years and older. In males, a smaller size catheter is recommended and thus a number 5 Foley catheter, or a number 8 feeding tube, is used up to 1 year of age; a number 8 Foley catheter between 1 and 3 years of age; and a number 10 Foley catheter for older boys. The intravesical location is ascertained by passage of urine through the catheter. Since the patient often voids prior to catheterization, urine may not be obtained and, in the female child, the correct placement of the Foley catheter can be determined by instilling normal saline. If the catheter is within the bladder, there will be free flow of the saline, whereas if it is in the vagina, there will be back leakage after instilling only a few milliliters.

Once the catheter is in place, saline warmed to body temperature is instilled up it preceded by a bolus injection of 1 mCi of ^{99m}Tc pertechnetate. It is not recommended that the radionuclide be administered via the saline bottle since only a fraction of the dose will be used in patients with small bladder capacities, in which case it is difficult to generate adequate images.

Essential to the success of the examination is the achievement of full bladder capacity. It has been determined that in each individual VUR is directly related to a certain bladder volume and that in some instances this

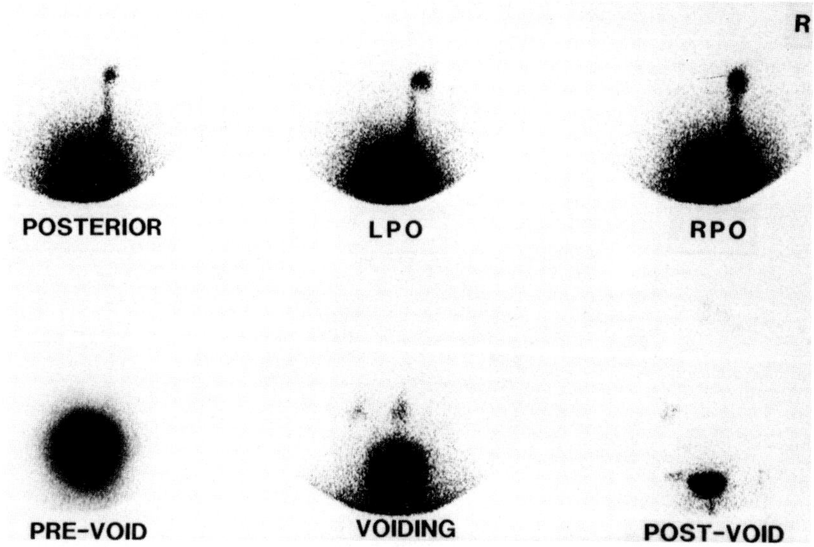

Fig. 2. A typical radionuclide cystogram demonstrating right VUR at low bladder volumes and pressure on the right side, and minimal left VUR during voiding. Of interest, the reflux activity on the left drained slowly after voiding.

volume is maximal bladder capacity [19, 22]. There are some signs which are helpful in determining when the latter is reached. Among these are: (1) Back-up of fluid in the infusing saline bottle and tubing. (2) Voiding around the catheter. (3) Patient protestation. (4) Exceeding the expected bladder capacity.

The normal full bladder capacity increases with age and correlates well with the following formula:

Normal bladder capacity (ounces) = age (years) + 2.

Such correlation has not only been observed in children with clinical bladder dysfunction, but also in infrequent, as well as frequent voiders [30].

Permanent images are recorded at bladder capacity and in the posterior and posterior-oblique projections (fig. 2). The patient then sits and voids into a bed pan or urinal while additional imaging of the upper urinary tracts is obtained at a high sensitivity setting to detect even small volumes of VUR which may occur during the higher pressures of voiding. The observed data are entered onto a worksheet (fig. 3) for subsequent calculation and reporting.

Name: ______________________________

Hospital number: ______________________________

Date: ______________________________

Dose: ______________________________

Right reflux at ____________________ ml

Left reflux at ____________________ ml

Total instilled ____________________ ml

Total abdominal counts: ____________________ Pre-void ____________________ Post-void

Voided urine volume: ____________________ ml

$$\text{Residual volume} = \frac{\text{voided volume x post-void count}}{\text{pre-void count} - \text{post-void count}}$$

Residual volume = ____________ x ____________ = ____________
—

Residual volume = ____________ ml

Bladder reflux volume calcuation

Total capacity = voided volume + residual volume

Total capacity = __________ + __________ = __________ ml

Urine prod. volume = Total capacity — total saline instilled

Urine prod. volume = __________ — __________ = __________ ml

Bladder reflux volume = patient volume + total saline instilled

Bladder reflux volume = R __________ + __________ = __________ ml

3a L __________ + __________ = __________ ml

The Radionuclide Cystometrogram

Recently there has been a heightened interest in the evaluation of bladder dysfunction with urodynamic measurements in recent years. These now include the evaluation of pressures within the bladder during filling and voiding together with the electrical potentials from the pelvic muscles as they relate to micturition. Bladder pressure measurements are easily achieved during radionuclide cystography by connecting a double lumen

Name ______________________________

Address ______________________________

____

____

Telephone ______________________________

Date ______________________________

Hospital No. ______________________________

Age ______ (years) ______ (months) ______

History

UTI yes no Last infection ______________________________

Incontinence yes no

Days – morning afternoon evenings __________ /day or week

Nights – __________ /day or week

Voiding pattern – urgency – frequency – straining

Stream – slow and intermittent

– full and continuous

Bowel movements – ______________ /day

Cystometrogram

Cooperation – excellent fair poor

Catheter size – 8 10 12 fr

Residual urine post-catheterization: ______________ ml

post-void ______________ ml

Bladder capacity: ______________ ml

Sensation, first feeling of fullness: ______________ ml

first feeling of urgency: ______________ ml

Uninhibited contractions: yes no

Reflux:

		Refluxing pressure	Reflux volume	
Left	________	________	________	ml
Right	________	________	________	ml

3b Impression:

Fig. 3.a, b Worksheet for radionuclide cystogram.

catheter to a sensitive pressure transducer and recording device [3, 20, 23]. Four pressure patterns are generally recognized as follows:

(1) The Normal Pattern. This consists of a gradual increase in pressure during filling until a steep pressure increment occurs at near bladder capacity (fig. 4). Of interest, sensations such as fullness, or urgency, are variably related to bladder capacity.

(2) The Spastic-Reflex Pattern. This is characterized by a steeper pressure increment terminating in a bladder capacity at a much smaller volume than expected (fig. 4). This pattern has been encountered in infants and patients with cystitis and often accompanies spinal cord abnormality or injury.

(3) The Flaccid-Paralytic Pattern. This is a very mild increase in pressure, while the bladder capacities achieved are much larger than expected (fig. 4). This pattern is frequently observed in children with infrequent voiding and also in those with spinal cord abnormality or injury. Either the spastic-reflex or flaccid-paralytic pattern may be observed in patients with meningomyelocele.

(4) Uninhibited Bladder Contractions. This is characterized by intermittent pressure peaks which occur during filling of the bladder, when pressures are generally low and volumes are less than capacity (fig. 4). The pressure peaks are unrelated to sensations of fullness or urgency. This pattern is commonly observed in children who have voiding dysfunction.

The radionuclide cystometrogram can be performed without preparation or sedation and therefore is suitable as an outpatient examination. The nuclear medicine study thus provides an inexpensive alternative to the standard inpatient cystometrogram. Studies which correlate bladder pressures, volumes, patient sensations and VUR are currently under way.

Efficacy of Direct Radionuclide Cystography

There are few reports which compare the sensitivity of direct radionuclide cystography with conventional radiographic cystography. They indicate that the former is as effective [4,6–8,11,16,17], if not more effective [29], than the latter in detecting VUR. Even without these reports it would be reasonable to assume that direct radionuclide cystography is more sensitive for detecting VUR than conventional cystography because the

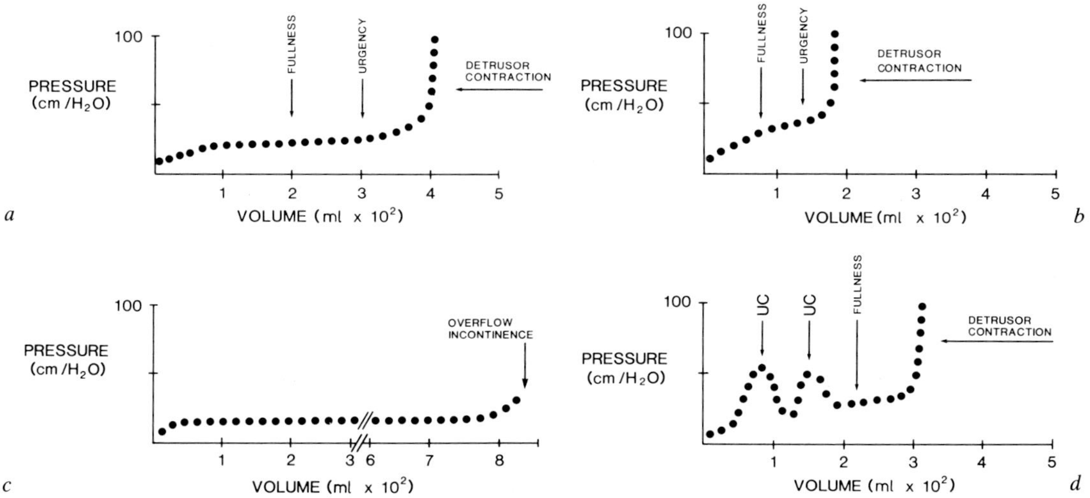

Fig. 4.a The normal cystometrogram pattern demonstrates a gradual increasing pressure increment until near bladder capacity, at which time the limits of bladder compliance are reached and pressure escalates markedly. *b* The reflex-spastic bladder pattern is similar to the normal one except for a much smaller capacity at which the limits of compliance are reached and pressure escalates. This pattern is typical of the infant without bladder control. *c* The paralytic-flaccid bladder pattern demonstrates a prolonged low pressure recording with increasing bladder capacity exceeding that expected. Oftentimes, only overflow and not detrusor action of the bladder occurs at capacity. This pattern or the spastic-reflex pattern is often found in patients with spinal cord abnormalities. *d* The uninhibited bladder contraction (uc) pattern illustrates several peaks of contraction which occur at low pressures and low bladder volumes and without sensations of fullness or urgency by the patient. Uninhibited bladder contractions are often found in patients with voiding dysfunctions.

radionuclide technique allows a longer continuous period of examination. Since VUR is a dynamic process which frequently appears and disappears during all phases of filling and emptying of the bladder, any process which allows continuous recording will be more effective. A number of studies have demonstrated that the great majority of VUR occurs at low pressures and small bladder volumes [27] and, in one study [15], VUR was documented in 23% of the patients prior to complete filling of the bladder or the start of voiding (fig. 5) while in 9% it was demonstrated only during the periods of higher pressure associated with voiding (fig. 6). Since X-ray studies do not routinely view the upper urinary tracts continuously during filling or voiding, and since interest is primarily focused upon the urethra during voiding, it can be expected that a significant amount of VUR is missed by these techniques.

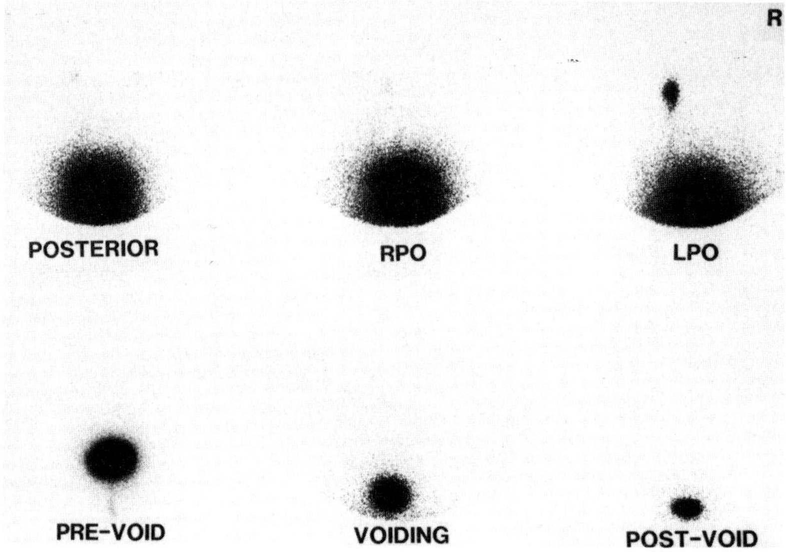

Fig. 5. An example of VUR at low bladder pressure and bladder volumes during filling, which disappears upon reaching the expected bladder capacity. Such VUR was found in 23% of the patients in one study [15]. Any technique which does not study all phases of bladder filling and emptying will not detect such VUR.

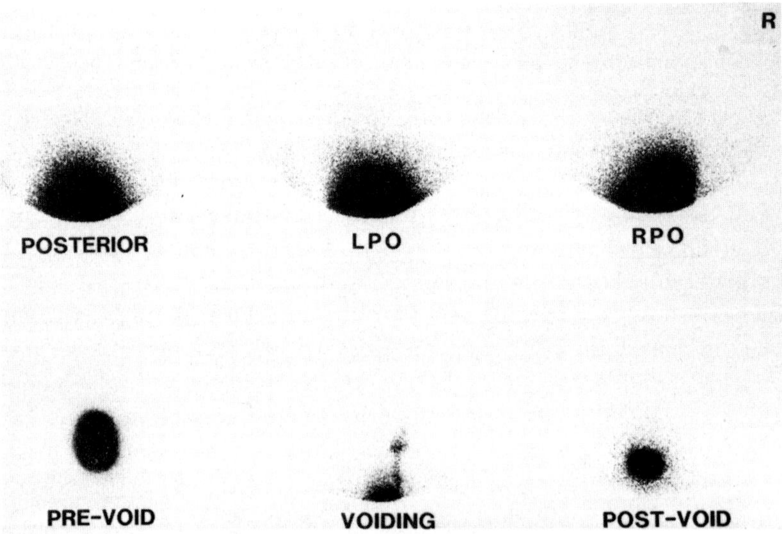

Fig. 6. An example of VUR which occurs only with the higher pressures during voiding. Again, techniques which do not visualize the upper urinary tracts during voiding might miss such VUR.

In those studies which compared conventional radiographic and direct radionuclide techniques, a significant percentage of VUR is limited to the lower ureters (grade I), is recognized only by the former and, less frequently noted with the radionuclide technique [4,8,11,16,17]. This may be due to poorer resolution, but such VUR may be iatrogenic, i.e. related to the contrast material used. As well, grade I VUR is discounted by most clinicians as being of no clinical significance.

Further evidence supporting the greater sensitivity of direct radionuclide cystography over radiographic cystography is derived from comparison between indirect radionuclide cystography and the latter. Unlike direct cystography, the indirect technique is at a disadvantage since it only records VUR during and after voiding [9, 10, 14, 15]. In spite of this, greater sensitivity for detecting VUR is claimed for the indirect radionuclide method than the conventional X-ray method [12, 21, 24, 28].

Thus, at one extreme, one can say that direct radionuclide cystography is of equal sensitivity to the radiographic VCU in detecting VUR, while at the other it probably detects 30% more VUR than the conventional method [15].

Quantitative Information

Residual Volume Determination

Radionuclide cystography lends itself to quantitation of a number of functional parameters. Among these are the accurate calculation of residual volume [33–35]. Residual volume has traditionally been measured by catheterization following voiding.

This is valid except in those patients who have VUR with dilatation of the upper urinary tracts and who have poor drainage and/or stasis. Significant volumes of urine can sequester in the upper urinary tracts, or in diverticula. This sequestered residual volume is not evident with the simple catheterization technique.

The radionuclide technique provides an accurate determination of residual volume. Calculation is based upon a simple dilution formula:

$$\text{Residual volume} = \frac{\text{voided volume} \times \text{residual count}}{\text{initial count} - \text{residual count}} .$$

There is 10% attenuation of photons per 100 ml bladder volume and this is a constant measure, i.e. 100 ml will calculate to be 90 ml. Any large residual volume is of little clinical significance since the patient may have hesitated to empty the bladder completely during the study, particularly in full view of an audience. The residual volume determination, however, can be used to calculate the total urinary tract capacity achieved during the study and the bladder volume at which VUR occurs. The urinary tract capacity is derived by adding the residual volume to the voided volume:

Urinary tract capacity = residual volume + voided volume.

Bladder Capacity

The expected bladder capacity in children has not been well documented. Only a few studies are reported and are in conflict. Perhaps the disparity is technique-related [36–39]. Recent work at the Children's Memorial Hospital [30] has shown a good linear correlation with the formula:

Bladder capacity (ounces) = age (years) + 2.

The importance of determining an expected bladder capacity is to provide a guideline for filling the bladder during radionuclide cystography. One wishes to achieve maximum fullness of the bladder without overflow or voiding around the catheter, since the quantitative data is invalidated by loss of urine. The expected bladder capacity is a goal which one attempts to achieve or surpass during the examination.

Prognostic Significance

The majority of children with VUR will undergo spontaneous resolution over a variable interval of time [40–42]. It would be of great value to be able accurately to predict which of these children will *not* experience resolution, since their recognition might lead to earlier surgical intervention and perhaps a reduction of renal function loss. The decision as to whether or not surgery is required has been based upon criteria which are primarily determined by the clinical course. The evidence of this clinical outcome has hitherto been centered on renal function loss as assayed by laboratory chemistry, a history of recurrent UTIs, and on the changing appearance of the kidneys on IVU. Unfortunately, these parameters are not predictive since both the biochemical and radiographic data must occur prior to their recognition. Thus, in reality, surgery to prevent VUR is more correctly directed to the prevention of additional function loss. Radionuclide cystography in contrast provides the opportunity for an early, accurate determination of clinical outcome, and thus can serve as a management tool before renal function loss occurs.

The individual grading of VUR especially by X-ray techniques is of questionable value since the volume of urine refluxed, and hence its grade, varies during the examination with changes in bladder volumes and pressures. This fact is demonstrated during radionuclide cystography by VUR occurring at low bladder pressures, and/or small bladder volumes, and subsequently disappearing when bladder capacity is reached. It is further substantiated by VUR which occurs only during the higher pressures of voiding. Any technique which does not examine all aspects of bladder filling and emptying will therefore miss both a significant incidence of VUR, and also fail to determine the volume of urine which is refluxed at any given time.

The grading system used for X-ray cystography is subjective and arbitrary. Indeed, as pointed out elsewhere in this volume, there are several grading systems and one can expect grading variations on both subjective and objective bases. For example, in one system grade 2B (filling of the calyces with slight dilatation) and grade 3 (filling of the calyces with greater dilatation) certainly must be considered subjective. Another example of how the grade can change during examination is the common observation of moderate to marked dilatation of the calyces from VUR during cystography which is immediately followed by normal-appearing calyces during the intravenous urography (IVU). This further indicates that the range of calyceal dilatation is very dependent upon the volumes and pressures achieved during filling and emptying of the bladder. The continuously changing relationship of pressures and volume within the bladder will result in a continuously changing volume of VUR during the examination and, depending upon when the X-rays are exposed, will determine the grade observed. Since most X-ray cystography studies evaluate the upper urinary tracts only after the bladder has been completely filled and after voiding, one should expect a limited success in recognizing VUR, let alone its maximum volume. The grading of VUR with this modality, as a consequence, may be of less significance than other parameters, such as the bladder volume and pressure at which VUR occurs [19, 22] or the time it takes for the refluxed urine to return to the bladder [27]. Such parameters and their significance are currently being evaluated.

One of them, the bladder volume at which VUR occurs during radionuclide cystography, is of significant prognostic value with regard to spontaneous resolution of VUR [19, 22]. 39 children with documented

VUR who had been examined with radionuclide cystography on 2 or more occasions over a 5-year interval were retrospectively evaluated for their clinical, laboratory and roentgenographic evidence of VUR resolution, and this was correlated with the bladder volume at which VUR occurred. A direct correlation (93%) between an *increase* in the bladder volume at which VUR occurred was observed in the clinically stable group. [This is *not* the same as maximum bladder capacity – *Editor*.] In the clinically unstable group there was a 77% correlation of *unchanged or decreasing* bladder volume at which VUR occurred.

The quantitative radionuclide cystogram provides an objective as opposed to subjective data base for management of patients with VUR. A much earlier decision regarding surgery can be reached, resulting in less renal function loss. Conversely, recognition of a trend predicting spontaneous resolution will obviate unnecessary surgery.

Thus, it is reasonable to perform radionuclide cystography during the initial evaluation of the patient with a urologic disorder. There is no question that X-ray cystography offers greater anatomic detail but it lacks the capability of functional information which assists in management decisions. The use of radionuclide cystography is particularly reasonable in patient groups who are susceptible to VUR such as the infant with meningomyelocele or children with functional bladder disorders.

Complications

Since 1970, approximately 3,500 radionuclide cystograms and cystometrograms were performed at the Children's Memorial Hospital. In that period, very few complications occurred. On a few occasions minor hematuria was observed during the first void following the procedure, and there were approximately 6 instances of documented cystitis seemingly related to the examination. This low incidence of complication and/or symptomatic UTI is surprising since many of the children had chronic occult UTI which was documented by urine cultures obtained during the study. The low incidence of symptomatic UTI is probably related to prophylactic antibiotics which are commonly administered to children being followed for urinary tract abnormality.

Mucosal disruption of the urinary tract is a possibility since occasionally significant levels of absorbed radionuclide can be recognized in the patient's blood following the examination. The stomach may even faintly visualize with the absorbed ^{99m}Tc pertechnetate on delayed imaging. Absorption of the radionuclide was particularly associated with patients who were

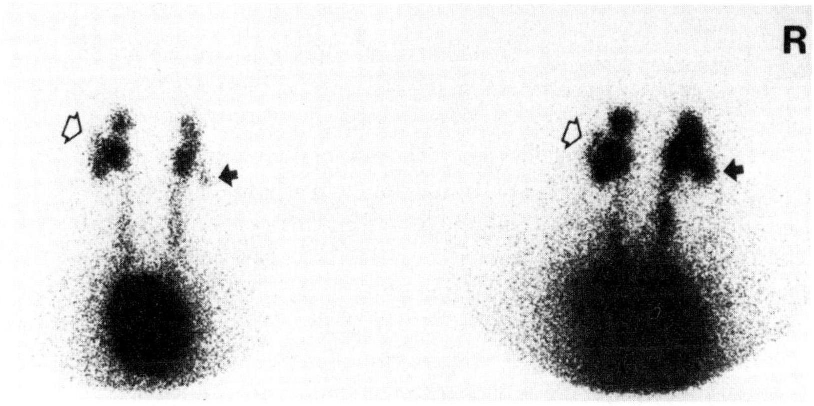

Fig. 7. The scintigrams suggest extension of radioactivity from the calyceal system (open and closed arrows) which might represent evidence of IRR. A later image, on the right, however, demonstrates a structure (closed arrow) having the appearance of a calyx which on the earlier image was only partially filled. The inherent resolution of scintigrams has prohibited the accurate identification of IRR. That such a phenomenon occurs is supported by a greater incidence of absorption of radionuclide into the blood stream by patients who have VUR as opposed to those who do not [8].

cystoscoped immediately prior to the study. There is also a higher incidence of absorption of radionuclide in those children who demonstrate VUR. In our initial report on radionuclide cystography, 8 of 16 (50%) blood samples in children with VUR and 8 of 40 (20%) blood samples in children without VUR had blood radioactivity levels significantly above background [8]. This suggests that some leakage of urine frequently occurs from the upper urinary tracts in patients with VUR and may provide circumstantial evidence of intrarenal reflux (IRR) in the kidney (fig. 7). Unfortunately, the current imaging resolution of gamma cameras mitigates against the actual demonstration of IRR with scintigraphy although this has been reported to occur in the pig kidney [16]. It has been suggested that retention of ^{99m}Tc sulfur colloid in the kidneys may be related to pyelolymphatic drainage [11].

Rupture or extravasation of radionuclide from the urinary tract has not been observed during radionuclide cystography, although bladder pressures in excess of 80 cm of water are frequently recorded during the examination.

Dosimetry

The radiation dose received from a diagnostic procedure should be of concern in those patients requiring repeated urologic studies and especially since most of these studies are performed in childhood. Traditionally, X-ray cystography has been the method of choice for the detection of VUR. X-ray techniques, however, allow only a brief interval viewing of the bladder and thus depict the dynamic functional aspects of the bladder in a static manner. X-ray fluoroscopy can be added to provide a better evaluation of the dynamic nature of VUR but only at the expense of considerably increased radiation burden to the patient. Depending upon the X-ray technique, the number of films obtained, the use of fluoroscopy, screen-film combinations, patient size and collimation, the radiation dose to the gonads of the child from X-ray ranges from 130 mrad to several rad per examination [31, 32]. Of concern is the performance of these studies on a sporadic basis in institutions that do not routinely deal with children. A persistent fluoroscopist and an obstreperous child can result in significant radiation from the X-ray study.

Radionuclide cystography has been estimated to deliver a radiation dose of approximately 30 mrad to the bladder wall over a 30-min interval. Consequently, there is a resultant dose to the female ovaries which is even lower [7, 8]. Less than 5 mrad is received by the male gonads [7]. The low radiation dose from radionuclide cystography is also more consistent from study to study, since the technique is more standardized. Radionuclide cystography is, therefore, a much more reasonable method of examination for those patients requiring multiple follow-up studies. A further reduction of radiation dose is achieved by draining the bladder via the catheter in those infants and children who cannot void on command. If the older child refuses to void following the procedure, fluids should be pushed. It is infrequent that the radioisotope remains within the bladder for longer than 1 h. Frequently, an inability to void is immediately corrected by a little privacy.

The radiation dose from indirect radionuclide cystography is greater than that from the direct techniques but is still generally less than X-ray techniques. The indirect technique is not advocated since it examines the process of VUR primarily during voiding and does not provide quantitative data regarding bladder function.

A comment, however, is in order. The radiation dose derived from any diagnostic study which is prudently performed has never been shown to cause significant genetic or somatic injury in man. The benefit/risk considerations far outweigh any concern for the radiation dose received during X-ray or nuclear diagnostic studies of the urinary tract. A conservative approach, however, would favor that technique which is the least invasive and delivers the lowest radiation dose for the same information.

Conclusions

This presentation is based upon a comprehensive clinical experience from over 3,500 radionuclide cystogram studies over a 12-year interval. The direct radionuclide cystogram has been determined to be as sensitive, if not more sensitive, than other techniques in detecting VUR. It can be modified to measure pressures during filling and emptying of the bladder and thus serves in evaluating functional bladder disorders. It delivers a significantly less radiation dose than X-ray techniques which is a desirable attribute for any test which is used repeatedly and primarily in the pediatric population group. The quantitative data derived during radionuclide cystography correlates well with the spontaneous cessation of VUR and therefore serves as a prognostic management tool. All of these factors warrant its routine use in the patient with a urinary tract disorder. It is recommended that it serve as an initial study in the patient with UTI and it can serve equally well as a screening tool for suspect population groups. Its simplicity allows utilization in any hospital or clinic with standard state of the art nuclear medicine imaging capability. A computer and sophisticated imaging is not required. Radionuclide cystography continues to have an immense research potential for defining the parameters affecting VUR. Radionuclide cystography has already impacted significantly on the practice of urology and will continue to do so in the future.

References

1 Winter, C.C.: A new test for vesicoureteral reflux: an external technique using radioisotopes. J. Urol. *81*: 105–111 (1959).

2 Dodge, E.A.: Vesicoureteric reflux. Diagnosis with iodine ^{131}sodium orthoiodohippurate. Lancet *i*: 303–304 (1963).

3 Aperson, J.W.; et al: The value of the isotope cystogram in determining pressure and volume at which ureteral reflux occurs. J. Urol. *89*: 405–413 (1963).

4 Blaufox, M.D.; Gruskin, A.B.; Sandler, P.; Ogwo, J.E.; Goldman, H.S.; Edelmann, C.M., Jr.: Detection of ureteral-vesical reflux in children with Tc-pertechnetate. J. nucl. Med. *11*: 622–623 (1970).

5 Corriere, J.N., Jr.; Sanders, T.P.; Kuhl, D.E.; Schoenberg, H.W.; Murphy, J.J.: Urinary particle dynamics and vesicoureteral reflux in humans. J. Urol. *103*: 599–602 (1970).
6 Erd, W.; Havranek, C.; Hofer, R.; Krepler, P.: Comparative studies with roentgencystometry and isotope cystography by means of an Anger Chamber in vesico-ureteral reflux. Mschr. Kinderheilk. *118*: 201, 203 (1970).
7 Blaufox, M.D.; Gruskin, A.; Sandler, P.; Goldman, H.; Ogwo, J.E.; Edelman, C.M., Jr.: Radionuclide scintigraphy for detection of vesicoureteral reflux in children. J. Pediat. *79*: 239–246 (1971).
8 Conway, J.J.; King, L.R.; Belman, A.B.; Thorson, T., Jr.: Detection of vesicoureteral reflux with radionuclide cystography. A comparison study with roentgenographic cystography. Am. J. Roentg. Rad. Ther. nucl. Med. *115*: 720–727 (1972).
9 Handmaker, H.; McRae, J.; Buck, E.G.: Intravenous radionuclide voiding cystography (IRVC). An atraumatic method of demonstrating vesicoureteral reflux. Radiology *108*: 703–705 (1973).
10 Conway, J.J.; Belman, A.B.; Kling, L.R.: Direct and indirect radionuclide cystography. Semin. nucl. Med. *4*: 197–211 (1974).
11 Servadio, C.; Nissenhorn, I.; Baron, J.: Radioisotope cystography using ^{99m}Tc sulfur colloid for the detection and study of vesicoureteral reflux. J. Urol. *111*: 750–754 (1974).
12 Hahn, V.K.; Eifsner, D.; Kerkmann, D.; Grimm, W.; Eisen, M.; Straub, E.: Die katheterlose Isotopenrefluxpruing mit ^{99m}Tc-Eisen-Komplex. Fortschr. Roentgenstr. *123*: 321–324 (1975).
13 Weiss, S.; Conway, J.J.: The technique of direct radionuclide cystography. Appl. Radiol. *4*: 133–137 (1975).
14 Conway, J.J.; Belman, A.B.; King, L.R.; Filmer, R.B.: Direct and indirect radionuclide cystography. J. Urol *113*: 689–693 (1975).
15 Conway, J.J.; Kruglik, G.D.: Effectiveness of direct and indirect radionuclide cystography in detecting vesicoureteral reflux. J. nucl. Med. *17*: 81–83 (1976).
16 Rothwell, D.L.; Constable, A.R.: Radionuclide cystography in the management of vesico-ureteric reflux. Br. J. Urol. *49*: 621–627 (1977).
17 Rothwell, D.L.; Constable, A.R.; Albrecht, M.: Radionuclide cystography in the investigation of vesicoureteral reflux in children. Lancet *May*: 1072–1074 (1977).
18 Hedman, J.K.; Kempi, M.; Voss, H.: Measurement of vesicoureteral reflux with intravenous ^{99m}Tc-DTPA compared to radiographic cystography. Radiology *126*: 205–208 (1978).
19 Nasrallah, P.F.; Conway, J.J.; King, L.R.; Belman, A.B.; Weiss, S.: Quantitative nuclear cystogram: an aid in determining spontaneous resolution of vesicoureteral reflux. Urology *12*: 654–658 (1978).
20 Maizel, M.; Weiss, S.; Conway, J.J.; Firlit, C.F.: The cystometric nuclear cystogram. AUA Courses in Urol. *1*: 239–245 (1979).
21 Merrick, M.V.; Uttley, W.S.; Wild, R.: A comparison of two techniques of detecting vesico-ureteric reflux. Br. J. Radiol. *52*: 792–795 (1979).
22 Nasrallah, P.F.; Conway, J.J.; King, L.R.; Belman, A.B.; Weiss, S.: The quantitative nuclear cystogram: an aid in determining the spontaneous resolution of vesicoureteral reflux. Trans. Am. Ass. Genito-Urinary Surg. *70*: 52–54 (1979).
23 Maizels, M.; Weiss, S.; Conway, J.J.; Firlit, C.F.: The cystometric nuclear cystogram. J. Urol. *121*: 203–205 (1979).

24 Pollet, J.E.; Sharp, P.F.; Smith, F.W.: Radionuclide imaging for vesico-ureteral reflux using intravenous ^{99m}Tc DTPA. Pediatr. Radiol. *8*: 165–167 (1979).

25 Meller, S.T.; Ward, B.C.H.; Eckstein, H.B.: Radionuclide cystography vs. micturating cysto-urethrography for diagnosing vesico-ureteric reflux in children. Br. J. Radiol. *53*: 262–263 (1980).

26 Merrick, M.V.; Wild, S.R.; Uttley, W.S.: Radionuclide cystography vs. micturating cysto-urethrography for diagnosing vesico-ureter reflux in children. Br. J. Radiol. *53*: 263 (1980).

27 Nissenkorn, I.; Gil, I.; Servadio, C.; Lubin, E.: Radionuclide cystography: the significance of retention time of the refluxed radioisotope. J. Urol. *126*: 448–451 (1981).

28 Pollet, J.E.; Sharp, P.F.; Smith, F.W.; Davidson, A.I.; Miller, S.S.: Intravenous radionuclide cystography for the detection of vesicorenal reflux. J. Urol. *125*: 75–78 (1981).

29 Nassrallah, P.F.; Nara, S.; Crawford, J.: Clinical applications of nuclear cystography. J. Urol. *128*: 550–553 (1982).

30 Berger, R.M.; Maizels, M.; Moran, G.G.; Conway, J.J.; Firlit, C.F.: Bladder capacity (ounces) = age (years) + 2 – predicts normal bladder capacity and aids diagnosis of abnormal voiding patterns. J. Urol. (accepted for publication, 1983).

31 Fendel, H.: Radiation exposure due to urinary tract disease. Prog. pediat. Radiol., vol. 3, 116–135 (Karger, Basel 1970).

32 Kaude, J.V.; Lorenz, E.; Reed, J.M.: Gonad dose to children in voiding urethrocystography performed with 70-mm image intensifier fluorography. Radiology *92*: 771–774 (1969).

33 Mulrow, P.J.; Havos, A.; Buchanan, D.L.: Measurement of residual urine with ^{131}I-labeled diodrast. J. Lab. clin. Med. *57*: 109 (1961).

34 Rosenthal, L.: Residual urine determination by roentgenographic and isotope means. Radiology *80*: 454 (1963).

35 Strauss, B.S.; Blaufox, M.D.: Estimation of residual urine and urine flow rates without urethral catheterization. J. nucl. Med. *11*: 81 (1970).

36 Starfield, B.: Functional bladder capacity in enuretic and non-enuretic children. J. Pediat. *5*: 557 (1982).

37 Muellner, S.T.: Development of urinary control in children. J. Am. med. Ass. *1972*: 7256 (1960).

38 Hallman, N.: On the ability of enuretic children to hold urine. Acta paediat. belg. scand. *39*: 87 (1950).

39 Esperanca, M.; Gerrard, J.W.: Nocturnal enuresis: studies in bladder function in normal children and enurethics. Can. med. Ass. J. *101*: 324 (1969).

40 King, L.R.: Current management of vesicoureteral reflux in infants and children. J. C. E. Urol. *1977*: 15–32.

41 Edwards, D.; Normand, I.C.S.; Prescod, N.; Smellie, J.M.: Disappearance of vesicoureteric reflux during long-term prophylaxis of urinary tract infection in children. Br. Med. J. *ii*: 285–288 (1977).

42 Wachsman, J.; Anderson, E.E.; Glenn, J.F.: Management of vesicoureteral reflux. J. Urol. *119*: 814–816 (1978).

James J. Conway, MD, Chairman, Department of Radiology,
Division of Nuclear Medicine, Chicago Children's Memorial Hospital,
2300 Children's Plaza, Chicago, IL 60614 (USA)

Contr. Nephrol., vol. 39, pp. 20–27 (Karger, Basel 1984)

2. ^{99m}Tc-DMSA Scanning and Segmental Renal Vein Renin Estimations in Children with Renal Scarring[1]

Michael J. Dillon, Isky Gordon, Vanita Shah

Renal Unit and Department of Radiology, The Hospital for Sick Children, London, England

Introduction

The commonest cause of severe hypertension in childhood is coarse renal scarring secondary to urinary tract infection (UTI) and vesico-ureteric reflux (VUR). Decisions concerning management are dependent on the degree of the hypertension, the extent of the scarring and the potential for surgical intervention. In terms of evaluating such children, intravenous urography (IVU) and ultrasonography provide useful information but have limited value in terms of function and can, at times, fail to demonstrate the full extent of the renal pathology. However, a combination of ^{99m}Tc-dimercaptosuccinic acid (DMSA) scanning plus segmental renal vein renin (RVR) estimations have proved invaluable in demonstrating local areas of parenchymal damage and of significant renin release. This paper describes the use of these techniques in 12 children with coarsely scarred kidneys and hypertension.

Patients and Methods

12 children with hypertension and coarsely scarred kidneys were studied. In 9 of these the aetiology of the scarring was considered to be 'chronic pyelonephritis' with preceding VUR and UTI. In 3 children, the scarring was initially thought to be due to chonic pyelonephritis but sebsequently shown to be due to renovascular disease.

[1] This work was supported by the Kidney Research Aid Fund.

All children were shown to be significantly hyper-reninaemic on peripheral venous sampling and underwent IVU and ultrasonography examination. Subsequently ^{99m}Tc-DMSA scanning and main and segmental RVR sampling were undertaken. The latter were performed since surgery was being considered as part of their blood pressure management.

The ^{99m}Tc-DMSA scan followed injection of isotope scaled down on body size basis from an adult dose of 2 mCi. Images were obtained 2–4 h after i.v. injection. Scans were performed on a Nuclear Enterprise Mark V HR gamma camera linked to a dedicated Informatek Simis 3 Computer [6, 8].

RVR sampling was undertaken as previously described [3–5] with 0.5–1 ml aliquots for plasma renin activity (PRA) estimation being obtained from the main and segmental renal veins plus the inferior vena cava below the renal veins. Segmental samples were taken from the upper, middle, and lower zones of each kidney; collected in pre-chilled plastic tubes containing 25 μl 0.3 *M* disodium ethylenediaminetetraacetic acid (EDTA) and transported to the laboratory under refrigeration. PRA was measured by radio-immunoassay of generated angiotensin I [2].

Results

IVU demonstrated unilateral scarring in 4 patients, bilateral scarring in 7 and no abnormality in 1. Ultrasonography was somewhat unsatisfactory but tended to echo the IVU appearances but with some difficulty, especially over the upper poles where rib acoustic shadows made interpretation impossible. The ^{99m}Tc-DMSA scans confirmed the presence of local areas of pathology seen on IVU and in 2 children, patients 10 and 11, showed scarring that had been entirely missed on IVU (table I). The RVR studies demonstrated locally increased PRA levels in blood from segmental veins draining areas of scarring when these could be entered. There were occasions when only a main renal vein, or perhaps one or two segmental veins could be entered in a kidney and hence on these occasions the study was incomplete. However, of potentially 72 segmental samples from the 24 kidneys studied, 63 were successfully obtained. No segmental samples were taken from the right kidney in patients 11 and 12; there was only one segmental sample on the right in patient 7 and two on the right in patient 10.

Representative Clinical Examples

Patient 1. A girl of 10 years presented with severe hypertension, having had a past history of UTI. Investigations demonstrated hyper-reninaemia, and IVU showed a small scarred right and an apparently normal left kidney (fig. 1). Micturating cystourethrogram showed no VUR, and a ^{99m}Tc-DMSA scan confirmed the small scarred right kidney (21% overall function) and the normal left (fig. 2). The renal vein renin studies demon-

Table I. IVU, ^{99m}Tc-DMSA and segmental renal vein renin (RVR) results in 12 children with hypertension and scarred kidneys

Patients	IVU	DMSA	RVR
1	R*	R*	R*
	L–	L–	L–
2	R*	R*	R*
	L–	L–	L–
3	R*	R*	R*
	L–	L–	L–
4	R**	R**	R**
	L*	L*	L*
5	R*	R*	R*
	L**	L**	L**
6	R*	R*	R*
	L**	L**	L*
7	R**	R**	R**
	L*	L*	L*
8	R**	R**	R**
	L*	L*	L*
9	R*	R*	R*
	L**	L**	L*
10	R–	R*	R*
	L–	L–	L–
11	R*	R**	R*
	L–	L*	L–
12	R*	R*	R**
	L*	L*	L*

R = right kidney; L = left kidney.
* Raised RVR; ** = RVR higher than on opposite side; – = no abnormality detected.

strated clear lateralization of renin release on the right side, and indeed to the upper and middle zones of that kidney, with a seemingly normal left side (fig. 3). Right nephrectomy entirely cured the girl's hypertension.

Patient 5. A girl of 9 years who presented with severe hypertension had a previous history of one confirmed UTI. Investigations showed her to be hyper-reninaemic, and on IVU a small scarred left and a duplex right kidney with a normal upper moiety and small scarred lower moiety were demonstrated (fig. 4). Micturating cysto-urethrography (MCU) showed

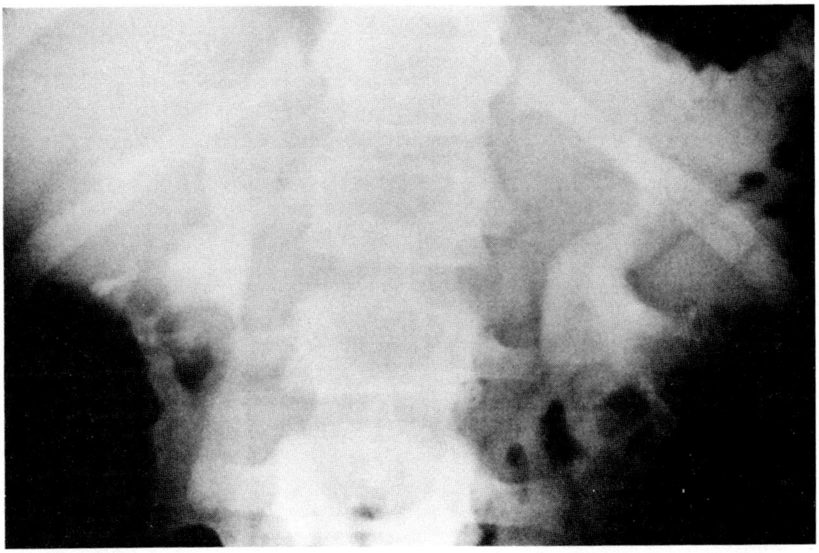

Fig. 1. Patient 1. IVU showing scarred right and normal left kidneys.

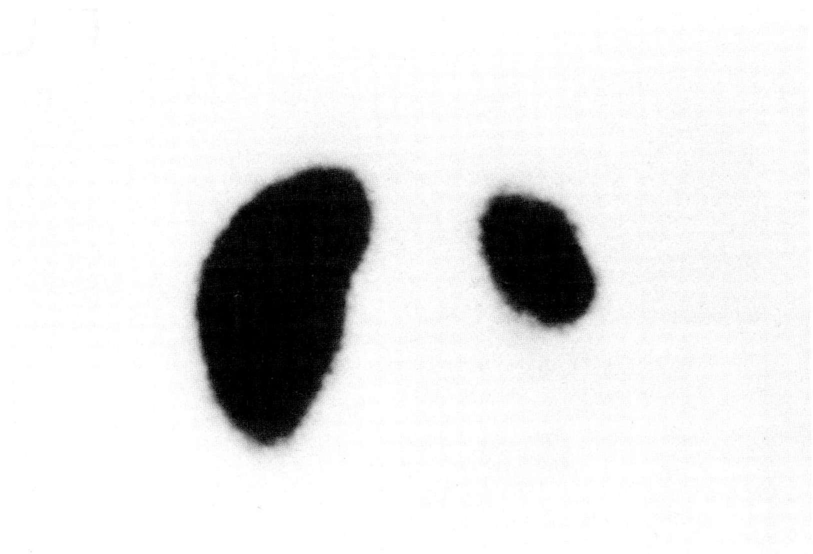

Fig. 2. Patient 1. ^{99m}Tc-DMSA scan (posterior view) showing small scarred right and normal left kidney. Right kidney contributed 26% to overall function.

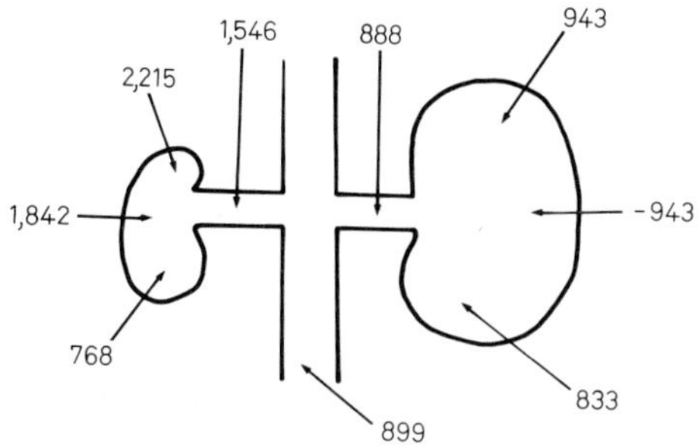

Fig. 3. Patient 1. Main and segmental renal vein renin measurements. PRA (in ng AI $l^{-1}\ h^{-1}$) in main renal veins, segmental renal veins and inferior vena cava (IVC), demonstrates lateralization of renin release to right kidney (right to left main renal vein ratio: 1.74) and suppression of left kidney (left main renal vein to IVC ratio: 0.99).

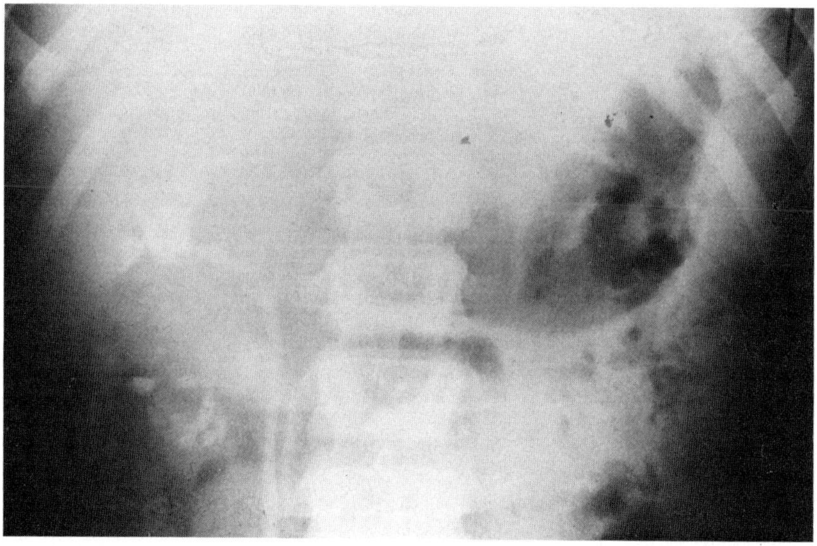

Fig. 4. Patient 5. IVU showing small scarred left kidney and a duplex right kidney with a normal upper and a scarred lower moiety.

VUR up three ureters. ^{99m}Tc-DMSA scan showed a normal right upper moiety and a small non-functioning lower one, with two small areas of isotope uptake on the left side, suggesting a duplex system here also (fig. 5). Differential function was 93% on the right and 7% on the left. Renal vein renin studies showed clear lateralization of renin release to the left

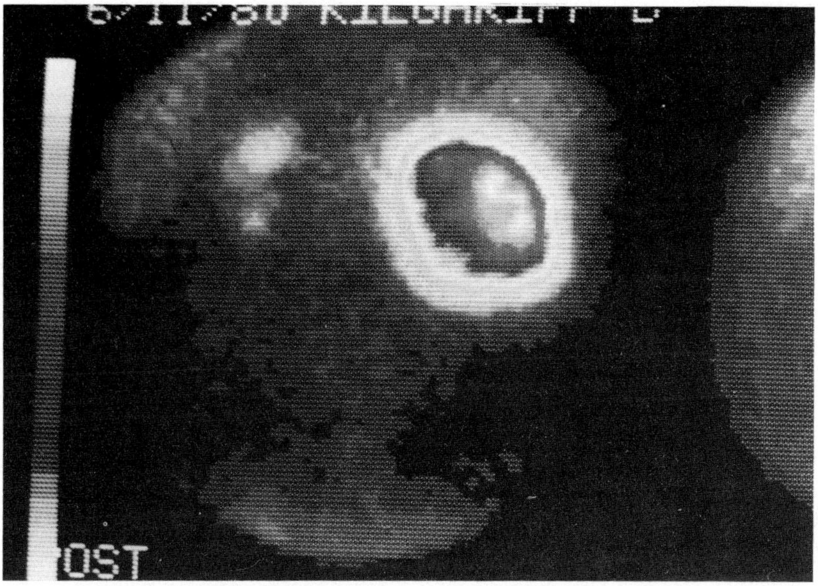

Fig. 5. Patient 5. ^{99m}Tc-DMSA scan (posterior view) showing a normal right upper, but a small scarred lower moiety, plus two small areas of isotope uptake on left suggesting a very small duplex kidney on that side. Differential function was 93% on right and 7% on left.

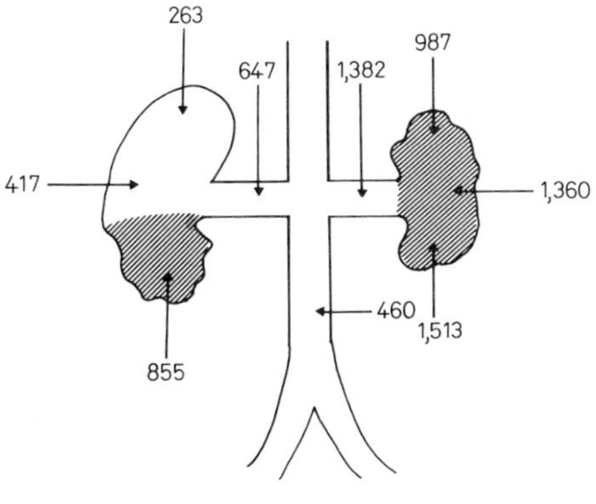

Fig. 6. Patient 5. Main and segmental renal vein renin measurements. PRA (in ng AI l^{-1} h^{-1}) in main renal veins, segmental renal veins and IVC. Demonstrates lateralization of renin release to the left kidney but also defines a local region of excess release in the lower duplex moiety on the right.

side, with a local excess from the right lower pole as well (fig. 6). A right lower pole heminephrectomy was undertaken, with improvement in blood pressure, but this only finally returned to normal without treatment after the left kidney was also removed.

Discussion

This study emphasizes the particular value of the ^{99m}Tc-DMSA renal scan in identifying areas of renal pathology that can be missed utilizing other investigative tools such as IVU and ultrasonography. Furthermore, even when confirming abnormal areas within the renal parenchyma seen on IVU and ultrasonography, the distinction between normal and abnormal kidney tissue, whether analysed by eye or with the aid of iso contours, was particularly striking.

We feel that a normal ^{99m}Tc-DMSA scan goes a very long way to exclude significant renal parenchymal disease and this has important implications when total or partial nephrectomy is being considered and there is a need to demonstrate normality in the tissue which is to remain. The value of ^{99m}Tc-DMSA scanning has been well shown in childhood renovascular disease, except in cases of main renal artery stenosis without intrarenal vessel anomaly [6, 8], where localized areas of ischaemia can be precisely located. Focal DMSA defects may reflect local hypoperfusion because the proximal tubules in the diseased areas extract a smaller proportion of DMSA relative to the adjacent normal parenchyma or, alternatively, local ischaemic tubular damage because the proximal tubules are incapable of taking up DMSA. Its value in identifying areas of renal damage in coarsely scarred kidneys has been previously well demonstrated [1, 7] and may have a similiar basis.

The combination of ^{99m}Tc-DMSA scans and segmental renal vein renin studies when investigating children with hypertension has already been applied in this institution to renovascular disease, where the correlation of ^{99m}Tc-DMSA scan findings, segmental renal vein renin results and arteriographic anomalies was very high [6, 8]. Potential for surgery may be more limited in chronic pyelonephritis. Unsuccessful surgical intervention in terms of blood pressure control is often due to false assumptions about the contralateral kidney's normality when using such techniques as IVU and main RVR sampling. Segmental RVR measurements identify local sources of renin release, eliminate false positive ratios in main veins, and can identify excess renin production within a kidney when a main vein ratio is negative. This, coupled with the ^{99m}Tc-DMSA scan, will allow rational decisions concerning treatment, advocating and, equally importantly, guarding against surgery if the latter is likely to be unsuccessful.

We would feel that no investigative protocols for hypertensive children are complete without a ^{99m}Tc-DMSA scan and, if the diagnosis remains unclear in a patient with increased PRA, or surgery is contemplated, this must be combined with a segmental RVR study.

References

1 Bingham, J.B.; Maisley, M.N.: An evaluation of the use of ^{99m}TC-dimercaptosuccinic acid (DMSA) as a static renal imaging agent. Br. J. Radiol. *51*: 599–607 (1978).

2 Dillon, M.J.: Measurement of plasma renin activity by semi-micro radioimmunoassay of generated angiotensin I. J. clin. Path. *28*: 625–630 (1975).

3 Dillon, M.J.: Renal vein renin determination in evaluating hypertensive children; in Gruskin, Norman, Pediatric nephrology, pp. 127–133 (Nijhoff, The Hague 1981).

4 Dillon, M.J.; Shah, V.; Barratt, T.M.: Renal vein renin measurement in children with hypertension. Br. med. J. *ii*: 168–170 (1978).

5 Gerdts, K.-G.; Shah, V.; Savage, J.M.; Dillon, M.J.: Renal vein renin measurements in normotensive children. J. Pediat. *95*: 953–958 (1979).

6 Gordon, I.; Stringer, D.A.; Bruyn, R. de; Vivian, G.; Haskell, C.; Dillon, M.: Technetium-99m DMSA scan – a sensitive index of renal perfusion in hypertension; in Joekes, Contable, Brown, Tauxe, Radionuclides in nephrology, pp. 205–209 (Academic Press, London 1982).

7 Merrick, M.V.; Uttley, W.S.; Wild, S.R.: The detection of pyelonephritic scarring in children by radioisotope imaging. Br. J. Radiol. *53*: 544–556 (1980).

8 Vivian, G.; Stringer, D.; Bruyn, R. de; Dillon, M.; Gordon, I.: ^{99m}Tc DMSA scans in renovascular hypertension in childhood; in Raynaud, Nuclear medicine and biology, pp. 2663–2666 (Pergamon Press, Paris 1982).

Dr. Michael J. Dillon, The Hospital for Sick Children, Great Ormond Street, GB-London WC1N 3 JH (England)

Contr. Nephrol., vol. 39, pp. 28–35 (Karger, Basel 1984)

3. Radionuclide Imaging of Acute Bacterial Nephritis

James J. Conway

Division of Nuclear Medicine, The Children's Memorial Hospital;
Northwestern University Medical School, Chicago, Ill., USA

Introduction

The clinical presentation of urinary tract infection (UTI) does not usually pose a difficult diagnostic problem. Flank pain and fever, bacteriuria and radiologic changes usually signal the site of abnormality. A positive urine culture and response to appropriate antibiotic therapy further substantiate the diagnosis. However, there are patients, particularly infants, who present less characteristically, and flank pain, fever and bacteriuria may be absent or unrecognized [1]. Frequently, the kidneys appear normal on the intravenous urogram (IVU). The infant may only exhibit irritability or failure to thrive. In some children, fever may be the only sign and in that instance the patient usually undergoes an extensive workup for fever of unknown origin.

The radiographic findings of acute renal infection are well-defined. They include focal swelling of the renal parenchyma, obliteration of the renal outlines, distortion of the calyces, decreased concentration of contrast material or delayed visualization of the kidney [2, 3] and loss of kidney mobility on inspiration/expiration double exposure X-ray films. Focal bacterial nephritis frequently involves the upper poles of the kidneys, an area difficult to evaluate in the child. Fat infrequently surrounds the kidney to outline its margins and gas within the bowel often obscures detail. Various measures can be undertaken to obtain adequate renal definition, but most pediatric radiologists agree that individual cases will defy all efforts completely to evaluate each kidney. The role of the IVU in UTI, particularly in infants and children, has thus been questioned in recent years because of the success of other imaging modalities. These include ultrasound

[4, 5, 7], computed X-ray tomography [4–6], and nuclear medicine [7–11]. This presentation emphasizes the use of infection-seeking and cortical-imaging radiopharmaceuticals. Nuclear medicine techniques are recommended as the method of choice when routine IVU fails to define an abnormality adequately.

Patients and Methods

This study consists of 8 patients examined at the Children's Memorial Hospital from July 1981, to March 1983. There were 7 children and 1 adult ranging in age from 4 months to 19 years, who presented with varying complaints. The most common presenting sign was fever of unknown origin. Several patients complained of abdominal or flank pain. All 8 underwent radionuclide imaging studies and all demonstrated abnormalities primarily characterized by focal or diffuse defects in the kidneys on cortical imaging with ^{99m}Tc-glucoheptonate. 2 patients studied with ^{67}Ga-citrate also demonstrated focal sites of infection within the kidneys. In each instance the site and extent of infection was accurately defined by isotope imaging; 5 of the 8 demonstrated more than one lesion in the kidney or kidneys. Poor renal perfusion, or ischemia, was detected at the sites of infection with radionuclide angiography, and a loss of local segmental function was noted, with subsequent scarring over a short interval. Of note, 2 patients initially had negative urine cultures, although 1 had received an antibiotic 10 days prior to admission for otitis media.

Of importance, IVUs were abnormal in only 4 of 7 patients so studied. Renal ultrasound was abnormal in only 4 of 7 instances, even when the locus of abnormality was known from a previous radionuclide study. Only one study with computed tomography was obtained and that was normal.

Case Report 1

This 8-month-old female presented at another hospital with a high fever of several days duration. The patient had not received antibiotics, an IVU was normal, the urinalysis did not demonstrate bacteriuria, and urine as well as blood cultures were normal. The infant was discharged from the hospital after 2 days with a diagnosis of acute viral infection. Intermittent fever persisted for 2 weeks precipitating admission to the Children's Memorial Hospital. On admission the patient appeared chronically ill with evidence of a chronic anemia. Bone marrow, blood and stool cultures were negative. A ^{67}Ga-citrate scan was performed for fever of unknown origin and demonstrated two foci of abnormal localization in the upper and lower poles of the right kidney (fig. 1). The renal localization was further documented with ^{99m}Tc-glucoheptonate cortical scintigraphy. Ultrasound and computed tomography examination of the kidney failed to define any abnormalities. Suprapubic urine cultures documented 80,000 and subsequently greater than 100,000 colonies of *E. coli*/ml. The patient was then treated with appropriate antibiotics with an excellent result. Cystography was not performed.

Case Report 2

This 7-year-old female experienced intermittent episodes of fever and flank pain for 6 weeks prior to admission. An initial culture grew greater than 100,000 colonies of *E. coli*. She

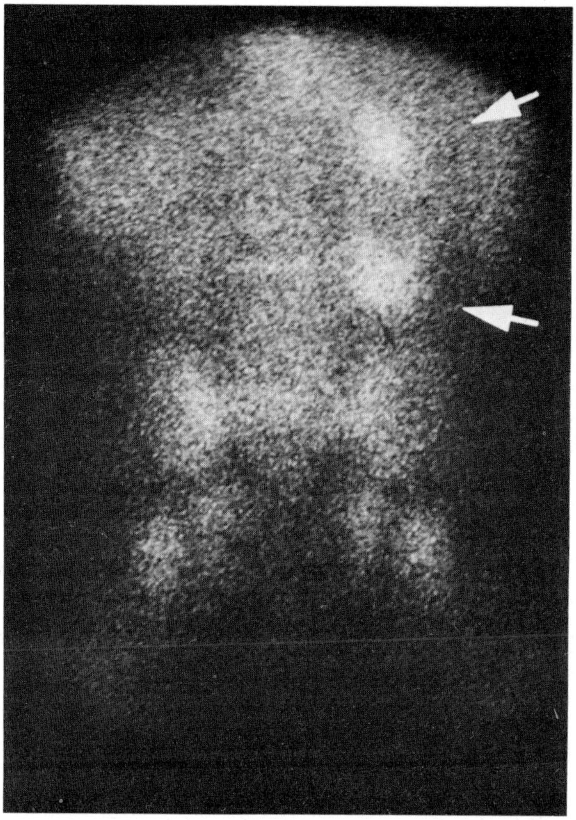

Fig. 1. A posterior ^{67}Ga-citrate image of the abdomen in this 9-month-old female with fever of unknown origin depicts two foci of abnormal localization (arrows) which are in the upper and lower poles of the right kidney.

was treated with oral ampicillin with an excellent response. 2 weeks prior to admission fever up to 40°C recurred at night. Repeat urine cultures again demonstrated greater than 100,000 *E. coli*. The patient was treated with oral gantrisin with good response. 3 days prior to admission, flank pain and fever of 40°C recurred. Upon admission, an IVU demonstrated duplication of the kidney, but otherwise a normal appearance (fig. 2). Ultrasound was also normal. X-Ray as well as nuclear cystograms did not demonstrate VUR. A cortical scintigram using ^{99m}Tc-glucoheptonate demonstrated a focal area of abnormality in the anterior lower third of the right kidney (fig. 3a). She was treated with i.v. Ceftriaxone for 10 days and became afebrile. She has continued to do well after discharge. Subsequent ^{99m}Tc-glucoheptonate scintigraphy follow-up at 9 months demonstrated cortical scarring with decrease in the size of the focal defect in the kidney (fig. 3b).

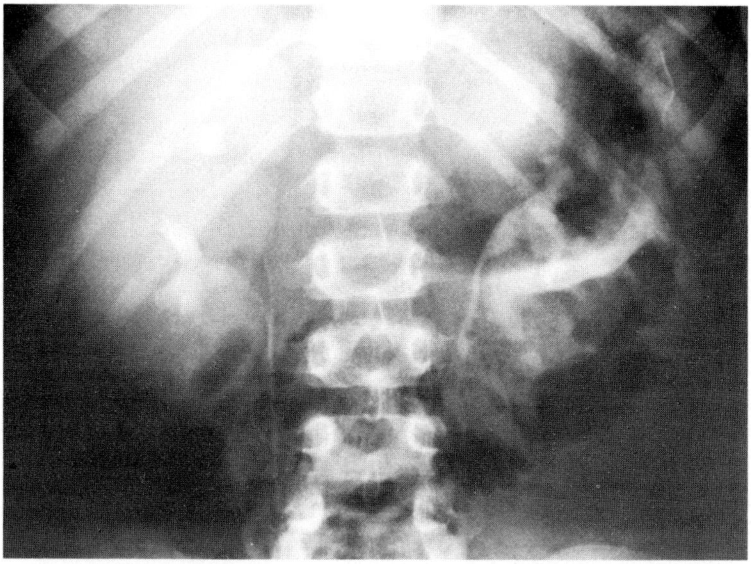

Fig. 2. An intravenous urogram demonstrates duplication of the right kidney but no other abnormality.

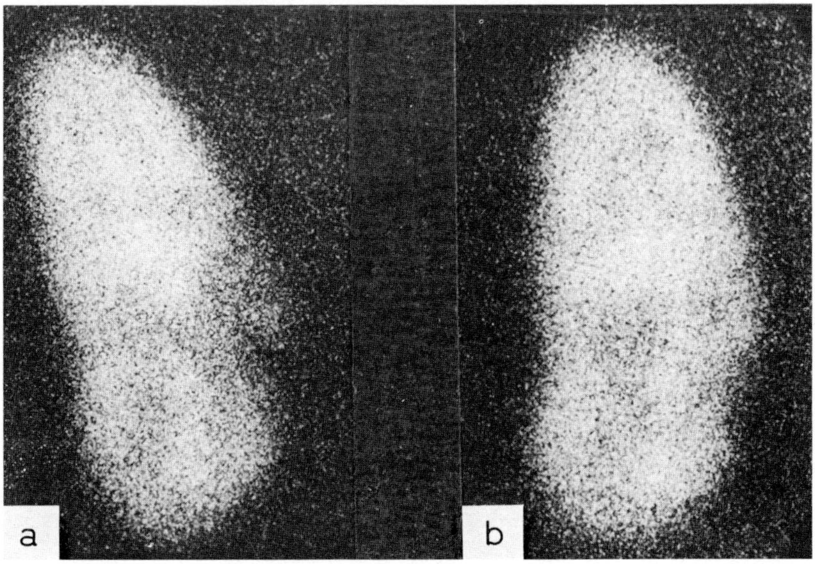

Fig. 3a. A focal defect is illustrated in the anterior mid to lower third of the right kidney on this ^{99m}Tc-glucoheptonate right posterior oblique scintigram. *b* Follow-up right posterior oblique ^{99m}Tc-glucoheptonate scinitgram, 9 months later demonstrates scar formation, with a decrease in the size and extent of the previous defect.

Discussion

It is dangerous to derive conclusions from a limited anecdotal experience. However, the enigma of UTI of the 'focal bacterial nephritis' variety warrants speculation regarding its etiology and evolution. The newer cortical imaging radiopharmaceuticals now available in nuclear medicine provide an excellent noninvasive method for measurement of renal perfusion on a segmental basis, and allow repeated parenchymal visualization to follow the evolution of scarring. The IVU is insensitive to segmental perfusion changes other than those that are moderate or severe. When the remaining function is good, the pyelogram demonstrates the collecting systems adequately. However, focal parenchymal abnormalities can exist, which include contusion, laceration and infection, and which may not visualize on the urogram. Ultrasound has contributed significantly to the advancement of urinary tract diagnosis in recent years but may be limited in its ability to recognize parenchymal abnormalities such as focal bacterial nephritis, particularly in small children. Continued evaluation of this modality to determine its role is recommended. Computed tomography has also demonstrated focal nephritis in adults, but is at a disadvantage because of its cost and limitations as a screening modality and the problem of exposure time in infants. As well examination with and without contrast material, with its inherent increased morbidity, is required.

That nuclear medicine imaging can serve in the diagnosis of acute bacterial nephritis is now established. Parenchymal imaging agents such as ^{197}Hg-chlormerodrin [16, 17] and ^{99m}Tc-dimercaptosuccinc acid (DMSA) [12, 13] have been demonstrated to be effective in evaluating the substance of the kidneys, but with the disadvantage of a relatively higher radiation dose to the kidneys than for other radiopharmaceuticals. Although such radiation doses have not been shown to result in adverse effects in man, one commonly adopts a conservative attitude that prefers the examination which delivers the same or more information for less radiation.

This information can be derived with the use of ^{99m}Tc-glucoheptonate, which received the Food and Drug Administration's (FDA) approval for routine use in 1978. Subsequently it has had limited use for parenchymal imaging of the kidneys in infection. It delivers a gonadal radiation dose which is significantly less than that of IVU utilizing multiple views and/or tomography [14, 15]. Its images, as with other imaging modalities, are nonspecific, since similar findings, namely diminished perfusion and a focal defect within the kidney, can be derived from neoplastic disease. Conversely, demonstrating function within a possible 'mass lesion' indicates its normal nature [16, 17]. A major advantage of renal cortical imaging is its noninvasive nature, which allows serial examination, and which has been shown to be effective in defining the evolution of scarring within the kidney due to focal bacterial nephritis. Patients are easily studied on an outpatient basis.

Our limited experience provides reason for speculation on the etiology and evolution of focal bacterial nephritis in the kidney. 2 patients presented without initial bacteriuria. Sporadic use of antibiotics theoretically might clear the collecting system of bacteria. The interval of treatment and recurrent symptomatology in several of our patients was of such duration that this seems unlikely. In one instance no antibiotics had been administered. The origin of infection by hematogenous routes to bone, heart, brain, liver and other organs is well-established. The potential for hematogenous spread of infection to the kidneys should be considered. Such infection, originating and localizing in the medulla or cortex of the kidney, would result in focal ischemia and loss of function, which is well-demonstrated with the ^{99m}Tc-glucoheptonate studies. A lack of function and urine output might explain the absence of bacteriuria since the bacteria are not washed downstream. More important is the recognition that focal ischemia and lack of function will compromise the eradication of the disease process with routine antibiotic therapy, since effective therapeutic dose requirements may not be achievable in the presence of ischemia. This perhaps is an explanation for the recurrent nature of this disease process, as illustrated in case report 2 in spite of routine antibiotic therapy. As in osteomyelitis, prolonged intravenous antibiotic therapy may be required. Renal parenchymal imaging may thus provide an indication for prolonged antibiotic therapy if ischemia is demonstrated. A rapid return of perfusion and function to the affected area would document an effective therapy regimen.

^{67}Ga-Citrate has been demonstrated effective in the recognition of occult infectious and/or inflammatory processes [7-9]. Normal localization of ^{67}Ga-citrate in the kidneys on early imaging and in the gastrointestinal tract on delayed imaging limits slightly its efficacy. The delay in diagnosis required for ^{67}Ga-citrate imaging is another factor which limits its utilization in the actuely ill patient. Most diagnoses, however, are readily made within 8–24 h from injection of the radionuclide. Localization occurs at sites of infection in spite of immediate response to antibiotic therapy. The examination is costly and technically difficult, particularly in small children, where collimation of the radionuclide limits resolution. As a result, ^{67}Ga-citrate imaging is reserved for those patients in whom the etiology of fever of unknown origin has not been determined by other studies. Early renal visualization with ^{67}Ga-citrate should be expected. The kidneys in children are normally visualized up to 48 h in contrast to adult kidneys, which seldom show up after 24 h. In most instances bacterial nephritis is of a focal nature and is recognized on the early and delayed ^{67}Ga-citrate images as a focal area of increased uptake within the kidney.

When renal infection is known or suspected, the patient should be studied with ^{99m}Tc-glucoheptonate cortical imaging and, if that is unrewarding, then ^{67}Ga-citrate can be injected immediately for imaging on the following morning.

Conclusions

A limited anecdotal experience with cortical renal radiopharmaceuticals and infection-localizing radiopharmaceuticals is presented to define their role in the diagnosis and management of acute focal bacterial nephritis. In the patient with normal or equivocal diagnostic studies, which include IVU and ultrasound, the next study of choice is ^{99m}Tc-glucoheptonate renal scintigraphy. ^{67}Ga-Citrate has been demonstrated effective in diagnosing urinary tract infection when totally unsuspected.

Speculation is offered proposing a hematogenous spread of focal bacterial nephritis in some children and the suggestion made that intravenous antibiotic therapy may have to be prolonged in the presence of ischemia and/or loss of renal function in the area affected. (Dr. Conway now has records of over 20 similar cases, about 75% with VUR. Others are being found elsewhere. Ed.)

Acknowledgement

The stimulation and interest of *Howard S. Traisman*, MD, who referred several of his patients for study, was instrumental in the initiation of this report and its findings.

References

1 Friedland, G.W.: Recurrent urinary tract infections in infants and children. Radiol. Clin. N. Am. *XV*: 19–35 (1977).

2 Davidson, A.J.; Talner, L.B.: Urographic and angiographic abnormalities in adult-onset acute bacterial nephritis. Radiology *106*: 249–256 (1973).
3 Davidson, A.J.; Talner, L.B.: Late sequelae of adult-onset acute bacterial nephritis. Radiology *127*: 367–371 (1978).
4 Lee, J.K.T.; et al: Acute focal bacterial nephritis: emphasis on gray scale sonography and computed tomography. Am. J. Roentg. *135*: 87–92 (1980).
5 Hoddick, W.; et al: CT and sonography of severe renal and perirenal infections. Am. I. Roentg. *140*: 517–520 (1983).
6 Hoffman, E.P.; et al: Computed tomography in acute pyelonephritis associated with diabetes. Radiology *135*: 691–695 (1980).
7 Rosenfield, A.T.; et al: Acute focal bacterial nephritis (acute lobar nephronia). Radiology *132*: 553–561 (1979).
8 Brugh, R., III; et al: Gallium 67 scanning and conservative treatment in acute inflammatory lesions of the renal cortex. J. Urol. *121*: 232–235 (1979).
9 Frankel, R.S.; et al: Renal localization of gallium 67 citrate. Radiology *114*: 393–397 (1975).
10 Kumar, B.; Coleman, R.E.: Significance of delayed ^{67}Ga localization in kidneys. J. nucl. Med. *17*: 872–875 (1976).
11 McAfee, J.G.: Radionuclide imaging in the assessment of primary chronic pyelonephritis. Radiology *133*: 203–206 (1979).
12 Enlander, D.; et al: Renal cortical imaging in 35 patients: superior quality ^{99m}Tc DSMA. J. nucl. Med. *15*: 743–749 (1974).
13 Handmaker, H.; et al.: Clinical experience with ^{99m}Tc DMSA (dimeraptosuccinic acid), a new renal-imaging agent. J. nucl. Med. *16*: 28–32 (1975).
14 Leonard, J.C.; et al.: Glucepate renal imaging. Clin. Pediat. *19*: 615–619 1980.
15 Leonard, J.C.; et al: Renal cortical imaging and the detection of renal mass lesions. J. nucl. Med. *20*: 1018–1022 (1979).
16 Braunstein, P.; et al: Scintiscan evaluation of prominent renal columns. Radiology *104*: 103–106 (1972).
17 Pollack, H.M.; et al: Radionuclide imaging in renal pseudotumors. Radiology *111*: 639–644 (1974).

James J. Conway, MD, Chief, Division of Nuclear Medicine,
The Children's Memorial Hospital, 2300 Children's Plaza, Chicago, IL 60614 (USA)

Contr. Nephrol., vol. 39, pp. 36–39 (Karger, Basel 1984)

Discussion on Chapters 1–3

Dr. *J. Conway*: One of the things that has startled me is the amount of quantitative data that we have already accumulated from these techniques which is not being utilized or understood. For example, since it was my observation over the years that patients who had unilateral vesico-ureteric reflux (VUR) and had the affected ureter reimplanted, often later developed VUR on the other side, we quickly looked through our data last week. There were 59 children who had had unilateral reimplantations, and of these, 22% later showed VUR on the other side where it had not been previously demonstrated. In all of these patients this 'opposite' VUR disappeared within a period of 3 months to 3 years.

Dr. *W. Asscher*: Dr. *Conway*, with regard to the technique of cystography: do such factors as the rate of infusion, the temperature of the infused fluid and sedation have any effect on the result:

Dr. *J. Conway*: We use no sedation whatsoever. We find that most children tolerate this examination, although there are problems with small babies. But what is one to do? Sedation adds a parameter that may change your functional measurements, and any data derived from sedation studies may be valueless. Under the standard conditions of cystography, the infusion rate is related mainly to the size of the catheter.

Dr. *W. Asscher*: Not to the pressure?

Dr. *J. Conway*: It has some relation to pressure, of course, but only when bladder filling is completed. Before this point, varying the height of the infusion reservoir has little effect on the pressure in the bladder. The latter is dictated by the muscular tone of the bladder walls. In other words, bladder wall compliance continues until the full capacity of the bladder is reached, then the pressure rises rapidly and can reach the height of the infusion reservoir.

Dr. *J. Winberg*: Was there a higher incidence of VUR in those children who were infrequent voiders?

Dr. J. Conway: Those data we don't have, but we can extract that very rapidly. That would be very simple to do.

Dr. *J. Winberg*: We find VUR very often in the frequent voiders, even in the absence of UTI.

Dr. *P. Kincaid-Smith*: What do you mean by the term 'reflux bladder volume'? Is that the volume at which VUR occurs?

Dr. *J. Conway*: That is the volume at which, when we distend the bladder, VUR occurs. It is fairly constant in each individual. We have studied patients at short intervals, and if VUR occurs at, say, 120 ml on one occasion it will do so again at the next examination. Obviously, one may consider that there is an anatomic principle involved in this observation and this appears likely, because the refluxing volume changes as the patient grows.

Dr. *P. Kincaid-Smith*: Another point: a couple of years ago some people in our unit did a study that showed the occurrence of VUR during cystography was clearly dependent on the degree of diuresis present. In other words, the grade of VUR was dependent on the amount or urine being formed.

Dr. *J. Conway*: Yes, but I have no data on this point available. High grades of VUR can occur at low pressures and in the absence of voiding. The present parameters, based on ureteral dilatation, are valueless in our experience because these grades are inconstant in every patient. The VUR grade is an X-ray perception obtained at the particular point in time that a film was taken. It may have nothing to do with the maximum grade reached at another point in time.

Dr. *P. Ransley*: Has the change in reflux bladder volume in two studies spaced apart enabled you to predict with any sort of accuracy the likely time when VUR will cease spontaneously?

Dr. *J. Conway*: Yes. We now believe that we can predict, within 6 months, when VUR will end in the majority of cases. Such forecasting is not 100% accurate, because events that affect the patient in between studies are what determine in many instances whether VUR will disappear; e.g. urinary tract infections (UTIs), changes in voiding patterns, states of hydration at the time of examination and so on. There are many, many different factors which affect the outcome.

Dr. *R. Bailey*: Do you rate your technique of catheterization as being less invasive than injecting the radionuclide suprapubically:

Dr. *J. Conway*: I have not used the suprapubic route. I can't imagine that passing a needle into the abdomen can be classified as being non-invasive.

Dr. *R. Bailey*: Well, suprapubic aspiration (SPA) is just so simple in the neonate and infant, and usually less disturbing than catheterization.

Dr. *J. Conway*: I understand. But again, I don't know if we could obtain all the quantitative information, such as the residual volumes, etc., that we get now by our method. And until SPA becomes a common practice in the USA, I don't think we shall be able to compare the two approaches.

Dr. *P. Ransley*: Now we can discuss the relative merits and harmful effects of isotopes used for renal parenchymal imaging. It is an important matter, the question of radiation and the relative diagnostic potential of dimercaptosuccinic acid (DMSA) and ^{99m}Tc-glucoheptonate which are becoming such valuable imaging agents in the care and handling of this type of case.

Dr. *J. Conway*: I don't think that there is any difference in the quality of the images obtained by DMSA and ^{99m}Tc-glucoheptonate. Dr. *Dillon* was discussing their use as functional imaging modalities and perhaps in this glucoheptonate has the edge. But I know of no publication dealing with this point. The relative radiation problems can be overcome by halving the dose and doubling the imaging time. In our hands the dosage to the kidney is about equivalent to a standard urogram, say 1.0–1.5 rad. At least, these are the estimated levels as published in the literature.

Dr. *R. Bailey*: The diagnosis of UTI must surely depend on bacteriology not on any imaging modality. The second comment I have is that we have found isotope studies to give excellent data relating to kidney function as well as parenchymal integrity. As a result, renal function studies based on ureteric catheter specimens have been superceded.

Dr. *P. Kincaid-Smith*: I want to ask Dr. *Dillon* what percentage of the scarred kidneys that he investigated had high renal vein renin levels? He seemed to imply that virtually all of them had.

Dr. *M. Dillon*: In answer, it's fair to say that the only children that were investigated were those in whom we anticipated a possible need for surgery. This was therefore a highly selected group, and all its members had raised peripheral renin or other criteria for a renin component to their blood pressure. But it is true that zones of renin release within a kidney may not be dominant in comparison with other zones, and so give rise to a false negative result.

Dr. *P. Kincaid-Smith*: So virtually all scars in this group of hypertensive children produced excess renin?

Dr. *M. Dillon*: In general that is right. But it is hard to know where scars begin and end. Segmental veins don't necessarily allow sampling from the precise areas the DMSA or other imaging modality is identifying.

Dr. *J. Hodson*: So far we have been hearing of the 5- to 10-year age group. But by this time the damage is usually done. What about imaging a baby's kidneys by isotopes? What about the problem of movement?

Dr. *J. Conway*: Even if our babies don't move, their kidneys do! There is no control over that. One can 'gate' the radiation from a certain area but this greatly prolongs the time required to obtain an adequate image. Both DMSA and glucoheptonate can equally well identify scars and the extent of these has shown a remarkable correlation with hypertension, but of course they do not indicate whether renin is being produced or not.

One further point is that DMSA and other imaging agents have been shown to produce results which bear some relationship to function; although they have a very poor correlation when it is poor and only questionable correlation when it is good. But the preferable agents for functional measurements are, of course, diethylenetriaminepentaacetic acid (DTPA), iodohippurate, and ^{51}Cr-ethylenediaminetetraacetic acid. They have similar results and involve a lot less radiation than DMSA or glucoheptonate.

Dr. *P. Ransley*: In our hands DTPA has been successful in determining renal function in small children with dilated urinary tracts and diminished renal blood flow, particularly in the first few weeks of life, and in following renal function in the first few months of life. But one cannot exclude scarring with either DMSA or glucoheptonate in babies although one may, of course, define it.

Dr. *M. Dillon*: I would support that. I want to take slight exception to the comment that scarring as demonstrated by glucoheptonate or DMSA does not indicate the release of renin from those areas; I am sure the speaker meant that these modalities have no bearing on renin production. I don't believe that release of renin from a scarred area necessarily causes immediate hypertension, but with time it may develop in some cases. There may be increased renin being released that one can identify, but it may not be enough to cause hypertension. I have evidence that renin behaves differently in children with scarred kidneys and normal blood pressure than in children who have normal kidneys.

Dr. *P. Ransley*: Another matter that has been touched on today is the question of renal surgery for scarring. We have had success with a number of Dr. *Dillon*'s patients and have relieved their hypertension. But this is an area the exploration of which is only just beginning. Simple procedures like nephrectomy on one side and heminephrectomy on the other are already straightforward. But we may now be advancing to the stage when we are able to offer segmental scar excision in order to control hypertension?

Dr. *W. Asscher*: Dr. *Dillon*, do you do any other workup, other than radiology, isotope imaging and renin estimations, before you decide on surgery?

Dr. *M. Dillon*: We are now quite convinced about the value of peripheral renins in treating hypertension. Our previous experience showed that a peripheral renin assay under controlled conditions was extremely helpful in defining a renin-dependent situation. In a non-treated child, if we have doubts, we have used the response to either saralasin or captopril. We sometimes found this helpful. But in general we tend to use the peripheral renin level compared with our normal range as our identifying factor.

Dr. *J. Winberg*: Dr. *Conway*, I was fascinated to see your slides of children with acute pyelonephritis. Have you ever seen such big lesions heal completely if they are properly and promptly treated?

Dr. *J. Conway*: I have not enough experience to answer that question reliably.

Dr. *R. Bailey*: We've certainly shown that.

Dr. *P. Ransley*: That they can heal completely? That type of lesion, with the large circumscribed ischemic area?

Dr. *R. Bailey*: Yes, histologically it is typical of acute pyelonephritis; a focal lesion of the kidney.

Dr. *J. Hodson*: And it heals completely?

Dr. *R. Bailey*: Usually.

Dr. *P. Ransley*: As shown by DMSA or intravenous urography (IVU)?

Dr. *R. Bailey*: IVU mainly, but also by DMSA and computerized tomography which gives even better images.

Dr. *J. Winberg*: That is certainly the clinical impression and it is very valuable to have it demonstrated.

Dr. *P. Ransley*: I don't think that in children I've seen a large lesion like this heal without leaving some trace behind on the DMSA scan.

Dr. *J. Conway*: In a comparison study between DMSA scans and IVUs by Dr. *McAfee*'s group in Cleveland on adult patients, all in this group returned to normal [Radiology *133*: 203–206, 1979].

Dr. *P. Ransley*: This has been a mind-boggling session because, in the first half, we turned the conventions upside down and showed that totally new criteria were now indicated for assessing VUR and predicting its consequences. And in the second half we have been shown a new imaging approach which makes it difficult to maintain any enthusiasm for the results of the studies of VUR and reflux nephropathy over the last 25 or 30 years.

Section II: Clinical Aspects

Contr. Nephrol., vol. 39, pp. 40–51 (Karger, Basel 1984)

4. Familial and Genetic Data in Reflux Nephropathy

Ross R. Bailey, Edward Janus, Kevin McLoughlin, Kelvin L. Lynn, George D. Abbott

Departments of Nephrology, Pediatrics and Immunohematology, Christchurch Hospital, Christchurch, New Zealand

Primary vesico-ureteric reflux (VUR) is a congenital lesion, and in some instances is familial and inherited. In this study we have documented our own and the published familial and genetic data for patients with VUR and reflux nephropathy (RN).

Family Studies

Introduction

Since *Stephens* et al. [1] reported VUR in identical twins there have been several further sets of identical twins documented [2–6]. At the Bermuda Workshop on Reflux Nephropathy *Heale* et al. [7] reported on a study undertaken in this hospital between 1969 and 1971 on 15 families with RN. These 15 families came to attention on casual enquiry of 213 patients investigated with RN. Radiologic abnormalities of the urinary tract were found in 67 (38%) of 175 relatives of the 15 propositi. In 12 of these 15 families there was a hereditary pattern, suggesting an autosomal dominant inheritance with variable penetrance. There was no evidence that VUR was sex-linked.

At the same workshop [8] I briefly reported on 56 further families investigated in Christchurch since 1971 and noted that in 17 (30%) of these families there were one or more affected members. A positive family history was more frequent (50%) in those families where the propositus had renal failure. In 15 of the 17 families there was transmission across a generation.

Table I. Summary of 88 families investigated

Group	Number of families investigated	Number of family members investigated (excluding propositus)	Number of families affected	
			n	%
Requiring renal replacement therapy	18	43	5	28
Renal failure	2	4	1	50
Normal renal function	68	195	24	35
Total	88	242	30	34

Table II. Details of all 88 families investigated

Group (number of families)	Family members affected (number/total)			
	siblings	offspring	parents	others
Requiring renal replacement therapy (18)	4/8	5/21	1/10	2/4
Renal failure (2)	1/1	0/3	0/0	0/0
Normal renal function (68)	9/43	12/108	4/26	10/18
Total number	14/52	17/132	5/36	12/22
%	27	13	14	55

Results

Familial Data. Since the Bermuda Workshop we have extended the number of families studied to 88. The results are summarized in tables I and II. There were 18 families in which the propositus reached end-stage RN. In 5 of these there were a total of 12 additional family members with VUR or RN (table III).

Table III. Details of 30 families with 1 or more affected members with VUR or reflux nephropathy

Group (total number of families)	Number of affected families	Family members affected (number/total)			
		siblings	offspring	parents	others
Requiring renal replacement therapy (18)	5	4/4	5/10	1/1	2/3
Renal failure (2)	1	1/1	0/0	0/0	0/0
Normal renal function (68)	24	9/26	12/38	4/10	10/15
Total	30	14/31	17/48	5/11	12/18

Overall 30 of the 88 (34%) families investigated had more than 1 affected subject. The data for these are summarized in table III. In figure 1 the pedigrees of a number of the families are shown. In 21 of them VUR or RN was detected in 2 or more consecutive generations. Details of the 32 transfers across a generation are included in table IV, and compared with a series collected from the literature by *Lewy and Belman* [9]. There was no evidence of sex-linked transmission. The large number of mothers shown relates to their diagnosis during pregnancy and the subsequent investigation of their new-born children. In 6 families there were 3 generations affected (examples in fig. 1).

Genetic Mechanisms. Evidence for the genetic mechanism involved was obtained firstly from an inspection of the family trees and tables, and secondly from formal testing using an appropriate computer mode.

Inspection of the data suggested a Mendelian dominant mode of inheritance with incomplete penetrance. The evidence for this was as follows:

(1) In the 30 families with more than 1 affected case there were 90 first-degree relatives (i.e. parents, siblings and offspring) investigated. 36 were affected and 54 were not (table III). In 4 instances apparently non-affected relatives were likely asymptomatic carriers of the gene as they had both affected children and an affected parent (family 31, fig. 1; and 2 other families), or affected children plus an affected sibling (family 24, fig. 1). In the case of a Mendelian dominant gene with complete penetrance the ratio of affected to non-affected would be 1:1 and our 36:54 (or 40:50) was close

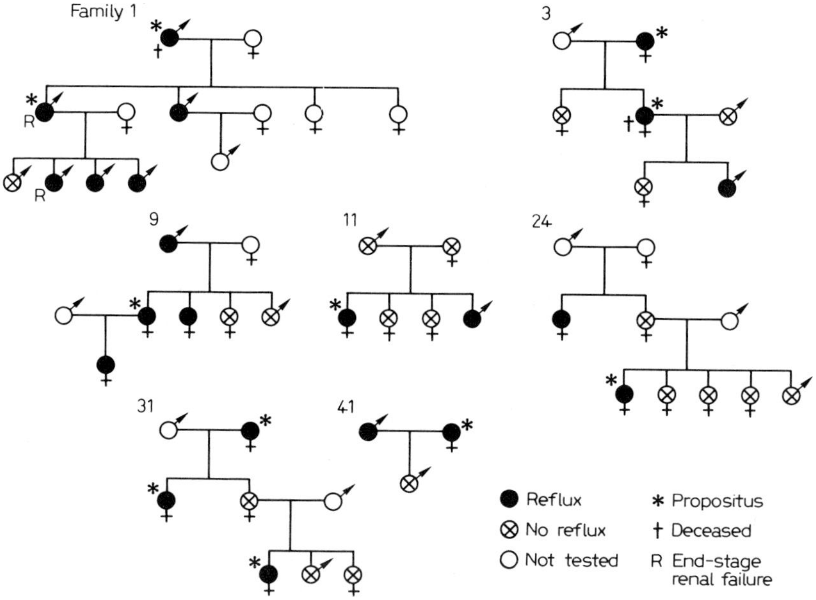

Fig. 1. Pedigrees of some of the families in which more than 1 member had VUR or reflux nephropathy. The data are consistent with an autosomal dominant mode of inheritance with incomplete penetrance.

Table IV. VUR or RN in 2 consecutive generations

		Christchurch	Reference 9
Mother	daughter	13	8
Mother	son	8	3
Father	daughter	4	5
Father	son	7	1
Total		32	27

to this. (2) 3 generations were affected in 6 families and 2 generations in a further 15 families. (3) In 4 families first-degree relatives (siblings) of the propositus transmitted the gene to their offspring (not shown). (4) There was no evidence of sex linkage (table IV). (5) In 1 family both parents were affected, but the only child was unaffected (family 41, fig. 1). This was consistent with a dominant, but not with a recessive, mode of inheritance.

It was important to eliminate bias from the data and so, in the formal testing using a computer model, all 88 families were included in the analysis. The model used was that of the Population Genetics Laboratory of the University of Hawaii. It assumed a population prevalence of VUR in 1%. The 3 possible sources of variation were a single major locus, polygenic variation and random environment.

The results will be published in detail elsewhere, but in summary our data were best explained on the basis of an uncommon autosomal dominant (gene frequency about 1 in 200) with some random environment component. Sporadic cases were accounted for within the model and did not require an additional explanation. The results indicated that the possibilities of no genetic effect or of recessive inheritance could be rejected. Polygenic inheritance fitted the data somewhat better, but nowhere near as well as autosomal dominant transmission.

Conclusion

These studies confirmed our earlier observations that VUR may be inherited [7, 8]. An editorial in 1975 [10] reviewed the familial occurrence of VUR, but noted no uniform inheritance pattern. Table V outlines most of the published literature, which is summarized in table VI. The distribution of affected individuals in most reported families has suggested a dominant gene. However, affected offspring have been found in families of 2 non-affected parents, suggesting a dominant gene with incomplete penetrance. The latter is compatible with the variable failure of the development of a vesico-ureteric junction. *Burger and Burger* [29] concluded that VUR was a multifactorial, genetically controlled anomaly of the vesico-ureteric junction, and that the functional expression depended on a number of other local or environmental factors. *De Vargas* et al. [6] have reached a similar conclusion. However, analysis of our data has strongly suggested inheritance on the basis of an autosomal dominant gene with incomplete penetrance.

It remains our strong recommendation that all infants born to parents with known VUR or RN, or who have siblings with this abnormality, should be investigated as soon after birth as possible. This is particularly important if the propositus has renal failure. The initial investigation for new-born children should be a micturating cysto-urethrogram. Clinicians should be aware that VUR may be familial, and have a high index of suspicion in siblings, parents and offspring of patients with VUR or RN.

Table V. Published literature of familial VUR

Reference No.	Number of families (n = 212)	Suggested transmission
1–6	6	identical twins
11	2	familial tendency
12	1	possible female sex-linked
13	9	NS
14	2	NS
15	3	NS
16	5	NS
17	8	NS
18	7	polygenic multifactorial
19	10	dominant gene with incomplete penetrance
20	9	NS
21	1	polygenic multifactorial
22	20	NS
23	1	single gene inheritance with variable expression and occasional lack of penetrance
24	8	polygenic inheritance and undefined environmental factors
25	8	NS
9	1	autosomal dominant with incomplete penetrance
26	1	sex-linked
27	40	NS
28	10	autosomal dominant with variable penetrance
6	39	multifactorial
7	15	autosomal dominant with variable penetrance

NS = Not stated.

Table VI. Review of published literature

27 reports ⟶ 212 affected families

Suggested transmission:

Autosomal dominant with incomplete penetrance;
5 reports ⟶ 37 families
Polygenic multifactorial; 4 reports ⟶ 55 families
Sex-linked; 2 reports ⟶ 2 families
Not stated; 16 reports ⟶ 118 families

Genetic Studies

Introduction

As the pattern of aggregation of VUR in our studied families suggested an inherited basis, attention was given to possible genetic markers. Early studies in this unit showed that HLA-B12 was significantly more frequent in patients reaching end-stage RN compared with those entering our dialysis-transplant programme from all other causes [30]. We suggested that HLA-B12 may prove useful as a genetic marker for primary VUR.

Sengar et al. [31] studied the histocompatibility antigens of 36 unrelated French Candian children (34 girls) with a history of at least 2 *E. coli* UTIs and found HLA-AW32 to be present in 6 of the 16 with VUR, compared with 0 of 20 without VUR. These workers suggested that a gene (or genes) other than those governing the HLA was responsible for the genesis of VUR. However, these would be in close linkage with the major histocompatibility complex, and may be in linkage disequilibrium with AW32. *McDonald* et al. [32] suggested HLA-A3 may be more frequent in those with VUR.

In a detailed study by *Torres* et al. [33] the frequency of 40 HLA antigen specificities was determined in 44 American patients with end-stage RN and compared with those observed in 526 blood donors. Higher than normal frequencies were observed for HLA-B12 in female patients and HLA-B15 in both sexes. In addition, there was an increase in the frequency of the combinations A9/B8, A9/BW15, A1/A9 and B8/BW15 in the male patients. There was no increase in HLA-AW32 or HLA-A3. The authors concluded that the major histocompatibility antigens may be in linkage disequilibrium with a gene (or genes) determining the susceptibility to renal damage by VUR, and that this linkage, or its clinical expression, may be influenced by variations in relation to the sex of the patients.

Present Study

Patients and Methods. Our preliminary findings [30] have been extended to 33 patients with end-stage RN, 108 patients with end-stage renal failure from all other causes and compared with 179 healthy volunteers, most of whom were blood donors.

Comparisons of HLA antigen and HLA haplotype frequencies in patients and controls were made. The method of analysis used was that reported by *Svejgaard* et al. [34], using *Woolf*'s [35] method and *Haldane*'s [36] correction for small sample sizes. This method produces a conservative χ^2 figure for significance, and provides a relative incidence ratio which

Table VII. HLA antigen frequency in controls versus patients with end-stage RN (entries are percentages of healthy subjects or patients with a particular antigen)

	Males and females			Male			Female		
Antigen	control (n = 179)	RN (n = 33)	RI	control (n = 48*)	RN (n = 16)	RI	control (n = 42*)	RN (n = 17)	RI
A1	32	27	0.8	21	25		38	29	
A2	48	45	0.91	48	50		43	41	
A3	27	24	0.88	42	25		31	24	
A9	14	30	2.84[a]	13	25	2.35[b]	21	35	1.99[b]
A10	12	9	0.85	10	13		17	6	
A11	13	12	1.02	15	13		7	12	
A28	6	–	0.22	4	–		12	–	
A29	7	3	0.62	6	6		5	–	
A30/31		3	3	1.46	–	6		2	–
A32	4	3	0.93	10	6		2	–	
B5	8	9	1.31	8	6		7	12	
B7	28	39	1.64	29	38		26	41	
B8	17	24	1.57	13	38	4.05[b]	26	12	0.44[b]
B12	39	36	0.88	42	44		33	29	
B13	3	–	0.4	2	–		5	–	
B14	6	9	1.68	6	13		5	6	
B15	11	9	0.94	15	13		7	6	
B16	4	–	0.3	4	–		2	–	
B17	11	3	0.36	8	6	24	–		
B18	5	–	0.27	8	–		7	–	
B21	4	–	0.3	6	–		5	–	
B22	6	12	2.24[b]	6	13		10	12	
B27	9	9	1.07	4	6		10	12	
B35	16	6	0.4	17	6		21	6	
B37	3	–	0.47	4	–		–	–	
B40	14	12	0.92	17å 6		10	18		

RI = Relative incidence by *Woolf*'s [35] method using *Haldane*'s [36] correction.
^{a}p < 0.05; ^{b}0.05; * Sex was not recorded on some of the normal controls;
–<antigen not found and therefore percentage not calculated.

can be used as a useful scanning guide. No value of the relative incidence can be stated as an absolute indicator, but values <0.5 or <1.5 can be used as a warning level at which further calculations may prove useful. The estimation of haplotype (the unit of inheritance of the HLA system) frequency was based on data from a Caucasian population published by *Albert* et al. [37].

Table VIII. Frequency of HLA haplotypes in end-stage RN (entries are percentage of healthy subjects and patients with a particular HLA haplotype

Haplotype	RN (n = 33)	Controls (n = 179)	RI
A1–B8	15	16	1.03
A2–B7	9	7	1.48
A2–B8	9	3	3.52*
A2–B12	12	20	0.6
A3–B7	15	16	0.99
A9–B12	12	6	2.38*

RI = Relative incidence by *Woolf*'s [35] method using *Haldane*'s [36] correction.
*$p < 0.05$.

Results. The HLA antigen frequency in the control subjects versus patients with end-stage RN are included in table VII. Only for HLA-A9 was there significantly higher incidence in the patients compared with the controls. When the patients were subdivided according to sex the trend persisted, but statistical significance was lost.

The HLA haplotypes which showed an obvious percentage difference between the patients with end-stage RN and the controls are included in table VIII. The relative incidence of the combination HLA-A9-B12 picked out a difference which may have been noted as an HLA-B12 preponderance in our earlier report [30]. The combination HLA-A2-B8 also showed an increased relative incidence in the patients compared with the controls, but neither combination was statistically significant.

When patients with end-stage RN were compared with those reaching end-stage chronic renal failure from all other causes some differences were apparent (table IX). The relative incidence of the haplotypes HLA-A2-B8 and HLA-A9-B12 was significantly more frequent in those patients with end-stage RN.

Discussion

In our earlier study [30] we showed that HLA-B12 was more frequent in patients with end-stage RN compared with those reaching end-stage renal failure from all other causes. At that time there was no evidence that HLA-B12 was more frequent in those with end-stage RN compared with the normal population.

Table IX. Frequency of HLA haplotypes in end-stage RN compared with all other causes of end-stage renal failure (entries are percentage of patients with a particular HLA haplotype)

Haplotype	RN (n = 33)	Other cause of RF (n = 108)	RI
A1–B8	15	26	0.55
A2–B7	9	9	1.08
A2–B8	9	2	4.89*
A2–B12	12	17	0.75
A3–B7	15	11	1.49
A9–B12	12	2	6.5*

RI = Relative incidence by *Woolf*'s [35] method using *Haldane*'s [36] correction.
*$p < 0.05$.

Between the HLA-B and -DR loci on chromosome 6 there are 5 other polymorphic regions, 1 or 2 of which may prove to be as diverse as HLA itself. It may be that the tenuous associations between HLA and disease that we are able to demonstrate are merely indicators to the true markers. Indeed, it may be that there are several interactions between the genes of a whole segment, and that the present findings indicate a haplotypic linkage disequilibrium. Rather than thinking of haplotypes it may be better to think of supertypes and, in investigations like this, to assay markers such as 21-hydroxylase, C2, C4a, C4b and Bf, in addition to HLA.

Conclusion

In this study HLA-A9 was significantly more frequent in patients with end-stage RN compared with normal subjects. This association has not been reported previously. Certain haplotypes (HLA-A2-B8 and HLA-A9-B12) were more frequent in patients with end-stage RN than those with all other causes of end-stage renal failure.

Since the haplotype is the unit of inheritance of the HLA system it is necessary to consider the distribution of HLA genes in a population in terms of the haplotype frequencies [38]. It is hoped that other investigators with larger numbers of patients and greater expertise in this area will be encouraged to pursue this very important line of investigation. Clearly the search must go on for the genetic marker(s) for RN.

Acknowledgements

We wish to thank Dr. *Cyril Chapman*, Medical Geneticist, Wellington Hospital, Wellington, New Zealand, for undertaking the computer analysis of the family data.

References

1 Stephens, F.D.; Joske, R.A.; Simmons, R.T.: Megaureter with vesicoureteric reflux in twins. J. Urol. *108*: 635 (1972).

2 Mebust, W.K.; Foret, J.D.: Vesicoureteral reflux in identical twins. J. Urol. *108*: 635 (1972).

3 Pochaczersky, R.; Nayson, P.; Ratner, H.: Congenital non-obstructive hydronephrosis and bilateral vesicoureteral reflux in identical twins. Am. J. Roentg. *120*: 398 (1974).

4 Hampel, N.; Levin, D.R.; Gersh, I.: Bilateral vesico-ureteric reflux with pyelonephritis in identical twins. Br. J. Urol. *47*: 535 (1975).

5 Redman, J.F.: Vesicoureteral reflux in identical twins. J. Urol. *116*: 792 (1976).

6 De Vargas, A.; Evans, K.; Ransley, P.; Rosenberg, A.R.; Rothwell, D.; Sherwood, T.; Williams, D.I.; Barratt, T.M.; Carter, C.O.: A family study of vesico-ureteric reflux. J. med. Genet. *15*: 85 (1978).

7 Heale, W.F.; Shannon, F.T.; Utley, W.L.F.; Rolleston, G.L.: Familial and hereditary reflux nephropathy; in Reflux nephrotaphy, pp. 48–52 (Masson, New York 1979).

8 Bailey, R.R.: An overview of reflux nephropathy; in Reflux nephropathy, pp. 3–13 (Masson, New York 1979).

9 Lewy, P.R.; Belman, A.B.: Familial occurrence of nonobstructive, non-infectious vesicoureteral reflux with renal scarring. J. Pediat. *86*: 851 (1975).

10 Editorial: Vesicoureteral reflux and its familial distribution. Br. med. J. *ii*: 726 (1975).

11 Stephens, F.D.; Lenaghan, D.: The anatomical basis and dynamics of vesicoureteral reflux. J. Urol. *87*: 669 (1962).

12 Tobenkin, M.I.: Hereditary vesicoureteral reflux. Sth. med. J., Nashville *57*: 139 (1964).

13 Baker, R.; Maxted, W.; McCrystal, H.; Kelly, T.: Unpredictable results associated with treatment of 133 children with ureterorenal reflux. J. Urol. *94*: 362 (1965).

14 Ambrose, S.S.: Reflux pyelonephritis in adults secondary to congenital lesions of the ureteral orifice. J. Urol. *102*: 303 (1969).

15 Mulcahy, J.J.; Kelalis, P.P.; Stickler, G.B.; Burke, E.C.: Familial vesicoureteral reflux. J. Urol. *104*: 762 (1970).

16 Simpson, J.L.; German J.: Familial urinary tract anomalies. J. Am. med. Ass. *212*: 2264 (1970).

17 Amar, A.D.: Familial vesicoureteral reflux. J. Urol. *108*: 969 (1972).

18 Burger, R.H.: A theory on the nature of transmission of congenital vesicoureteral reflux. J. Urol. *108*: 249 (1972).

19 Miller, H.C.; Caspari, E.W.: Ureteral reflux as genetic trait. J. Am. med. Ass. *220*: 842 (1972).

20 Schmidt, J.D.; Hawtrey, C.E.; Flocks, R.H.; Culp, D.A.: Vesicoureteral reflux. An inherited lesion. J. Am. med. Ass. *220*: 821 (1972).

21 Mobley, D.F.: Familial vesicoureteral reflux. Urology *2*: 514 (1973).

22 Zel, G.; Retik, A.B.: Familial vesicoureteral reflux. Urology *2*: 249 (1973).
23 Frye, R.N.; Patel, H.R.; Parsons, V.: Familial renal tract abnormalities and cortical scarring. Nephron *12*: 118 (1974).
24 Bois, E.; Feingold, J.; Benmaiz, H.; Briard, M.L.: Congenital urinary tract malformations: epidemiologic and genetic aspects. Clin. Genet. *8*: 37 (1975).
25 Bredin, H.C.; Winchester, P.; McGovern, J.H.; Degnan, M.: Family study of vesicoureteral reflux. J. Urol. *113*: 623 (1975).
26 Middleton, G.W.; Howards, S.S.; Gillenwater, J.Y.: Sex-linked familial reflux. J. Urol. *114*: 36 (1975).
27 Dwoskin, J.Y.: Sibling uropathology. J. Urol. *115*: 726 (1976).
28 Atwell, J.D.; Cook, P.L.; Strong, L.; Hyde, I.: The interrelationship between vesicoureteric reflux, trigonal abnormalities and a bifid pelvi-calyceal collecting system: a family study. Br. J. Urol. *49*: 97 (1977).
29 Burger, R.H.; Burger, S.E.: Genetic determinants of urologic disease. Urol. Clins. N. Am. *1*: 419 (1974).
30 Bailey, R.R.; Wallace, M.: HLA-B12 as a genetic marker for vesicoureteral reflux? Br. med. *i*: 48 (1978).
31 Sengar, D.P.S.; McLeish, W.A.; Rashid, A.; Wolfish, N.M.: Histocompatibility antigens in urinary tract infection and vesicoureteral reflux: a preliminary communication. Clin. Nephrol. *10*: 166, 1978.
32 McDonald, I.M.; Dumble, L.J.; Kincaid-Smith, P.S.: HLA-A3, vesicoureteric reflux and analgesic abuse. 1st Int. Symp. on HLA and Disease, Paris. Abstract book, 1976, p. 255.
33 Torres, V.E.; Moore, S.B.; Kurtz, S.B.; Offord, K.P.; Kelalis, P.P.: In search of a marker for genetic susceptibility to reflux nephropathy. Clin. Nephrol. *14*: 217 (1980).
34 Svejgaard, A.; Jersild, C.; Nielsen, L.S.; Bodmer, M.F.: HL-A antigens and disease statistical and genetical considerations. Tissue Antigens *4*: 95 (1974).
35 Woolf, B.: On estimating the relation between blood group and disease. Ann. hum. Genet. *19*: 251 (1955).
36 Haldane, J.B.S.: The estimation and significance of the logarithm of a ratio of frequencies. Ann. hum. Genet. *20*: 309 (1955).
37 Albert, E.D.; Scholz, S.; Bertrams, J.; Ewald, R.W.; Seidl, S.; Ratschko, W.; Westphal, E.: Representative HL-A haplotype frequencies of several german populations. Z. ImmunForsch. exp. Ther. *148*: 367 (1975).
38 Albert, E.D.; Scholz, S.: The biology of the major histocompatibility complex in man. Behring Inst. Mitt. *62*: 21 (1978).

Ross R. Bailey, MD, Departments of Nephrology, Pediatrics and Immunohematology, Christchurch Hospital, Christchurch (New Zealand)

Contr. Nephrol., vol. 39, pp. 52–67 (Karger, Basel 1984)

5. Reflux Nephropathy: The Clinical Picture in South Brazilian Children

N.P. Goldraich, I.H. Goldraich, O.E. Anselmi, O.L. Ramos

Centro de Nefrologia Infantil, Porto Alegre, RS Brazil

Introduction

Reflux nephropathy (RN) is a disease normally assessed in vivo by its radiological aspects [5]. However, there is often difficulty in defining the renal outlines during intravenous urography [IVU] in infants and pre-school children due to the presence of gas in the bowel, a prerequisite to identifying the scarring of RN. Also, children with primary vesicoureteric reflux (VUR) need a long-term follow-up, with repeated IVUs and their cumulative radiation doses. Therefore, it is preferable to find an alternative method of evaluating the kidneys which involves less radiation.

^{99m}Tc-Dimercaptosuccinic acid (^{99m}Tc-DMSA), introduced in 1974 by *Lin* et al. [28], is a cortical marker which provides both functional (individual, and total renal function) and anatomical (presence of scars and/or contraction of the whole kidney) information and, further, allows the quantification of individual renal function [1, 10, 25]. This is particularly important in a disease such as RN in which, even when bilateral, the renal damage is always asymmetrical. Also, recent reports [9, 30] have shown that the ^{99m}TC-DMSA renal scan is a more sensitive method than IVU of detecting scars in the kidney.

Primary VUR is thought to be an anomaly which is present from birth. In this study untreated VUR was defined as the period from birth to the time VUR was diagnosed which, of course, corresponded to the child's age.

RN is an important cause of hypertension [3, 13, 22, 45] and chronic renal failure [7, 16] in children. To establish the prevalence of these two complications in pediatric patients we reviewed our records over the last 4.5 years and found that it was responsible for 10 of the 32 (30%) cases of severe and persistent hypertension (diastolic blood pressure 120 mm Hg or more) and for 9 of the 63 (15%) cases of chronic renal failure in children aged 0 to 15 years.

Considering that in our country VUR is still usually diagnosed at a late stage, the population we studied presents a few specific aspects: (a) there are still untreated individuals in all three age groups considered (infants, pre-school and school-age); (b) those with very severe renal damage were naturally excluded from the study either by death or because renal function was grossly impaired; (c) since the renal damage in RN is asymmetrical, we could only study severely damaged kidneys if the function on the opposite side was sufficient, through compensatory hypertrophy, to meet our criteria. Such discrimination was made possible by the use of ^{99m}Tc-DMSA, which allows the estimation of individual renal function without resorting to such invasive methods as ureteral catheterization; (d) the follow-up of these patients will permit us to assess the effectiveness of conservative treatment of VUR and to establish at what age it must be started in order to modify the natural history of RN.

The objectives of the present study, therefore, were: (a) to establish the prevalence of RN, using ^{99m}Tc-DMSA renal scan in patients with VUR; (b) to study the influence on its prevalence of the duration and grade of untreated VUR; (c) to determine the prevalence of renal function impairment at diagnosis using the ^{99m}Tc-DMSA renal function index; (d) to follow both structural and functional progress under conservative treatment by means, again, of assessment by ^{99m}Tc-DMSA studies.

Patients and Methods

Criteria. The criteria for including patients in this prospective study, begun in January 1978, were: (a) presence of VUR on micturating cystourethrography (MCU); (b) age between 0 and 14 years; (c) at least one documented episode of urinary tract infection (UTI) before VUR was diagnosed; (d) serum creatinine below 3 mg/dl; (e) proteinuria below 200 mg/24 h; (f) no previous radiologic, endoscopic or surgical procedure on the urinary tract; (g) adequate subsequent conservative treatment of VUR, including medical visits either monthly or at short time intervals; if UTI recurred, monthly urine cultures, continuous prophylactic therapy and 6-monthly scans with ^{99m}Tc-DMSA. Only patients who were able to submit to these conditions were included and kept in the study.

Patients. Between January 1978 and August 1982, 142 children were entered into the study. There were 23 males and 119 females. They were classified into 3 age-groups: (a) infants: 1 month to 2 years (n = 38); (b) pre-school: 2–6 years (n = 60); (c) school-age: 6–14 years (n = 44) (table I).

Table I. Distribution of VUR patients according to age and sex

Age groups	Males		Females		Total		Ratio M/F
	n	%	n	%	n	%	
Infants	10	43.5	28	23.5	38	26.8	1:2.8
Pre-school	9	39.1	51	42.9	60	42.2	1:5.7
School-age	4	17.4	40	33.6	44	31.0	1:10.0
Total	23	100.0	119	100.0	142	100.0	1:5.2

Table II. Distribution of renal units according to age groups and VUR grades

PVUR	Infants		Pre-school		School-age		Total	
	n	%	n	%	n	%	n	%
Slight	33	55.0	45	54.2	40	59.7	118	56.7
Severe	27	45.0	38	45.8	27	40.3	92	43.8
Total	60	100.0	83	100.0	67	100.0	210	100.0

In the whole group, 210 kidneys had refluxing ureters; 60 in group 1; 83 in group 2, and 67 in group 3 (table II). VUR was slight in 118 ureters and severe in 92. The distribution of the kidneys according to age groups and VUR grade is shown in table II. During the follow-up, the VUR ceased in 65.2% of all positive ureters; in 77.9% of those with slight, and 48.9% of those with severe VUR.

VUR Diagnosis. This was made by MCU, performed without sedation and/or anesthesia. All children had sterile urine for at least 4 weeks before the radiological study was done. VUR was classified in two grades, according to the findings at MCU: *Slight*: Incomplete or complete filling of urinary tract without dilatation; corresponding to grades I and II of the classification by *Smellie* et al. [44]. *Severe*: Complete filling of the upper urinary tract with dilatation of different intensities: corresponding to grades III and IV of the same classification.

VUR Follow-Up. VUR was considered cured when it was absent in two consecutive MCUs or on indirect radionuclide cystography. Up to January 1981 the MCU was repeated every 2 years. From then on, it was replaced by indirect radionuclide cystography with ^{99m}Tc-DTPA, which is repeated annually.

^{99m}Tc-DMSA Renal Scan. The radionuclide renal study was done injecting DMSA (CEA-Sorin Laboratory) labelled with technetium and utilizing a gamma camera connected to a computer. All children had sterile urine for a period of at least 4 weeks before the scan was carried out. The dose injected was 1 mCi and the children were scanned 8 h later.

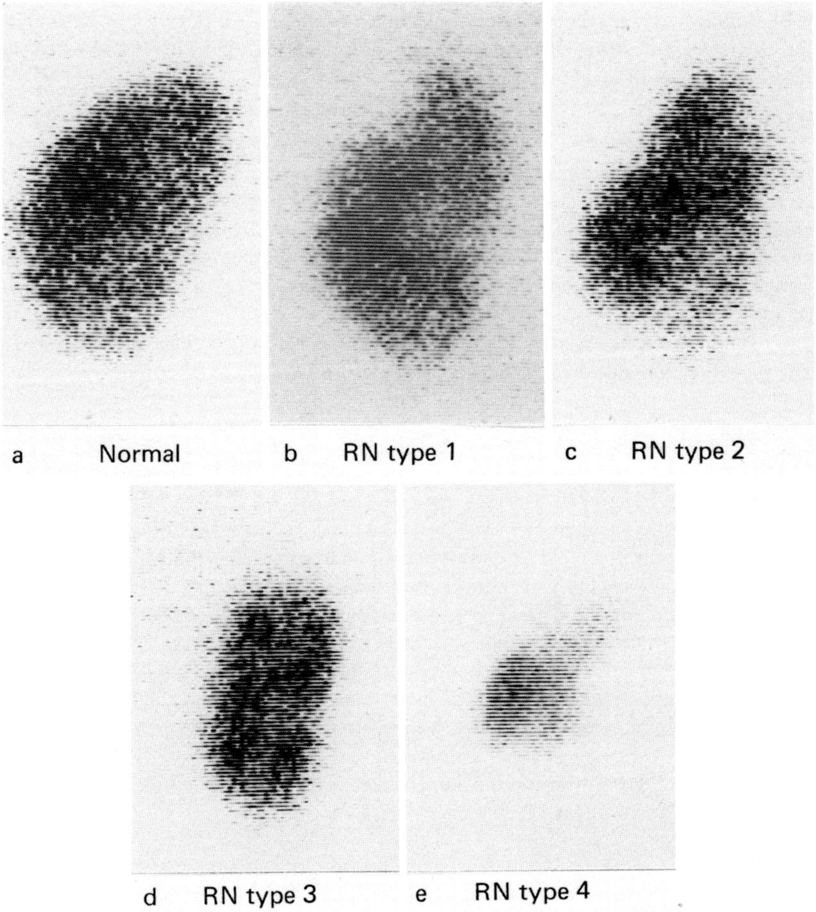

Fig. 1. Classification of the kidneys according to the aspect at ^{99m}Tc-DMSA renal scan. From the left to the right: normal kidney and kidneys with RN type 1, type 2, type 3 and type 4.

Static Images. The scan was performed obtaining posterior and two oblique views. These three views provided the anatomical information. A scar was defined as a defect in the kidney outline with no ^{99m}Tc-DMSA uptake. RN was identified by the presence of scars or by contraction of the whole kidney. Depending on the absence or presence of these findings, the renal units were classified as *without RN, (normal)*, or *with RN*.

Smellie et al. [42] proposed a 4-grade classification for RN based on the IVU appearance, which was adopted by the International Reflux Study Committee [24]. We employed a modification of this adapted to the findings of the ^{99m}Tc-DMSA scan (fig. 1): Type 1 – no more than 2 scarred areas. Type 2 – more than 2 scars with some areas of normal parenchyma between the scars. Type 3 – generalized damage to the whole kidney, similar to obstructive nephropathy, i.e. contraction of the whole kidney without, or with very few, scars in the outline. Type 4 – end-stage, shrunken kidney with little or no uptake of ^{99m}Tc-DMSA, i.e. less than 10% of overall renal function.

Functional Index. The renal areas were scanned in the posterior position. The results were expressed as a percentage of the dose administered taken up by each kidney, and termed ^{99m}Tc-DMSA renal function index. This index expresses the absolute function of each kidney. The technique used is similar to that described by *Raynaud* [33] to establish the individual renal function with ^{197}Hg-chlormerodrin. In computing results, the following factors were considered: (a) renal depth; (b) background radiation; (c) decay of radioactivity in the standard.

The formula proposed by *Raynaud and Knipper* [34] was used to calculate renal depth. The renal function index was calculated according to the following formula:

$$^{99m}\text{Tc-DMSA renal function index (\%)}: \frac{\text{LK or RK radioactivity}}{\text{CS radioactivity} \times \text{k}} \times 100,$$

where LK or RK radioactivity = left or right kidney radioactivity, obtained by subtracting background radioactivity from the value corresponding to radioactivity in each renal area; CS radioactivity = radioactivity of the corrected standard, achieved by dividing the standard by the dose injected into the patient; k = correction factor of the radioactivity of the standard for renal depth calculated according to a decreased exponential curve obtained by plotting a series of measurements of the standard against increasing thickness of plexiglass cover [35].

The function index was measured in 98 kidneys of 49 normal children (table III). The average value for the normal paediatric control group, as established in our laboratory, is 33.4 ± 3.3% [14].

The reproducibility of these results was assessed by repeating the scan on each of 13 patients at 0, 2 and 6 weeks. The

$$\text{variation coefficient} = \frac{\text{standard deviation}}{\text{mean}} \times 100$$

so obtained was 3.6% [15].

Renal function impairment evaluated by the functional index was defined as 2 SD or more below the mean and hypertrophy as 2 SD or more above it.

Conservative Treatment. This consisted of continuous low-dosage prophylactic chemotherapy, usually nitrofurantoin, with adequate fluid intake and regular bowel habits. The medication was maintained until two MCU's, or indirect radionuclide cystographies were negative for VUR. Children with sphincter control were put on a regimen of frequent and complete voiding, with double micturition at least once a day. Blood pressure was measured regularly and, when elevated, prompt treatment with antihypertensive drugs was instituted.

Follow-Up of Conservative Treatment. Urine cultures were repeated monthly, and also whenever there was any evidence of a breakthrough UTI. Urine was obtained by

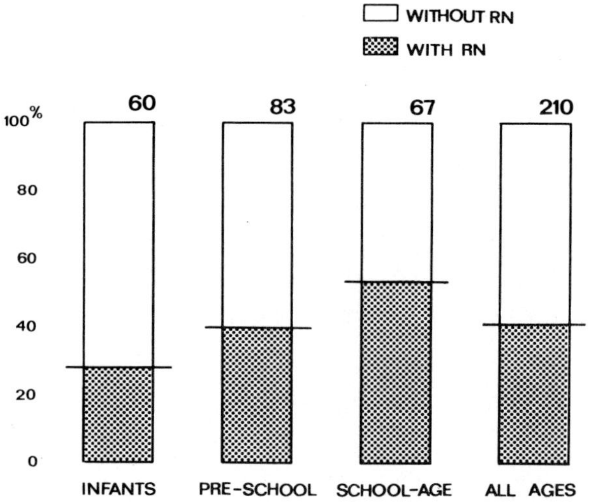

Fig. 2. Distribution of renal units according to age groups and the presence of RN.

suprapubic aspiration in all cases and was inoculated in both aerobic and anaerobic media. The presence of proteins and leukocyte counts were determined on the same urine specimen. The time interval between a recurrence of symptomatic UTI and a modification in treatment was always less than 7 days; whereas in the case of asymptomatic UTI it was always less than 40 days. The ^{99m}Tc-DMSA renal scan was repeated every 6 months and at that time a quantitative 24-hour protein excretion estimation was performed. Blood pressure was measured at each visit.

Results

The ^{99m}Tc-DMSA scan showed RN in 86 refluxing renal units in these 142 children (fig. 2). There was a significant association between the presence of RN and the age when VUR was first diagnosed, and UTI first treated. In all three age groups there was a significant association between the grade of VUR and the presence of scars in the ^{99m}Tc-DMSA scan (fig. 3).

As shown in figure 4, 52 of the 210 kidneys presented with renal functional impairment. In table III are seen the means of the ^{99m}Tc-DMSA renal function index in kidneys with slight and those with severe VUR. A significant association was found between the grade of VUR and impairment of renal function, but there were no significant differences between the means of the same grade of VUR among the three age groups. It is

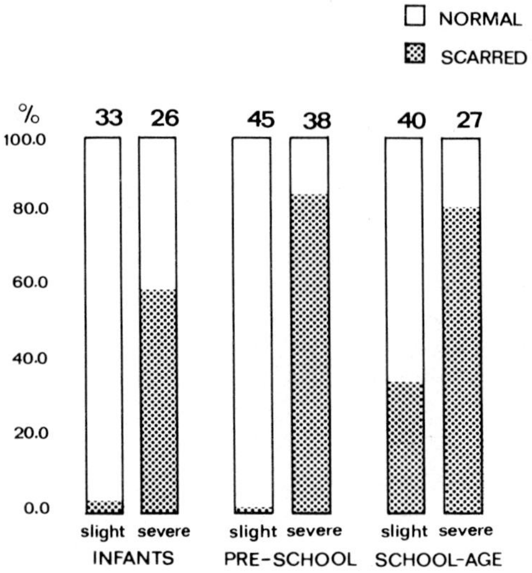

Fig. 3. Proportion of normal kidneys to scarred kidneys according to grade of VUR in the three age groups.

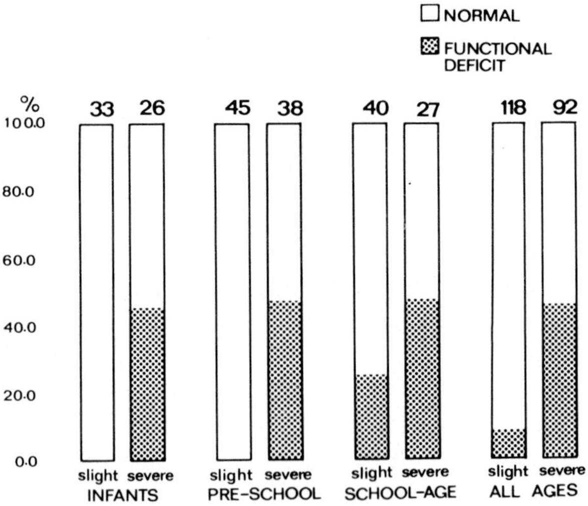

Fig. 4. Ratio of normal kidneys to kidneys with functional deficit according to grade of VUR in the three age groups.

Table III. ^{99m}Tc-DMSA renal function index at the time of VUR diagnosis and in normal children

VUR	Infants	Pre-school	School-age
Slight	34.2 ± 5.1[a] (33)	33.0 ± 3.5[a] (45)	31.6 ± 11.1[a] (40)
Severe	25.7 ± 9.7[b] (27)	27.3 ± 9.1[b] (38)	23.8 ± 13.4[b] (27)
Normal	32.8 ± 3.3[a] (32)	33.9 ± 3.3[a] (34) normal kidneys: 33.4 ± 3.3[a] (98)	33.4 ± 3.2[a] (32)

Number of renal units given in parentheses.
a × b: $p < 0.05$. a × a; b × b: $p > 0.05$.

Table IV. Proportion of renal units in the various functional indices according to anatomical aspects at scan in the three age groups

	Infants			Pre-school			School-age		
	↑	N	↓	↑	N	↓	↑	N	↓
Scan									
Normal	2	41	0	3	47	0	5	26	0
Scarred	0	5	12	1	15	17	2	11	23
Total	2	46	12	4	62	17	7	37	23

↑ = Increased; N = normal; ↓ = decreased.

worth noting that the prevalence of functional impairment was 24.8%, whereas the prevalence of RN was 41%. The combination of anatomical and functional information supplied by the ^{99m}Tc-DMSA renal scan is presented in table IV.

The 4.5-year follow-up on conservative treatment of these 210 kidneys with VUR showed neither a decrease in the means of the ^{99m}Tc-DMSA renal function index nor the development of new scars. No initially normal kidney developed scars. No patient presented persistent proteinuria. In some, using semiquantitative methods, up to 2+ of protein was detected in urine when there was a symptomatic recurrence of UTI, but this disap-

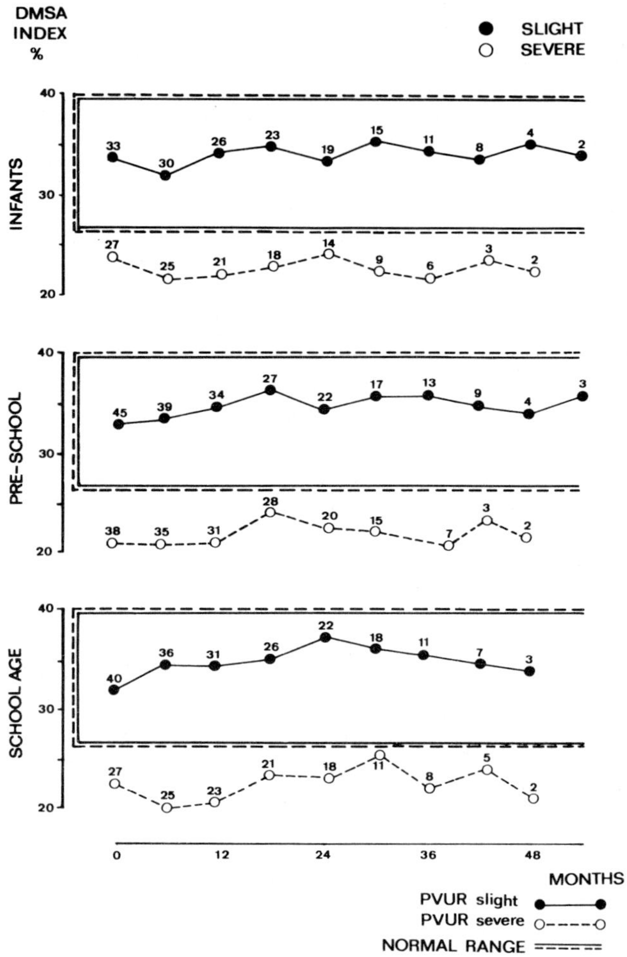

Fig. 5. ^{99m}Tc-DMSA renal function indices means every 6 months during conservative treatment of PVUR in the three age groups.

peared after bacteriuria was cleared. In figure 5, the means and the number of kidneys in each group are shown at 6-monthly intervals.

Discussion

Due to our climate we have a high incidence of respiratory infections; most of them, at least initially, viral in nature. High fevers are frequent findings, especially among infants and pre-school age children. As a result it is unusually difficult to identify the first episode of UTI because pyrexia in children is often treated with antibiotics, or only with antipyretics, without a urine culture. There is also a tradition of postponing the investigation of UTI, even in children under the age of 5 who are most at risk of developing renal scars [18, 23, 39, 42].

A careful history of the children in this study shows that most had at least one well-defined febrile episode before the age of 6 months. Since we are nephrologists and not pediatricians, and therefore are not involved in the primary care of children, the patients included in this study were referred to us either after presenting with febrile episodes or because they had several symptomatic recurrences of UTI.

Thus, our material, which included children in whom VUR had not yet been diagnosed, provided us with an opportunity of studying the natural history of untreated VUR and its effects on the kidney, as described by *Hodson and Edwards* [20], both using the ^{99m}Tc-DMSA renal scan which has become available since their time. Certainly the vast majority of these children received antibiotics for short periods, since they had presented with pyrexia, but none of them was given continuous low-dosage prophylactic therapy, such as proposed by *Normand and Smellie* [31]. As well, as pointed out by *Asscher* [4], short periods of treatment with antibiotics in patients with VUR and UTI may lead to reinfection of the urinary tract with different organisms, thereby disrupting the equilibrium established between the bacteria and the host and thus increasing the possibility of kidney damage. In the literature, it is clearly demonstrated that intermittent antibacterial treatment does not prevent scar formation in children with symptomatic UTIs [12, 27].

Hodson [18] had already indicated in 1964 that the renal lesions in RN can progress without any clinical signs to indicate how severely the kidneys have become compromised. If all children were screened at birth and for the first few months of life for UTI by some simple method, the first UTI might well be detected at a stage when it can be treated successfully and before irreversible renal damage has occurred [17, 43]. This idea is corroborated by the experimental study of *Ransley and Risdon* [38] who were able to demonstrate that the effective eradication of UTI, 1 week after it began, limited the degree of permanent scarring in a pig model.

In the three age groups that we studied, the females predominate, as reported elsewhere in the literature [6, 11]; and this trend increases with age. And this fact is almost certainly due to the higher incidence of UTI in girls after the first year of life [46].

Table V. Distribution of kidneys with RN according to age groups and type of renal lesion

RN	Infants		Pre-school		School-age		Total	
	n	%	n	%	n	%	n	%
Type 1	5	29.4	14	42.5	17	47.2	36	41.9
Type 2	3	17.6	8	24.2	4	11.1	15	17.4
Type 3	9	53.0	10	30.3	11	30.6	30	34.9
Type 4	0	0.0	1	3.0	4	11.1	5	5.8
Total	17	100.0	33	100.0	36	100.0	86	100.0

As shown in figure 2, there was an increased prevalence of RN in older children with VUR, from which we may infer that there is an association between the period of exposure to untreated VUR and the development of RN.

In all age groups there was a significant association between the grades of VUR and the presence of RN in the ^{99m}Tc-DMSA scans (fig. 3). But also in all three age groups, normal kidneys were still present in association with severe VUR. This finding can be explained on the basis of intrarenal reflux and the type of renal papillae present [21, 36, 37, 39]. In school-age children, there is a higher incidence of RN associated with lower grades of VUR. But the natural history of VUR shows a spontaneous decrease in the grade of VUR with age [6, 11]. Thus, this VUR now identified as 'slight' was in all probability 'severe' at an earlier age, and it was at this time that the renal damage was established.

Several reports [19, 40, 43] suggest the possibility of two forms of RN, defined according to the pattern of scar distribution and the mechanisms by which damage occurs in the kidneys: (a) focal: coarse scars, usually polar; (b) generalized: indistinguishable from obstructive nephropathy.

As mentioned by others [40, 42, 43] based on the radiological findings, and establishing a direct correlation with those of the ^{99m}Tc-DMSA scans, we find that in our patients the generalized form (type 3 of the classification we proposed) was the most common form of RN in infants (table V).

It is also noteworthy that in 9 of the 17 kidneys with VUR and RN in our infants, severe renal damage was already present. According to the 'big bang' theory, kidneys possessing many compound papillae which allow of intrarenal reflux, would be prone to this form of damage of the time of their first UTI [36]. This emphasizes still further the need for a simple and effective method of making a diagnosis of this entity, at a stage when treatment might be efficacious.

It has been shown before that the appearance of new, usually polar, scars is related to the occurrence of UTI and VUR, especially in the first 5 years of life [2, 12, 23, 32, 42]. This was also our experience, comparing the marked increase of type 1 scarring between infants and pre-school children, with the insignificant difference between the pre-school and school-age groups.

End-stage kidneys (type 4) were found in both pre-school and school-age children, and this may indicate a long-term evolution of severely damaged kidneys which continued to be drained by refluxing ureters and in which UTI was superimposed. Certainly, the criteria we used for inclusion in our study, which barred patients with either a serum creatinine higher than 3 mg/dl and/or proteinuria above 200 mg/24 h, modify the overall figures at the time of VUR diagnosis, as they exclude some severely damaged kidneys in both age groups. This would explain the apparently paradoxical finding that severe lesions (type 3) were significantly more frequent in infants, and highlights the fact that during the 4 years of this study 9 children with RN entered the renal failure program.

The renal scan showed the prevalence of RN to be 41% and that of renal impairment, as assessed by the functional index, to be 24.8%. Compensatory hypertrophy of unaffected areas of the kidney probably accounts for this difference between the two results and indicates that it is necessary to combine both anatomical and functional information fully to evaluate the effects of VUR on the kidney.

When VUR is only slight, as illustrated in figure 3, a significant prevalence of impaired renal function (25%) is found only in the school-age group (fig. 4). To explain this finding it is reasonable to assume that what is now slight VUR must have been severe VUR in the past, and function was thereby impaired. Particularly as in 78 kidneys drained by ureters with slight VUR in other children of the same age, no impairment of function occurred.

When the DMSA scan was normal, we never found decreased function (table IV). But when there was a normal or hypertrophied renal function index, a scan might reveal either a normal or a scarred kidney. In kidneys with normal function, scars were less common in infants (10.9%), but equally frequent in pre-school (24.2%) and school-age children (29.7%).

Thus, in the absence of scars it is unnecessary to perform a functional assessment and, conversely when scarring is present, it is *indispensable* to evaluate renal function in order to establish the prognosis.

In the follow-up, no normal kidney developed scars. The Cardiff-Oxford Bacteruria Study Group [8] found the same, although a different population from ours, consisting of children over 5 years of age but with *covert* bacteriuria, was studied. Likewise, no deterioration of function was documented during the follow-up. We may conclude therefore that with adequate treatment there is no decrease in function or appearance of new scars in any of the age groups. The proof of completely effective treatment will be the same prevalence of scars (28.3%) in our infants when they reach pre-school and school-age as there is now.

Because of the statistically significant differences between the prevalence of scarring in the three age groups (28.3% in infants, 39.8% in pre-school and 53.7% in school-age children), we may conclude that the disease is progressive in the absence of treatment, whereas through the 4.5 years of this study its course has been essentially benign.

In both the reports of the European Dialysis and Transplantation Association [7], and in other studies [16, 26, 29, 41], as well as our own, there is evidence that RN is an important cause of chronic renal failure in pediatric patients and young adults, which seems contrary to the results of our own follow-up. But all our patients were closely followed and, furthermore, all those in whom the time between the onset of symptomatic UTI and its treatment was longer than 7 days, and those whose urine cultures could not be repeated monthly, were excluded from the study, since its object was to assess the effect of treatment of UTI on the progress of kidneys subjected to VUR. The strict control of blood pressure by anti-hypertensive therapy whenever a significant increase was detected must also have contributed to a favorable outcome in these patients.

Conclusion

The prevalence of RN, as defined by the presence of scars and/or contraction of the whole kidney by ^{99m}Tc-DMSA scanning, was 41%. There was a significant association between the time during which the kidneys were subjected to untreated VUR (the child's age at the time VUR was identified) and the presence of RN.

The prevalence of renal function impairment assessed by the ^{99m}Tc-DMSA renal function index was 24.8%. No significant differences were found between the functional index among age groups, in spite of differing prevalences of RN, indicating that compensatory hypertrophy of undamaged parenchyma can mask the effects of VUR on kidney function.

There was a significant association between the grade of VUR, (classified as slight and severe) and the presence of RN at scan, and also of functional impairment, as measured by the ^{99m}Tc-DMSA renal function index.

During the follow-up with conservative (non-surgical) management, no further significant functional or structural changes developed, even in children with severe VUR, thus indicating that conservative treatment can modify the course of the disease at these ages.

For an adequate assessment of the effects of VUR on the kidney, it is indispensable to combine anatomical evaluation (detection of scars and contraction) with functional information. The renal uptake of ^{99m}Tc-DMSA provides a simple means of achieving these requirements.

Acknowledgments

We are grateful to Prof. *Edgar Mario Wagner* for his help and statistical analysis in the preparation of this paper.

References

1 Abbou, C.C.; Moretti, J.L.; Chopin, D.; Sanabria, E.; Msallag, M.; Nebout, T.; Auvert, J.: La scintilographie au dimercaptosuccinate de technetium: DMSA ^{99m}Tc. Apport dans l'évaluation de la fonction rénale separée. Nouv. Presse méd. *10*: 1475–1478 (1981).

2 Acton, C.M.; Drew, J.H.: Reflux nephropathy; Chap. 7, pp. 62–69 (Masson, New York 1979).

3 Andersen, H.J.; Jacobsson, B.; Larsson, H.; Winberg, J.: Hypertension, asymmetric renal parenchymal defect, sterile urine, and high *E. coli* antibody titre. Br. med. J. *iii*: 14-18 (1973).

4 Asscher, A.W.: The challenge of urinary tract infections, pp. 112-128 (Academic Press, London 1980).

5 Bailey, R.R.: The relationship of vesico-ureteric reflux to urinary tract infection and chronic pyelonephritis – reflux nephropathy. Clin. Nephrol. *1*: 132-141 (1973).

6 Baker, B.; Maxted, W.; Maylath, J.; Shuman, I.: Relation of age, sex and infection to reflux: data indicating high spontaneous cure rate in pediatric patients. J. Urol. *95*: 27–32 (1966).

7 Broyer, M.; Donckerwolcke, R.A.; Brunner, F.P.; Brynger, H.; Jacobs, C.; Kramer, P.; Selwood, N.H.; Wing, A.J.; Blake, P.H.: Proceedings of the European Dialysis and Transplant Association, vol. 18, pp. 60–87 (Pitman, London 1981).

8 Cardiff-Oxford Bacteriuria Study Group: Sequelae of covert bacteriuria in schoolgirls. Lancet *i*: 889–893 (1978).

9 Chrispin, A.R.; Gordon, I.; Hall, C.; Metreweli, C.: Diagnostic imaging of the kidney and urinary tract in children, pp. 62–73 (Springer, Berlin 1980).

10 Daly, M.J.; Henry, R.E.: Defining renal anatomy and function with ^{99m}technetium dimercaptosuccinic acid: clinical and renographic correlation. J. Urol. *126*: 5–9 (1981).

11 Edwards, D.; Normand, I.C.S.; Prescod, N.; Smellie, J.M.: Disappearance of vesicoureteric reflux during long-term prophylaxis of urinary tract infection in children. Br. med. J. *ii*: 285–288 (1977).

12 Filly, R.A.; Friedland, G.W.; Govan, D.E.; Fair, W.R.: Development and progression of clubbing and scarring in children with recurrent urinary tract infections. Radiology *113*: 145–153 (1974).

13 Gill, D.G.; Mendes da Costa, B.; Cameron, J.S.; Joseph, M.C.; Ogg, C.S.; Chantler, C.: Analysis of 100 children with severe and persistent hypertension. Archs Dis. Childh. *51*: 951–959 (1976).

14 Goldraich, N.P.; Goldraich, I.H.: Reflux nephropathy: assessment using DMSA renal uptake. Int. J. Pediat. Nephrol. *3*: 120 (1982).

15 Goldraich, N.; Sigulem, D.; Goldraich, I.; Almeida, J.; Ramos, O.: ^{99m}Tc-DMSA, a peritubular function marker: study in human and isolated perfused rat kidney (IPRK). Abstracts. 8th Int. Congr. Nephrol., Athens 1981, pp. 59.

16 Habib, R.; Broyer, M.; Benmaiz, J.: Chronic renal failure in children: causes, rate of deterioration and survival data. Nephron *11*: 209–220 (1973).

17 Hodson, C.J.: Focal scarring and renal reflux. Lancet *ii*: 784 (1978).

18 Hodson, C.J.: Pyelonephritis in children. Ann. Radiol. *7*: 355–359 (1964).

19 Hodson, C.J.: Reflux nephropathy: a personal historical review. Am. J. Roentg. *137*: 451–462 (1981).

20 Hodson, C.J.; Edwards, D.: Chronic pyelonephritis and vesicoureteric reflux. Clin. Radiol. *11*: 219–231 (1960).

21 Hodson, C.J.; Maling, T.M.J.; McManamon, P.J.; Lewis, M.G.: Reflux nephropathy. Kidney int. *8*: S50–S58 (1975).

22 Holland, N.H.; Kotchen, T.; Bhathena, D.: Hypertension in children with chronic pyelonephritis. Kidney int. *8*: S243–S251 (1975).

23 Hugosson, C.O.; Chrispin, A.R.; Wolverson, M.K.: The advent of the pyelonephritic scar. Ann. Radiol. *19*: 1–6 (1976).

24 International Reflux Study Committee: Medical versus surgical treatment of primary vesicoureteral reflux: a prospective international reflux study in children. J. Urol. *125*: 277:283 (1981).

25 Kawamura, J.; Hosokawa, S.; Yoshida, O.; Fujita, T.; Ishii, Y.; Torizuka, K.: The validity of ^{99m}Tc dimercapto-succinic acid renal uptake for an assessment of individual kidney function. J. Urol. *119*: 305–309 (1978).

26 Kincaid-Smith, P.; Becker, G.J.: Reflux nephropathy; Chap. 3, pp. 21–28 (Masson, New York 1979).

27 Lenaghan, D.; Whitaker, J.G.; Jensen, F.; Stephens, F.D.: The natural history of reflux and long-term effects of reflux on the kidney. J. Urol. *115*: 728–730 (1976).

28 Lin, T.H.; Khentigan, A.; Winchell, H.S.: A ^{99m}Tc-chelate substitute for organoradiomercurial renal agents. J. nucl. Med. *15*: 34–35 (1974).

29 MacGregor, M.E.: Pyelonephritis lenta: consideration of childhood urinary infections as the forerunner of renal insufficiency in later life. Archs. Dis. Childh. *45*: 159–172 (1970).
30 Merrick, M.V.; Uttley, W.S.; Wild, S.R.: The detection of pyelonephritic scarring in children by radioisotope imaging. Br. J. Radiol. *53*: 544–556 (1980).
31 Normand, C.; Smellie, J.: Reflux nephropathy; 2nd ed., pp. 281–286 (Masson, New York 1979).
32 Randolph, M.F.; Morris, K.E.; Gould, E.B.: The first urinary tract infection in the female infant; prevalence, recurrence and prognosis: a 10-year study in private practice. J. Pediat. *86*: 342–348 (1975).
33 Raynaud, C.: A technique for the quantitative measurement of the function of each kidney. Semin. nucl. Med. *4*: 51–60 (1974).
34 Raynaud, C.; Knipper, M.: The renal uptake of radioactive mercury ($^{197}HgCl_2$): method for testing the functional value of each kidney, technique, results, and clinical application in urology and nephrology, pp. 62–64 (Thomas, Springfield 1976).
35 Raynaud, C.; Ricard, S.: The renal uptake of radioactive mercury ($^{197}HgCl_2$): method for testing the functional value of each kidney, technique, results, and clinical application in urology and nephrology, pp. 65–68 (Thomas, Springfield 1976).
36 Ransley, P.G.: Vesicoureteral reflux: continuing surgical dilemma. Urology *21*: 246–255 (1978).
37 Ransley, P.G.: Risdon, R.A.: Reflux and renal scarring. Br. J. Radiol. *14*: suppl. pp. 1–35 (1978).
38 Ransley, P.G.; Risdon, R.A.: Reflux nephropathy: effects of antimicrobial therapy on the evolution of the early pyelonephritic scar. Kidney int. *20*: 733–742 (1981).
39 Rolleston, G.L.; Maling, T.M.J.; Hodson, C.J.: Intrarenal reflux and the scarred kidney. Archs Dis. Childh. *49*: 531–539 (1974).
40 Rolleston, G.L.; Shannon, F.T.; Utley, W.L.F.: Follow-up of vesico-ureteric reflux in the newborn. Kidney int. *8*: S59–S64 (1975).
41 Salvatierra, O., Jr.; Kounts, S.L.; Belzer, F.O.: Primary vesicoureteral reflux and end-stage disease. J. Am. med. Ass. *226*: 1454–1456 (1973).
42 Smellie, J.M.; Edwards, D.; Hunter, N.; Normand, I.C.S.; Prescod, N.: Vesico-ureteric reflux and renal scarring. Kidney int. *8*: S65–S72 (1975).
43 Smellie, J.M.; Normand, I.C.S.: Pediatric nephrology, pp. 149–153 (Nijhoff, The Hague 1981).
44 Smellie, J.M.; Pursell, R.; Prescod, N.; Brumfitt, W.: Urinary tract infecton, pp. 31–38 (Oxford University Press, London 1973).
45 Still, J.L.; Cotton, D.: Severe hypertension in childhood. Archs Dis. Childh. *42*: 34–39 (1967).
46 Winberg, J.; Andersen, H.J.; Bergstrom, T.; Jacobsson, B.; Larson, H.; Lincoln, K.: Epidemiology of symptomatic urinary tract infection in childhood. Acta paediat. scand. suppl. 252: 3–20 (1974).

N.P. Goldraich, MD, Centro de Nefrologia Infantil, Praça Dom Feliciano 78 conj. 410, 90000 Porto Alegre RS (Brazil)

Contr. Nephrol., vol. 39, pp. 68–80 (Karger, Basel 1984)

6. Peripheral Plasma Renin Activity, Hypertension and Renal Scarring in Children[1]

Michael J. Dillon, Jean M. Smellie

Renal Unit, The Hospital for Sick Children, and Department of Paediatrics, University College Hospital, London, England

The relationship between plasma renin and hypertension was perhaps first alluded to by *Bright* [3] in 1836 when he reported left ventricular hypertrophy in patients dying of chronic glomerulonephritis and implied that there was something in the blood causing vasoconstriction and hence requiring greater cardiac action to maintain the circulation. Since then considerable evidence has accrued to implicate the role of the renin-angiotensin system in various types of renal hypertension including that associated with pyelonephritic scarring (reflux nephropathy, RN) [13, 18] although some still doubt the relationship [1]. The studies outlined in this paper go some way to establish the role of renin in the hypertension of children with RN and emphasize the value of peripheral and renal vein renin measurements in investigation and treatment.

Peripheral Plasma Renin in Normotensive Children with RN

5 years ago 100 normotensive children were studied aged 2–15 years (group A) with radiologically demonstrable RN associated with previous vesico-ureteric reflux (VUR) in an attempt to evaluate the role of peripheral plasma renin activity (PRA) in predicting which patients might subsequently develop hypertension [16]. This was felt to be of relevance, since 10% of children with evidence of RN appear to develop hypertension [21] which carries with it serious implications in terms of morbidity and mortal-

[1] This work was supported by the Kidney Research Aid Fund. PRA measurements were undertaken by Mrs. *Vanita Shah*.

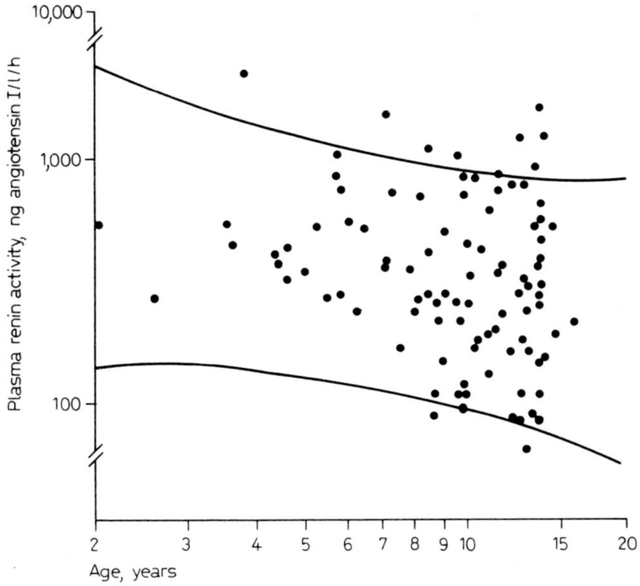

Fig. 1. PRA levels in 100 normotensive children with RN (group A). Solid lines indicate the upper and lower limits of the normal range [from ref. 16, with permission].

ity [6]. The already published findings revealed that 8 of the 100 children had PRA values above the normal range (fig. 1), and the negative correlation between PRA and age was much weaker than in normal children (fig. 2) ($r = -0.267$, $p < 0.01$, for the normotensive scarred group, and $r = -0.635$, $p < 0.001$, for the normal children). The difference was significant ($p < 0.001$) but there was no clear correlation between PRA and urine sodium creatinine ratio, plasma creatinine, blood pressure and severity of RN.

These children are currently being re-examined to establish their present PRA and blood pressure status but unfortunately there are no meaningful results available to date. However, 26 other normotensive children with RN (group B) have been examined at the Hospital for Sick Children recently and of these 5 (19.2%) had PRA above the normal range for age (fig. 3, 4). Comparing this normotensive group of children with RN, in terms of PRA, with a similarly aged group of normal controls (group C), there was a significant difference ($p < 0.05$); the negative correlation between PRA and age was weaker than in normal children ($r = -0.21$) and of the same order as found in the previous study.

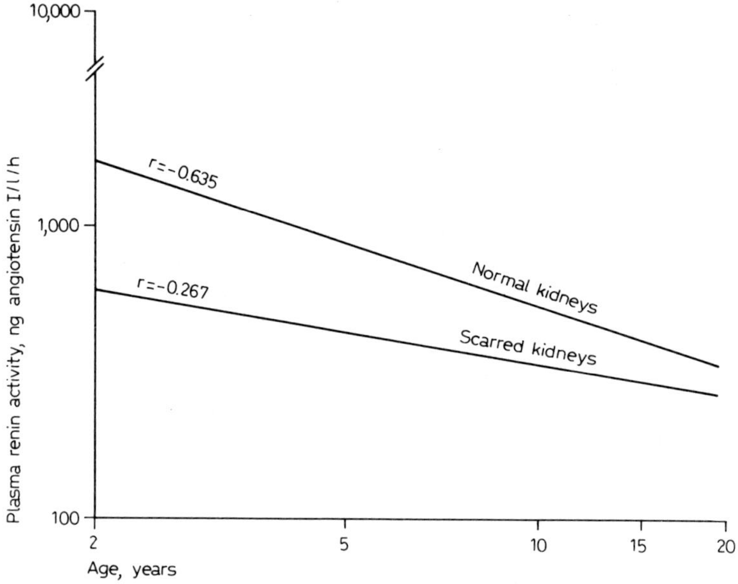

Fig. 2. PRA/age regression lines for normal and RN (groups A and C) [from ref. 16, with permission].

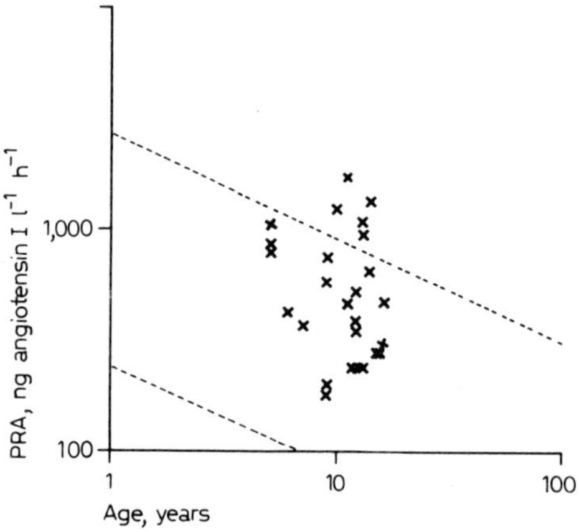

Fig. 3. PRA levels in 26 normotensive children with RN (group B). Dotted lines indicate upper and lower limits of the normal range.

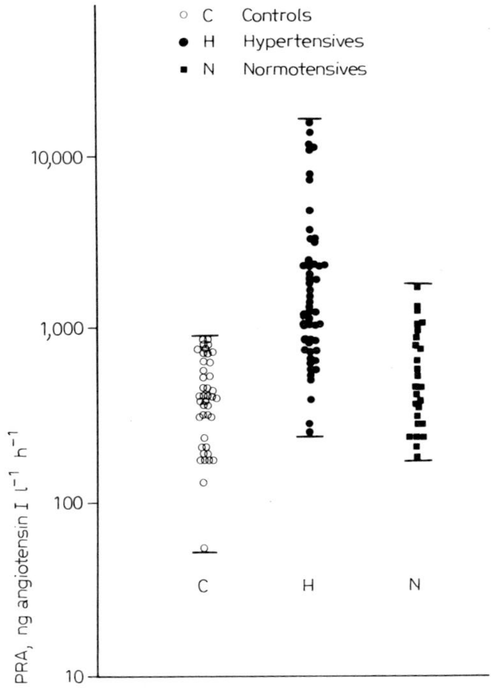

Fig. 4. PRA levels in healthy control children (group C) (C), hypertensive children with RN (group D) (H), and normotensive children with RN (group B) (N).

Peripheral Plasma Renin in Hypertensive Children with RN

We have previously shown that in children with significant hypertension associated with RN PRA is increased above the normal range in the majority of cases [7, 16]. This observation has been confirmed in a further 51 children with RN kidneys and significant, but non-malignant, hypertension studied at the Hospital for Sick Children (group D). In 36 children PRA was markedly above the normal range, and in 15 others the values were within this range but above the mean (fig. 4, 5).

PRA of this group of hypertensive patients (group D) was very significantly increased compared to age-matched controls (group C) ($p < 0.001$) but was also significantly increased compared to normotensive patients with RN ($p < 0.005$) (group B). What is more, the negative correlation between PRA and age for group D patients was weaker than seen in group B; with an r value of -0.19.

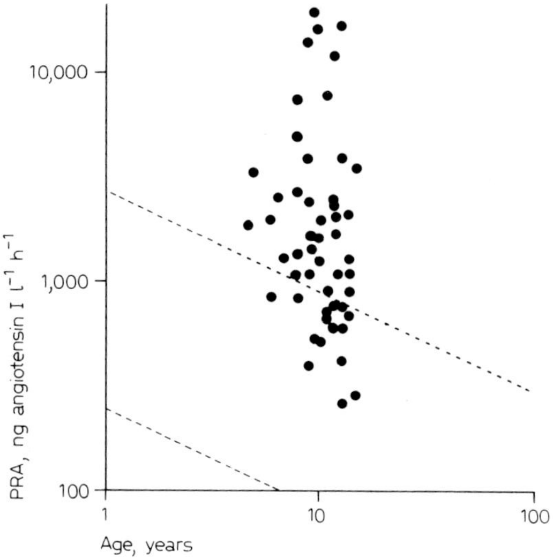

Fig. 5. PRA levels in hypertensive children with RN (group D). Dotted lines indicate upper and lower limits of the normal range.

Mixed (Hypertensive and Normotensive) Children with RN Scarred Kidneys

In comparison with the aforementioned, a further group of patients with RN and VUR was studied. This was composed of 47 children and young adults on prophylactic urinary antiseptics attending University College Hospital who had been followed carefully for many years by one of us. On these patients, 62 PRA measurements were undertaken; in 13 patients duplicate samples were obtained on separate occasions and, in one, PRA was estimated 3 times on separate occasions.

The patients were divided into 2 groups: children aged 5–15 years (group E), and young adults (group F) (fig. 6, 7). There was no significant difference in terms of PRA between the younger patients (5–15 years) and age-matched controls (group B). But in the older patients (group F), the PRA was significantly increased compared to controls, and 9 of them were hypertensive as defined by blood pressure measurements > +2 SD above the mean of the Task Force Report on Blood Pressure Control [2]. When followed graphically (fig. 7), 7 PRA values from 6 patients were above the normal range, and among whom 4 were marginally hypertensive (blood pressure 130/80 to 140/90 mm Hg). However, there were 9 other patients

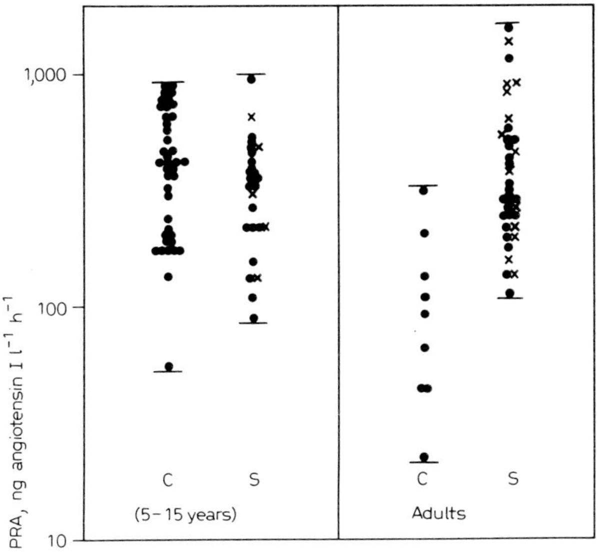

Fig. 6. PRA levels in healthy control children and young adults (group C) (C), and children with RN (groups E and F) (S). The latter are divided into groups by age and also by the presence (X) or absence, (●) of hypertension. (The symbols represent PRA measurements including duplicates.)

in whom the blood pressure was increased slightly, yet their PRA levels were within the normal range. Of these, 4 were in the 5–15 year age group. The negative correlation between PRA and age in this group as a whole was obliterated, with r = +0.1, which is significantly different to the findings in controls.

Indirect Means of Detecting Renin-Dependent Hypertension

Pharmacological means of blocking the action and production of angiotensin II (AII) are now available, and have some diagnostic and therapeutic implications. Saralasin (Sar^{1}-Ala^{8}-AII) is a competitive angiotensin II inhibitor which can cause a significant decrease in blood pressure on controlled i.v. infusion in hypertensive states in which there is a major 'angiotensiogenic' component [20]. Interpretation can be difficult in childhood [10], but in several hypertensive patients with RN who were not salt-depleted we found a hypotensive response correlated with pre-infusion

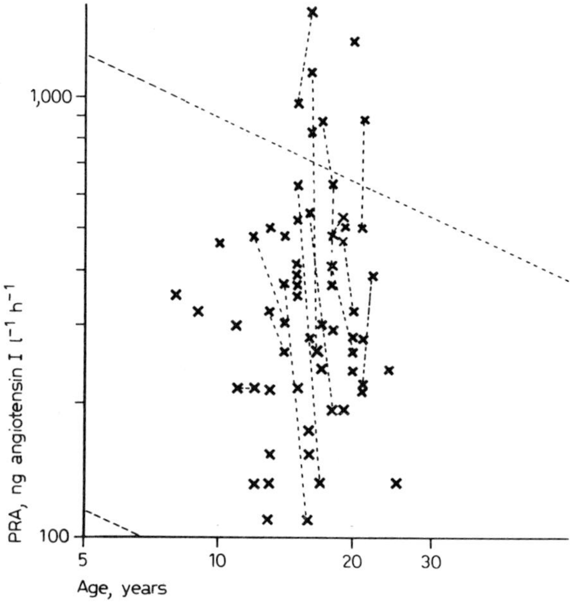

Fig. 7. PRA levels in children with RN (groups E and F). Dotted lines indicate upper and lower limits of normal range. Values joined by further dotted lines indicate duplicate results in the same child at different times.

PRA. However the test did not appear to offer a distinct advantage over peripheral renin measurements.

Similarly, attempts have been made to use captopril, a converting enzyme inhibitor, diagnostically in renin-dependent hypertensive states. Unfortunately the drug is capable of lowering the blood pressure in a variety of hypertensive situations and some have suggested that its action may be largely independent of circulating renin [4]. However, its hypotensive effect in hyper-reninaemic hypertensive children can be very pronounced and this phenomen has been utilized diagnostically in children following a single oral dose [12].

Renal Vein Renin Measurements

Determination of bilateral renal venous renin levels has been established as a diagnostically acceptable procedure in identifying surgically curable forms of renal hypertension [19] and this technique has been applied

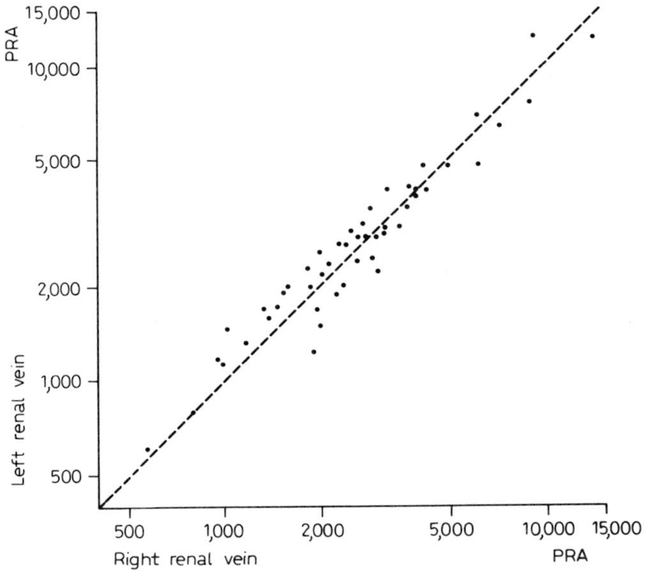

Fig. 8. Relationships between PRA (ng angiotensin I l^{-1} h^{-1}) in the left renal vein and right renal vein in normotensive children without kidney disease. Dashed line indicates line of identity [from ref. 11, with permission].

successfully to the investigation of hypertensive children [8, 9]. However, until relatively recently, a reference range of renal vein PRA ratios did not exist, although there were some reports on ratios in adult patients with essential hypertension and apparently normal kidneys [14, 17].

Renal Vein Renin Measurements in Normotensive Children without Kidney Disease. 3 years ago, *Gerdts* et al. [11] at the Hospital for Sick Children established a reference range of renal venous PRA ratios in normotensive children free of renal disease by studying 49 children undergoing routine cardiac catheterization. PRA levels did not differ significantly between both renal veins (fig. 8), with a mean right-to-left ratio of 1.03 and a mean higher-to-lower renal vein ratio of 1.16. Utilizing the latter ratios the 95% confidence limit was 1.41. There was a constant mean ratio of 1.21 between the renal veins and the inferior vena cava (IVC) at low, intermediate and high absolute PRA levels (fig. 9), and a figure of 1.15 was found, when analysed in terms of the lower main vein PRA to IVC ratio. These observations supported a main vein PRA ratio of 1.5 as an accepta-

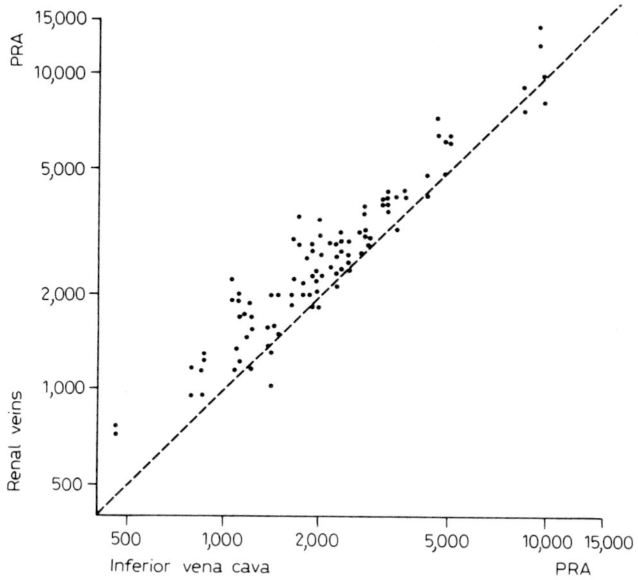

Fig. 9. Relationship between renal vein PRA (ng angiotensin I l^{-1} h^{-1}), both left and right, and inferior vena cava PRA in normotensive children without kidney disease [from ref. 11, with permission].

ble upper limit of normality, but interpretation of the contralateral kidney venous PRA to IVC ratio was less secure, since there was no pathological stimulus present to suppress renin release.

Renal Venous Renin Measurements in Hypertensive Children with Scarred Kidneys. During the past 8 years, 54 renal vein renin studies have been undertaken at the Hospital for Sick Children on 52 patients with RN and hypertension. In 21 patients the disease was unilateral, in 24 bilateral but asymmetrical, and in 7 bilateral and symmetrical. In 33 patients renal vein ratios were >1.5, and it is noteworthy that none of these had symmetrical renal disease. 13 patients with unilateral disease and 9 with bilateral asymmetrical disease underwent surgery. 14 were cured, and in 8 blood pressure control was significantly improved. There were 20 nephrectomies, 1 nephrectomy together with a partial nephrectomy, 1 partial nephrectomy, and the remainder were treated medically.

Segmental Renal Vein Sampling. A refinement on the main renal vein sampling technique is to obtain specimens for PRA analysis from the segmental veins within the kidneys. By so doing local sources of renin release can be identified that may be missed by main vein sampling. We have undertaken this type of study on 25 children with RN. Samples were obtained, when possible, from the upper, middle and lower zone segmental veins of each kidney in addition to the main renal vein and IVC specimens. In approximately half of these patients the data so obtained proved useful in terms of identifying sources of renin release that the main vein sampling had not detected.

Discussion

These peripheral plasma renin data strongly implicate renin in the hypertension seen in patients with RN and support our earlier similar findings, although at that time the number of children studied was limited [16]. However, though not all the PRA values in the hypertensive group of patients were above the normal range for age, they were probably inappropriately raised in relation to the blood pressure at the time. It could be argued that the physiological response to non-malignant hypertension is renin suppression, and any non-suppressed high normal range PRA is suggestive of a renin-dependent hypertensive state. Furthermore, the loss of the negative correlation of PRA with age in the hypertensive patients suggests a changed renin status which seems unlikely to be explained in terms of an epiphenomenon.

The use of agents which block the renin-angiotensin system, such as saralasin and captopril, has thrown some more light on the pathophysiology of the hypertension of children with scarred kidneys. In our limited experience, the hypotensive responses seen following controlled administration of these agents to children with hypertension and renal scarring have correlated with the preceding peripheral PRA values – namely a greater decrease in blood pressure in those with hyper-reninaemia. Undoubtedly a lowering of the blood pressure may result in circumstances other than those with renin excess [4, 10]., which can give rise to false-positive findings, but in spite of this the evidence adds some weight to the view that renin does have a role in the hypertension of renal scarring. The interesting observation that in our initial study of normotensive children (group A) with RN [16] 8% had PRA values above the normal range suggested a possible means of predicting those children at risk of subsequently developing hypertension. This was of particular relevance since approximately 10% of children and young adults with VUR and RN are hypertensive [21]. It remains to be seen whether the current review of these particular patients will confirm or refute this hypothesis.

The study of the second group of normotensive children (group B) supports this earlier view, as the findings that 5 of 26 children had PRA values above the normal range (19.2%) is clearly higher than those findings in group A and may possibly reflect more extensive RN in the children studied. Both groups A and B demonstrated a weaker negative correlation between PRA and age when compared to controls, suggesting a disturbance in the renin-angiotensin system contributing to the significantly reduced tendency of PRA to fall with age in the presence of renal scarring.

The findings of groups E and F tend to support a possible age factor in the evolution of hyper-reninaemia in children with RN. PRA in younger patients (group E) was not significantly different to that in age-matched controls, but in the young adults (group F) PRA was increased, and it was within this group that two thirds of the hypertensive patients were found. Taking groups E and F together, the overall incidence of hyper-reninaemia was 13%, which is similar to the original findings in group A, and about 8.5% of patients were hyper-reninaemic and also marginally hypertensive. With the overall incidence of hypertension, albeit mild, of 27.7% when groups E and F were combined, there were obviously some patients with high blood pressure yet normal peripheral PRA. As yet this finding remains unexplained. A possible explanation might be the so-called second pressor effect of angiotensin [5].

In the context of blood pressure measurements in groups B, E and F it is fair to say that the same stringent blood pressure recording protocol as used in group A was not employed. Blood pressure in these groups was taken by careful sphygmomanometry but without equipment to avoid observer bias or digit preference. However, undertaken appropriately we have shown that this method of blood pressure recording can be very accurate [15]; yet we accept its limitations in detecting minor blood pressure changes.

In our experience, the use of both main and segmental renal vein renin measurements has practical value in identifying local sources of renin release within kidneys, and is helpful in predicting success of surgical treatment of renal hypertension if this is considered feasible [8]. The establishment of a normal range of main renal vein renin ratios supports a renal vein PRA ratio of 1.5 as an acceptable upper limit of normality. This ratio has been used successfully in children to define asymmetric renin release and to predict a successful outcome to surgical treatment in terms of blood pressure control.

There are limited data on the use of these techniques in patients with scarred kidneys where the situation is not so well defined, as in, for example, renovascular disease. Nonetheless, in our large experience of renal vein renin measurements in children with hypertension and RN the 22 patients eventually treated surgically on the basis of a main vein renin ratio of >1.5 have been either cured or very significantly improved. Comparatively, as can be seen, the vast majority of cases have been managed medically because of bilateral disease with evidence of excess renin production in both kidneys. Segmental sampling may be a means of identifying local renin production in areas of scarring amenable to local surgical removal. However, although this may eventually be feasible the distinction betwen areas of scarring and normal kidney is far from clear and there is a long way to go before advocating this approach without serious reservations.

We find it difficult not to conclude that in hyper-reninaemic hypertensive individuals with RN, the high renin levels in main or segmental renal veins do indeed reflect increased renin release from those areas of kidney draining into them and that PRA measurements from these veins have a useful diagnostic role.

References

1 Bailey, R.R.; McCrae, C.U.; Maling, T.M.J.; Tisch, G.; Little, P.J.: Renal veing renin concentrations in the hypertension of unilateral reflux nephropathy. J. Urol. *120*: 21–23 (1978).

2 Blumenthal, S.; Epps, R.P.; Heavenrich, R.; Lauer, R.M.; Lieberman, E.; Mirkin, B.; Mitchell, S.C.; Naito, V.B.; O'Hare, E.; McFate Smith, T.; Tarazi, R.C.; Upson, D.: Report of the task force on blood pressure control in children. Pediatrics Springfield, *59*: suppl., pp. 797–820 (1977).

3 Bright, R.: Tabular view of the morbid appearances in 100 cases connected with albuminous urine with observations. Guy's Hosp. Rep. *1*: 380–400 (1836).

4 De Bruyn, J.H.B.; Wenting, G.J.; Man in 'T Veld, A.J. Derkx, F.H.M.; Schalekamp, M.A.D.H.: Captopril affects blood pressure equally in renovascular and essential hypertension and in the fluid-depleted anephric state. Clin. Sci. *59*: suppl. 6, pp. 83S–86S (1980).

5 Dickinson, C.J.; Lawrence, J.R.: A slowly developing pressor response to small concentrations of angiotensin. Its bearing on the pathogenesis of chronic renal hypertension. Lancet *i*: 1354–1356 (1963).

6 Dillon, M.J.: Recent advances in evaluation and management of childhood hypertension. Eur. J. Pediat. *132*: 133-139 (1979).

7 Dillon, M.J.: Application of study of renin-angiotensin system to pediatric pathology; in Giovannelli, New, Gorini, Hypertension in children andn adolescents, pp. 137–146 (Raven Press, New York 1981).

8 Dillon, M.J.: Renal vein renin determinations in evaluating hypertensive children; in Gruskin, Norman, Pediatric nephrology, pp. 127–133 (Nijhoff, The Hague 1981).

9 Dillon, M.J.; Shah, V.; Barratt, T.M.: Renal vein renin measurements in children with hypertension. Br. med. J. *ii*: 168-170 (1978).

10 Favre, L.; Boerth, R.C.; Braron, V.; Dean, R.H.; Hollifield, J.W.: Angiotensin II blockade by saralasin in the evaluation of hypertension in children. Kidney int. *15*: suppl. 9, pp. 75–82 (1979).

11 Gerdts, K.-G.; Shah, V.; Savage, J.M.; Dillon, M.J.: Renal vein renin measurements in normotensive children. J. Pediat. *95*: 953–958 (1979).

12 Goldraich, N.P.: Personal communication (1982).

13 Holland, N.H.; Kotchen, T.; Bhathena, D.: Hypertension in children with chronic pyelonephritis. Kidney int. *8*: suppl. 5, S243–S251 (1975).

14 Maxwell, M.H.; Marks, L.S.; Varady, P.D.; Lupu, A.N.; Kaufman, J.J.: Renal vein renin in essential hypertension. J. Lab. clin. Med. *86*: 901–909 (1975).

15 Savage, J.M.; Dillon, M.J.; Taylor, J.F.N.: Clinical evaluation and comparison of the Infrasonde, Arteriosonde, and Mercury sphygmomanometer in measurement of blood pressure in children. Archs Dis. Childh. *54*: 184–189 (1979).

16 Savage, J.M.; Dillon, M.J.; Shah, V.; Barratt, T.M.; Williams, D.I.: Renin and blood pressure in children with renal scarring and vesico-ureteric reflux. Lancet *ii*: 441–444 (1978).

17 Sealey, J.E.; Buhler, F.R.; Laragh, J.H.; Vaughan, E.D.: The physiology of renin secretion in essential hypertension. Estimation of renin secretion rate and renal plasma flow from peripheral and renal vein renin levels. Am. J. Med. *55*: 391–401 (1973).

18 Siegler, R.L.: Renin-dependent hypertension in children with refluy nephropathy. Urology *7*: 474 (1976).

16 Stockigt, J.R.; Noakes, C.A.; Collings, R.D.; Schambelan, M.; Biglieri, E.G.: Renal vein renin in various forms of renal hypertension. Lancet *i*: 1194–1198 (1972).

20 Streeton, D.H.P.; Anderson, G.H.; Freiberg, J.M.; Dalakos, T.G.: Use of an angiotensin II antagonist (saralasin) in the recognition of 'angiotensinogenic' hypertension. New Engl. J. Med. *292*: 657–662 (1975).

21 Wallace, D.M.A.; Rothwell, D.L.; Williams, D.I.: The long-term follow-up of surgically treated vesico-ureteric reflux. Br. J. Urol. *50*: 479–484 (1978).

Dr. Michael J. Dillon, The Hospital for Sick Children, Great Ormond Street, London WC1N 3JH (England)

Contr. Nephrol., vol. 39, pp. 81–93 (Karger, Basel 1984)

7. Vesicoureteral Reflux: A Comparison of Non-Surgical and Surgical Management

Mark F. Bellinger[a], *John W. Duckett*[b]

[a]The Pennsylvania State University, Director, Pediatric Urology, Milton Hershey Medical Center, Hershey, Pa.; [b]University of Pennsylvania Medical School, Director, Pediatric Urology. The Children's Hospital of Philadelphia, Philadelphia, Pa., USA

A vast and controversial body of literature has accumulated over the last several years concerning vesicoureteral reflux (VUR). Recent data concerning reflux nephropathy (RN), hypertension, and urinary tract infections (UTI) during pregnancy, with resultant fetal wastage [1], have underscored the importance of this disease to many segments of the medical community. In order to evaluate the success of our medical and surgical regimens, and to assess the factors that lead us to surgical intervention, we have reviewed the records of 392 patients treated for primary VUR at the Children's Hospital of Philadelphia from 1970 to 1979. During this period, 185 patients (47%) were treated non-surgically, while 207 (53%) underwent surgical correction of their VUR (table I). Patients with neuropathic bladders or dysfunctional voiding were excluded, as were those with obstructive uropathy.

Clinical Experience

The average age at presentation was 3.9 years in both non-surgical and surgical groups. Only 18% of the patients were males. UTI was the most common presentation, frequently with fever in the younger age group. Secondary enuresis was also a common presentation, indicative of UTI.

All patients were evaluated by intravenous urography (IVU) and voiding cystourethrography (VCU). Those in the non-surgical group had repeat studies at 12- to 18-month intervals unless more frequent follow-up was deemed necessary due to the age of the child or a marked degree of VUR. Those in the surgical group had follow-up IVUs and VCUs at 3

Table I. Patient population

Renal units	Non-surgical		Surgical		Total	
	n	%	n	%	n	%
Renal units	280		338		618	
Patients	185	47	207	53	392	
Male	30	16	39	19	69	18
Female	155	84	168	81	323	82

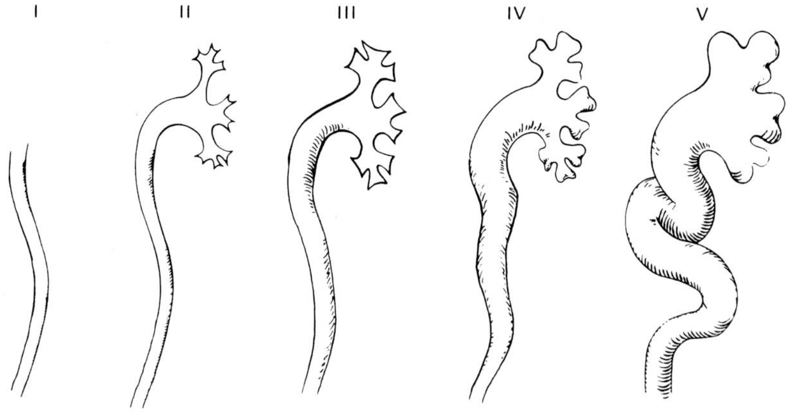

Fig. 1. Grades of reflux – International Study Classification: *I* Ureter only; *II* Ureter, pelvis and calices. No dilatation, normal caliceal fornices; *III* Mild or moderate dilatation and/or tortuosity of ureter and mild or moderate dilatation of renal pelvis but no or slight blunting of fornices; *IV* Moderate dilatation and/or tortuosity of ureter and moderate dilatation of renal pelvis and calices. Complete obliteration of sharp angle of fornices but maintenance of papillary impressions in majority of calices; *V* Gross dilatation and tortuosity of ureter. Gross dilatation of renal pelvis and calices. Papillary impressions are no longer visible in majority of calices.

months postoperatively, with subsequent IVUs at 1, 3, and 5 years to follow renal growth.

IVU demonstrated RN (i.e. chronic pyelonephritis, renal scarring) at presentation in 36 kidneys (13%) in the NS group and in 136 kidneys (40%) in the surgical group. VCU was performed on the awake patient, using bodytemperature contrast with judicious use of fluoroscopic monitoring, especially during the voiding phase. Small infant feeding tubes are used in all patients in preference to balloon catheters, to avoid overfilling and to

Table II. Cystographic grading at presentation in 618 renal units

	Non-surgical grade						Surgical grade					
	1	2	3	4	5	?	1	2	3	4	5	?
Unilateral VUR												
Left	8	26	9	3	1	1	0	13	17	17	6	1
Right	4	22	8	6	1	0	0	9	4	5	4	
Bilateral VUR												
Left	16	51	15	12	1	4	7	31	38	45	7	1
Right	12	47	16	11	0	6	5	27	43	48	9	1
Total	40	146	48	32	3	11	12	80	102	115	26	3

Table III. Cystoscopic Evaluation

Orifice Description	Non-surgical					Surgical				
	1	2	3	4	5	1	2	3	4	5
Normal	–	$\frac{5}{7}$	$\frac{0}{1}$	–	–	–	7	4	3	–
Moderately abnormal	$\frac{2}{3}$	$\frac{17}{30}$	$\frac{5}{15}$	$\frac{8}{14}$	$\frac{0}{1}$	1	27	15	37	3
Abnormal	–	–	$\frac{2}{9}$	$\frac{0}{3}$	$\frac{0}{1}$	–	13	28	37	5

$$\frac{\text{Numerator}}{\text{Denominator}} = \frac{\text{number ceasing VUR}}{\text{total number}}$$

allow for spontaneous voiding. We have graded VUR according the *Heikel and Parkkulainen* [2] system, recently refined and adopted by the International Reflux Study Committee [17] (fig. 1). The grades of VUR at presentation in our patients are seen in table II. 6 patients in the surgical group (not included in table II) developed contralateral VUR after unilateral reimplantation.

All patients in the surgical group were evaluated endoscopically prior to surgery. Selected non-surgical patients were also evaluated during their course of observation. Table III reflects the endoscopic findings in those patients whose records could be accurately evaluated.

Table IV. Renal scarring as to grade VUR

	Non-surgical group[1]									Surgical group[1]															
	2			3			4			2				3				4				5				?			
	a	b	c	a	b	c	a	b	c	a	b	c	d	a	b	c	d	a	b	c	d	a	b	c	d	a	b	c	d
Total scarred		10			12			12			12				26				74				22				3		
Unilateral scar		5			4			3			5				9				22				8				3		
	3	2	0	2	2	0	0	2	1	3	2	0	–	6	3	0	–	7	10	3	2	1	1	3	3	1	2	0	–
Bilateral scar	1	0		–	–	–	2	4	0	2	0	0	–	3	5	2	–	15	10	9	–	5	1	4	–	–	–	–	–
Unilateral scar with bilateral VUR		2			2			0			2				3				7				1				–		
VUR equal bilaterally	2	0	0	2	0	0	–	–	–	2	0	0	–	3	0	0	–	6	1	0	–	0	1	0	–				
Unequal VUR		2			4			2			2				4				11				4				–		
Worst side scarred	–	–	–	3	0	0	1	0	1	2	0	0	–	2	1	1	–	8	1	1	1	0	2	2	–	–	–	–	–
Unequal VUR		0			2			1			0				0				0				0				–		
Lesser side scarred	–	–	–	2	0	0	0	1	0	–	–	–	–	–	–	–	–	–	–	–	–	–	–	–	–	–	–	–	–
% scarring per grade		6			25			37			14				25				64				85						

[1]Numbers (2–5) = VUR grade; letters (a–d) = scarring grade.

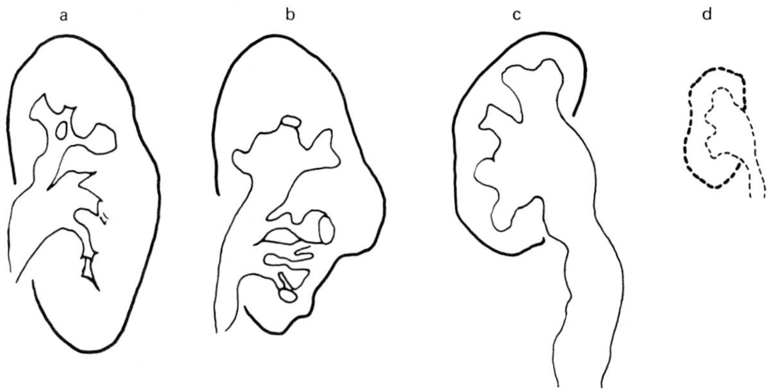

Fig. 2. Grading of parenchymal scarring: *a* Not more than 2 scars. *b* More than 2 scars plus areas of significant parenchymal thickness. *c* Diffuse thinness of parenchyma with generalized calicectasis. *d* Small kidney with insignificant parenchymal thickness. (From ref. 13, with permission).

Renal scarring (RN) was evaluated by assessment of the IVU. In the non-surgical group it was found in 6% of units with grade II reflux, 25% with grade III, and 37% of those with grade IV reflux (table IV). In the surgical group 14% of grade II, 25% of grade III, 64% of grade IV, and 85% of grade V had RN (table IV). We have also graded the degree of scarring according to the Smellie classification [9] (fig. 2).

Results of Non-Surgical Management

Of the 185 patients followed without surgical intervention, 48% had unilateral and 52% bilateral VUR. They were monitored closely, with frequent urine cultures, while being maintained on continuous suppressive doses of urinary antibacterials. Those who were lost to follow-up or who were followed less than 1 year were not considered in the spontaneous cessation rate (table V). Of the 165 units with VUR, it ceased spontaneously in 87% of grade I, 63% of grade II, 53% of grade III, and 33% of grade IV. Of the total group, 59% ceased; comprising 68% of grades I and II (undilated) and 47% of grades III and IV (dilated). The average age at which spontaneous cessation occurred was 6 years, and the mean period of follow-up between presentation and cessation was 3 years. At the end of the period of observation, 51% of the patients (41% of the renal units) con-

Table V. Spontaneous cessation of reflux in non-surgical group

	Grade				
	1	2	3	4	5
Number of renal units > 1 year in study	22	73	46	24	0
Cessation rate, %	87	63	53	33	–
Age at time of cessation, years	5.2	6.6	6.8	4.6	–
Time followed before cessation, years	2.3	3.3	3.9	1.8	–

tinued to reflux. Although 13% of the renal units demonstrated RN at presentation, only 1 patient (0.5%) developed further scarring during follow-up, after breakthrough UTI.

Results of Surgical Therapy

Of the 207 surgical patients, 77 (37%) had surgery recommended at the time of initial presentation to our institution. A number of these had been followed elsewhere before referral. The remaining 63% were followed for varying periods at our institution before undergoing surgery. Table II reflects that 42% of the patients had unilateral and 58% bilateral VUR. The primary success rate in preventing VUR was 95%, the overall one 98.5%. 6 patients (3%) developed contralateral VUR after unilateral reimplantation. Of these 1 resolved spontaneously, 2 have undergone reimplantation, and 3 continue to reflux. VUR was corrected by the techniques described by *Politano and Leadbetter* [3], *Glenn and Anderson* [4], and *Cohen* [5].

Cystoscopic evaluation prior to reimplantation was done in most cases and was considered an adjunctive measure to determine the need for reimplantation surgery and to assess the orifice of the contralateral ureter in children with unilateral VUR. 7% of the surgical group underwent bilateral reimplantation for unilateral VUR, the decision for this being primarily based on cystoscopic findings of a short contralateral submucosal tunnel. 7 patients underwent procedures other than ureteroneocystostomy; in 4, nephrectomy of a non-functioning kidney; in 1, heminephroureterectomy of the non-functional half of a duplicated system; and in 1, also with a duplicated system, ureteroureterostomy with excision of the refluxing renal seg-

Table VI. Surgical procedures in 207 patients

	%
Unilateral reimplantation	26
Bilateral reimplantation	63
Bilateral reimplantation for unilateral VUR	7
Contralateral reimplantation necessary after unilateral reimplantation	1
Procedure other than reimplantation	3

ment. 1 infant with severe VUR and sepsis underwent temporary diversion by vesicostomy, with later closure and bilateral reimplantation (table VI).

The surgical complication rate requiring reoperation was 5%, disregarding minor wound problems, transient VUR and transient obstruction (table VII). Of the 7 renal units developing postoperative obstruction, all had been reimplanted using the technique of *Politano and Leadbetter* [3]. Only 1 of these ureters had been tapered. Of the 9 units exhibiting postoperative ipsilateral VUR, 4 had been reimplanted using the technique of *Glenn and Anderson* [4], 4 using that of *Politano and Leadbetter* [3], and 1 using the Lich-Gregoire technique [6]. Surveillance of postoperative UTI was continued with routine cultures every 3 months for 2 years. Prophylactic medications were discontinued after the 3-month VCU was normal. In the group with grade II VUR, 3 patients had one postoperative UTI each, while 3 others had recurrent bouts of cystitis. In the grade III group, 2 had one UTI while 3 had recurrent UTIs; in the grade IV group, 3 had recurrent UTIs, and no UTI was documented in grade V. Thus, 7% of our surgical group had recurrent UTI while 1% (3 patients) had acute pyelonephritis in the immediate postoperative period (all 3 had their UTI detected only when the intraoperative culture results became available).

Discussion

Concepts in the treatment of VUR have undergone a continuous and, at times, confusing evolution as the traditional medical-surgical barriers be-

Table VII. Surgical complications in 338 renal units

Complication	Number of renal units	%
Obstruction		
Transient	1	0.3
Reoperation	7	2.0
VUR: Ipsilateral		
Transient	1	0.3
Persistent	2	0.6
Reoperation	7	2.0
VUR: Contralateral		
Transient	1	0.3
Persistent	3	1.0
Reoperation	2	0.6
Acute pyelonephritis	3	1.0
Hypertension	2	0.6

come less distinct and physicians concerned with the care of these children have begun to focus on RN and its pathogenesis. Most pediatric urologists and nephrologists consider that sterile VUR of moderate degree, and associated with normal renal growth does not require surgery. Severe VUR, recurrent UTI despite suppressive medication, RN, and non-compliance by the patient to medical therapy are considerations for surgery. Controversy still surrounds the non-surgical management of higher grades of VUR, the appropriate timing of surgical intervention in moderate VUR – if at all – and the efficacy of diagnostic methods in predicting the likelihood of spontaneous cessation.

The detection of a single proven UTI in a child requires radiologic investigation or other further work-up. Since 30–50% of children with UTI will be found to have VUR; and 80% of those with one UTI will suffer a recurrence, half of which will be asymptomatic [7], further delay in full evaluation is not warranted. Failure to thrive is a non-specific sign in infants and young children, typified by poor weight gain and a generally deficient metabolic state. Such children should always have their urine cultured, and if it is found positive, proceed to evaluation for VUR. IVU should be accompanied by an adequate VCU, as the former alone will not diagnose VUR. At the time of initial evaluation, we feel that contrast radiographic studies should be done in order to grade and delineate both anatomic and functional lesions. Subsequent follow-up by nuclear cystography has definite advantages. Renal scans have recently been shown to equal or surpass an IVU for sensitivity and specificity in the detection of renal scarring [16].

Endoscopy is not a routine screening procedure for the evaluation of VUR. Urethral dilatation has not been shown to be an effective treatment, so we do not think a patient with UTI need be subjected to an anesthetic for the purpose of cystoscopy and urethral dilatation. Endoscopic assessment of the ureterovesical anatomy is very subjective, the interpretation being modified by the degree of bladder filling and the experience of the observer in evaluating the trigone and ureteral orifices. In striving to define ureteral orifice location as described by *Mackie* et al. [8], and orifice configuration as outlined by *Lyon* et al. [9], we have been disappointed with our lack of consistency when several observers evaluate the same bladder. Therefore, we prefer a general orifice description, based on position and configuration, and labelled as normal, moderately abnormal, or abnormal (table III). In addition, the length of the submucosal tunnel seems an appropriate variable to record [10]. We can objectively measure this with a transilluminating ureteral catheter (such a product is now available from VanTech, P.O. Box 26, Spencer, IN 47460, USA). Other more subjective interpretations may be made with a calibrated ureteral catheter, or a more rigid No. 4F Bugbee electrode.

In our non-surgical group, half of the patients also had ureteral orifice assessment. Only 2 of the 13 recorded as abnormal have ceased their VUR (15%) while 32 of 63 recorded as moderately abnormal ceased (50%). In the surgical group, 179 of the 207 patients had adequately recorded criteria to assess their ureteral orifices. 46% were recorded as abnormal, 46% as moderately abnormal, and 8% as normal. In comparison, *Mulcahy and Kelalis* [11], using similar criteria, found that in a non-surgical group of 182 ureters VUR ceased in 25 (36%) of 69 severely abnormal orifices; in 17 (31%) of 55 moderately abnormal ones, and in 52% of the 58 recorded as normal. They further showed that the presence or absence of recurrent UTI did not seem to be a factor in the cessation rate. A review of these data leads one to conclude that there is probably no more than a 50% correlation between predictability of VUR cessation and orifice assessment.

7% of our surgical group underwent bilateral reimplantation for unilateral VUR. This was based on the endoscopic assessment that the contralateral orifice was abnormal. This probably accounts for our low (1.9%) contralateral VUR rate (table VII) in comparison with the 16% reported by others [12]. Again, however, cystoscopic evaluation probably has no more than a 50% accuracy in predicting VUR cessation. It may be that objective measurement of submucosal tunnel length using transillumination will be a refinement.

To further define the factors which influence the development of RN requires standardization of our investigative reports. To this end we are now designing a new recording system which encompasses the standardized grading systems advocated by the International Reflux Study Committee. By grading VUR according to *Heikel and Parkkulanien* [2], assessing parenchymal scarring by the method of *Smellie* et al. [13] and recording endoscopic findings at a standard 60 cm H_2O bladder pressure, we hope not only to minimize variables, but to provide a standardized record for effective later review.

Factors leading to our decision for surgical intervention are reviewed in table VIII. Radiographic evidence of scarring and the degree of VUR were most influential. Recurrent UTIs and cystoscopic confirmation of laterally placed orifices were additional factors in the majority of patients. It was clear that no single criterion was an indication for surgery. We do not feel that a rigorous point system as proposed by *Lyon* et al. [14] is justified.

The predictability of cessation of VUR remains a difficult problem. Our series, which includes a sizeable non-operative group to compare with those having surgical intervention, offers the best handle on this issue. Of patients followed non-operatively, 87% of grade I (19/22), 63% (46/73) of grade II, 53% (25/46) of grade III, and 33% (8/24) of grade IV ceased to reflux. The average length of time before cessation was approximately 3 years, and the patients were then about 6 years of age.

Surgical technique has changed over the years of this study. Initially, the Politano-Leadbetter method [3] was used and produced all of the obstructions (2%). Since most of these occurred in the early years, we anticipated that the advancement method as described by *Mathisen* [15] and advocated by *Glenn and Anderson* [4] in this country would avoid the potential kinking of the ureter during the creation of a new hiatus with the Politano-Leadbetter technique. We, however, failed to correct VUR in 4 patients using this technique. We are now pleased with the cross-trigonal advancement technique of *Cohen* [5] using the original ureteral hiatus (a modification of the Mathisen procedure), which will probably prove to be the most successful method, with the lowest complication rate.

Table VIII. Consideration for surgery in 207 patients

	At time of presentation		During medical regimen	
Abnormal X-ray	151		44	
RN		94		23
Poor renal growth		14		8
Severe VUR, blunting		43		13
Recurrent UTI	110		26	
Cystoscopy (abnormal orifice)	73		47	
Anatomic defect	39		5	
Paraureteral diverticulum		21		0
Ectopic or duplicate ureter		18		5
Child growing older with no change in VUR grade	0		23	
Failure to thrive	5		0	
Solitary kidney	4		1	
Poor renal function	1		1	
Pain	0		1	
Compliance	?		?	
Unknown	4		3	

Conclusions

Our objective in the management of VUR is to avoid progressive renal damage by the prevention of acute pyelonephritis and asymptomatic UTI. This may be achieved by continuous prophylactic antibacterial therapy, detecting asymptomatic UTI by close surveillance with routine urine cultures. Non-surgical management thus demands compliance to medication prescribed, complete understanding of the medical condition, and great patience over many years by the parents and primary care physicians. Periodic follow-up radiographic studies of various sorts are necessary to evaluate scarring and renal growth.

Likewise, these objectives may be achieved by the successful surgical correction of VUR. This is dependent on the skill and experience of the surgeon, on the state of the bladder, and on the degree of upper urinary tract dilatation. Surgical treatment carries the risk of postoperative obstruction which, if detected too late, may cause irreversible damage. With close postoperative surveillance, however, dangerous obstruction may be detected and corrected successfully. Persistent VUR after surgery can also be corrected successfully. All of our 7 obstructed units were successfully reimplanted a second time without suffering permanent damage. All have demonstrated normal renal growth after relief of obstruction.

Even with our secondary reoperation rate of 4% (2% obstruction and 2% VUR) of the total surgical group none are obstructed and only 1.5% of the renal units still show VUR. These patients are placed under the same close surveillance as those patients in the non-operative group. We thus have 100% preservation of renal tissue with a 98.5% cure of VUR including those who required secondary procedures. This was achieved in a selective group of patients, 72% having VUR with ureteral dilatation (grades 3, 4, 5) and 42% with severe dilatation (grades 4, 5). In this series, surgical management of the higher grades of VUR offers comparable results to those of all grades followed medically.

References

1 Naeye, R.L.: Causes of the excessive rates of perinatal morality and prematurity in pregnancies complicated by maternal urinary-tract infections. New Engl. T. Med. *300*: 819 (1979).

2 Heikel, P.E.; Parkkulainen, K.V.: Vesico-ureteric reflux in children: a classification and results of conservative treatment. Ann. Radiol. *9*: 37 (1966).

3 Politano, V.A.; Leadbetter, W.F.: An operative technique for the correction of vesicoureteral reflux. J. Urol. *79*: 932 (1958).

4 Glenn, J.F.; Anderson, E.E.: Distal tunnel ureteral reimplantation. J. Urol. *97*: 623 (1977).

5 Cohen, S.J.: Ureterozystoneostomie: eine neue Antirefluxtechnik. Akt. Urol. *6*: 1 (1975).

6 Lich, R.; Howerton, L.W.; Davis, L.S.: Recurrent urosepsis in children. J. Urol. *86*: 554 (1961).

7 Kunin, C.M.: Detection, prevention, and management of urinary tract infections; 3rd ed. (Lea & Febiger, New York 1979).

8 Mackie, G.G.; Awang, H.; Stephens, F.D.: The ureteric orifice: the embryologic key to radiologic status of duplex kidneys. J. pediat Surg. *10*: 473 (1975).

9 Lyon, R.P.; Marshall, S.; Tanagho, E.: The ureteral orifice: its configuration and competency. J. Urol. *102*: 504 (1969).

10 King, L.R.: Vesicoureteral reflux: history, etiology, and conservative management; in Kelalis, King, Clinical pediatric urology (Saunders, Philadelphia 1976).
11 Mulcahy, J.J.; Kelalis, P.P.: Non-operative treatment of vesicoureteral reflux. J. Urol. *120*: 336 (1978).
12 Bauer, S.B.; Willscher, M.K.; Zammuto, P.J.; Retik, A.B.: Longterm results of anti-reflux surgery in children; in Hodson, Kincaid-Smith, Reflux nephropathy (Masson, New York 1979).
13 Smellie, J.; Edwards, D.; Hunter, N.; Normand, I.C.S.; Prescod, N.: Vesico-ureteric reflux and renal scarring. Kidney int. *8*: 5–65 (1975).
14 Lyon, R.P.; Marshall, S.K.; Scott, M.P.: Treatment of vesicoureteral reflux. Urology *15*: 38 (1980).
15 Mathisen, W.: Vesicoureteral reflux and its surgical correction. Surgery Gynec. Obstet. *118*: 965 (1964).
16 Merrick, M.V.; Uttley, W.S.; Wild, S.R.: The detection of pyelonephritic scarring in children by radioisotope imaging. Br. J. Urol. *53*: 544 (1980).
17 International Reflux Study Committee: Medical versus surgical treatment of primary vesicoureteral reflux. Prospective International Reflux Study in Children. J. Urol. *125*: 277 (1981).

John W. Duckett, MD, The Children's Hospital of Philadelphia, 34th Street and Civic Center Blvd, Philadelphia, PA 19104 (USA)

Contr. Nephrol., vol. 39, pp. 94–101 (Karger, Basel 1984)

8. Reflux Nephropathy in the Adult

Priscilla S. Kincaid-Smith[a], *Marcus G. Bastos*[b], *Gavin J. Becker*[b]

[a]Department of Medicine, University of Melbourne;
[b]Department of Nephrology, The Royal Melbourne Hospital, Victoria, Australia

145 patients with reflux nephropathy (RN) aged 14–65 who presented to our unit over the past 10 years have been studied.

The group includes 123 women with a mean age of 30 years, and 22 males with a mean age of 27 years (fig. 1). Patients who presented with end-stage renal failure (ESRF) requiring dialysis have been excluded from this group because such patients represent a more selected series. The group of 145 patients does, however, include 7 who deteriorated to ESRF during follow-up. The 4:1 female:male sex ratio in this group is in keeping with previous studies in adults [1].

When one turns to patients with ESRF, on the other hand, the sex ratio is different (fig. 2, table I). A group of 82 such patients included 52

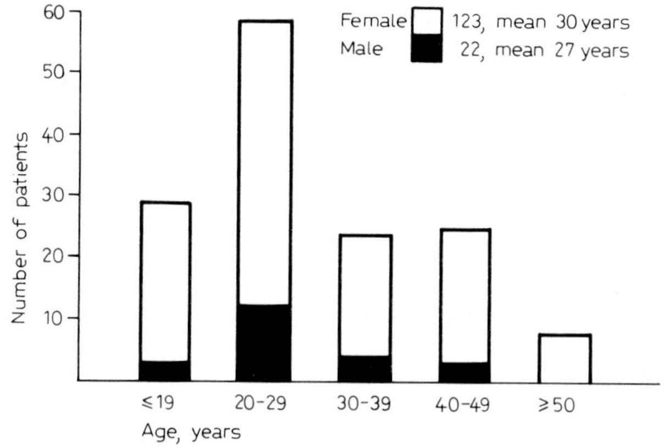

Fig. 1. Age and sex distribution in 145 adults with RN.

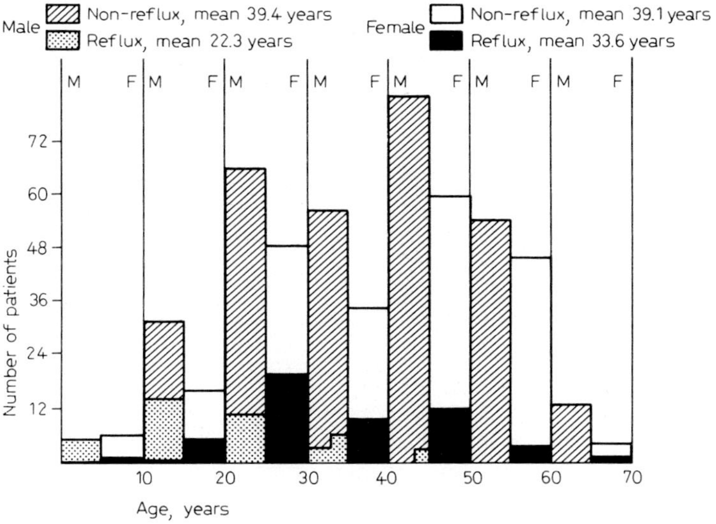

Fig. 2. Age and sex distribution of adults with RN presenting with ESRF.

Table I. End-stage renal failure

	1963–1972	1963–1982
Glomerulonephritis	76 (56%)	218 (41%)
Reflux nephropathy	25 (18.5%)[1]	82 (15.3%)[2]
Total	130	533

[1] Based on nephrectomy.
[2] Based on clinical and radiographic features.

women and 30 men, a ratio of less than 2:1 females to males. This same sex ratio in patients presenting with ESRF has been maintained over the 10-year period [2] and is clearly different from the sex ratio in the total group of adults with RN of all degrees. The mean age at which males with RN develop ESRF is 22 years, which is very significantly different from that of all males with ESRF of all categories treated in this unit, which is 39 years (fig. 2). For females, on the other hand, the same figures are 33 for those with ESRF from RN, compared with an age of 39 years for women with ESRF of all aetiologies; a difference of only 6 years.

Table II. Presenting findings[1] in 145 adults with reflux nephropathy

	Female (123)		Male (22)	
	n	%	n	%
UTI	62	50.4	4	18.1
Hypertension	26	21.1	5	22.7
Pregnancy-related abnormality	23	18.6	–	–
Proteinuria	4	3.2	11	50.0
Impaired renal function	5	4.0	2	9.0
Loin pain/abdominal pain	3	2.4	3	13.6
Microscopic haematuria	2	1.6	1	4.5
Family history alone	1	0.8	–	–

[1] Patients commonly had more than one abnormality.

Presenting features are also quite different in males and females with RN. 90% of women present in one of three ways: with urinary tract infection (UTI), hypertension, or pregnancy complications (table II). Males, on the other hand, most commonly present with proteinuria (50%) and are much more likely to present with impaired renal function. Hypertension was the presenting manifestation in 21.1% of females and 22.7% of males, but 45.3% of the overall group had a blood pressure over 140 systolic or 90 diastolic. 4.1% had accelerated hypertension with retinal haemorrhages and exudates, or papilloedema, or both at the same time. Malignant hypertension may cause rapid progression to renal failure.

The clinical feature which has the best predictive value for prognosis is proteinuria. Figure 3 shows the relationship between the degree of proteinuria and impaired renal function in males and females. It is noteworthy that only 3 of 22 males had a normal serum creatinine level at the time of presentation compared with 77.9% of 123 females. The relatively higher proportion of males developing ESRF due to RN reflect a much higher proportion with impaired renal function in the overall group.

At the time of first presentation as adults, a significant number of both males and females give a history of previous micturition abnormalities which could have led to earlier diagnosis. These are listed in table III. There is no doubt that symptoms such as loin pain during voiding, double micturition and frequency and dysuria should have been investigated during childhood and could have led to an earlier diagnosis. A history of enuresis was found in 21% of the patients. This is usually not investigated,

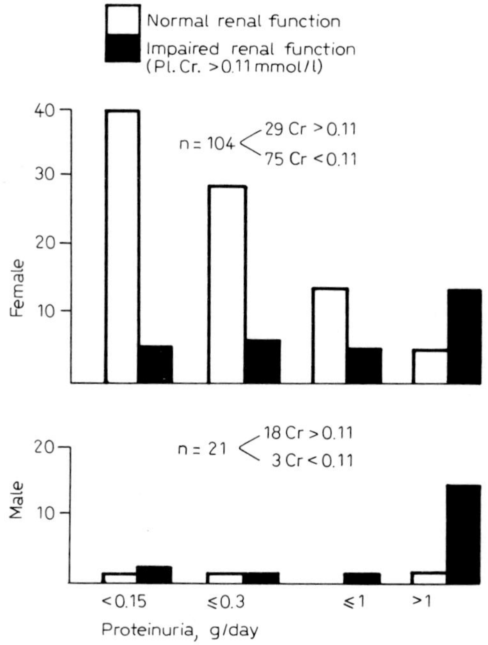

Fig. 3. The relationship between proteinuria and impaired renal function in 145 patients.

Table III. Significant past history in adult patients (n = 145) with reflux nephropathy

	Number	%
Frequency/dysuria	33	22.7
Enuresis	31	21.3
Loin pain during voiding	12	8.2
Double micturition	11	7.5
Childhood fevers	2	1.3

but perhaps with the development of new and less invasive tests, such as some of the radionuclide scanning procedures, it may be possible to investigate children with enuresis beyond the age of 4. Certainly all warrant a careful urine examination, including microscopy and culture; and the presence of protein, cells, casts or bacteria in abnormal numbers should prompt further investigation.

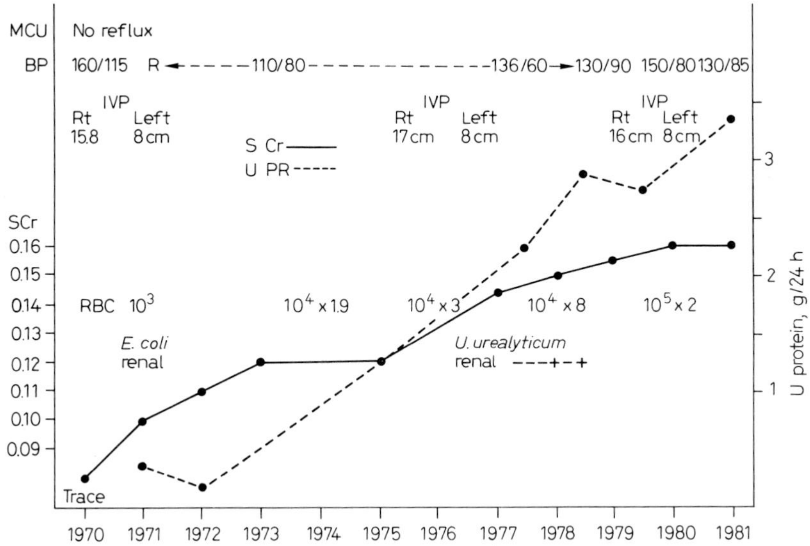

Fig. 4. Course over 11 years in a 27-year-old woman with unilateral coarse scarring on the left and a hypertrophied kidney with a normal outline and calyceal system on the right. The degree of microscopic haematuria and proteinuria has increased over 10 years. During this time the serum creatinine has risen from a strictly normal value below 0.09 to 0.16 mmol/l. Few UTIs were documented over this period – an *E. coli* in 1971 and two infections with *Ureaplasma urealyticum* in 1978. The blood presure has been well controlled since she first presented in 1970.

When proteinuria is present in an adult with RN it reflects the development of a glomerular lesion [3–11]. The reasons for the development of this glomerular lesion and its frequent progression are still unclear. The possibility that it is due to haemodynamic factors related to a reduced number of functioning nephrons should be considered, but the fact that the lesion may develop in a normal sized or hypertrophied kidney (fig. 4) makes this less likely. We have previously reported this glomerulopathy in the normal contralateral kidney in 4 patients [6] and figure 4 give details of a further one. In animals a progressive glomerular lesion is a regular finding with the 5/6 nephrectomy model [11], but whether unilateral nephrectomy can cause progressive glomerular lesions in man or animals is less certain. Focal glomerular sclerosis has recently been reported in unilateral renal agenesis [12]. This situation is, however, not analogous to that found in patients with RN in whom, despite a normal-sized kidney on one side, progressive impairment of renal function may lead to ESRF over 5–10

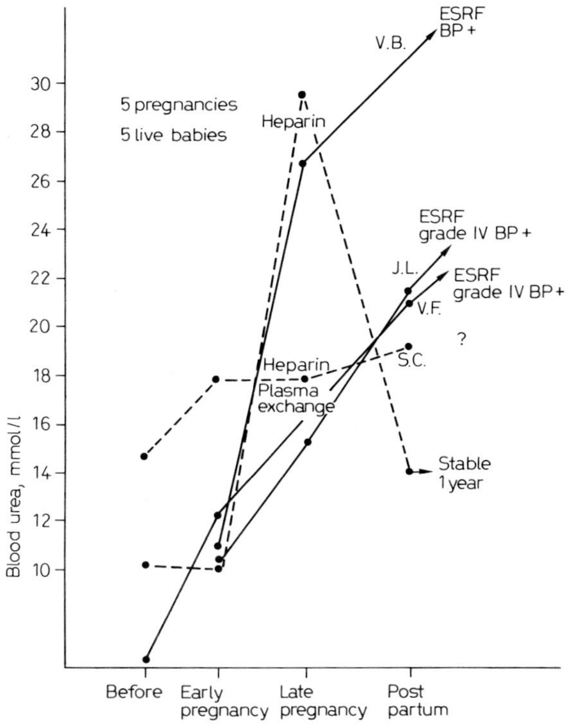

Fig. 5. Course during pregnancy, and after pregnancy, in 5 patients with impaired renal function in early pregnancy. All showed deterioration during pregnancy. 1 patient (S.C.), treated energetically during pregnancy using heparin and plasma exchange, deteriorated little during pregnancy, but like 3 others she deteriorated to ESRF within a few months of delivery. In each case this represents an accelerated course in comparison with the slowly progressive course which is usual in RN.

years. This means that either other factors contribute to progressive glomerular lesions in RN or that the apparently normal contralateral kidney is in fact not normal. There is some evidence that there may be a diffuse scarring process affecting the contralateral kidney in cases with RN and previous bilateral vesico-ureteral reflux, which could mean that far more nephrons have been lost from that kidney than is apparent from its normal or hypertrophied size and absence of coarse scars (see chapter 9).

The only other association which we have noted in patients with glomerular lesions is infection, often renal parenchymal infection, with atypical and fastidious micro-organisms [13]. Recent studies have shown that ureaplasmas [14] and *Gardnerella vaginalis* infections [15] are those most strongly associated with imparied renal function in RN.

Complications in pregnancy are a prominent feature in women with RN [1]. Patients with impaired renal function due to RN may run a greatly accelerated course to renal failure during pregnancy and in the early postpartum months (fig. 5).

Reflux nephropathy is not a benign disorder in adults. Children who have survived their early years without developing impaired renal function and even those with apparent unilateral coarse scars due to RN may still progress to renal failure as adults. The major prognostic feature is the onset of proteinuria which is invariably present in those who progress. Once proteinuria has developed, the course of progression to renal failure is normally gradual over 5–10 years. Malignant hypertension and pregnancy are two factors which may accelerate this course and result in rapid progression from mildly impaired renal function to ESRF over months.

References

1 Kincaid-Smith, P.; Becker, G.J.: Reflux nephropathy in the adult. Reflux nephropathy, pp. 21–28 (Masson, New York 1979).

2 Kincaid-Smith, P.: Pyelonephritis, chronic interstitial nephritis and obstructive uropathy. Nephrology, pp. 553–582 (Wiley & Sons, New York 1979).

3 Kincaid-Smith, P.; Mathew, T.H.; Becker, E.L.: Glomerulonephritis. Proc. Int. Symp. on Glomerulonephritis, p. 156 (Wiley & Sons, New York 1973).

4 Kincaid-Smith, P.: The prevention of renal failure. Proc. Vth Int. Congr. Nephrol. Mexico 1972, vol. 3, pp. 100–118 (1974).

5 Kincaid-Smith, P.: Advances in nephrology. Proc. VIth Int. Congr. Nephrol., Florence 1975, pp. 2–18 (1976).

6 Kincaid-Smith, P.: Glomerular lesions in atrophic pyelonephritis and reflux nephropathy. Kidney int. *8*: S81–S83 (1975).

7 Torres, V.E.; Velosa, J.A.; Holley, K.E.; Kelalis, P.P.; Sticker, G.B.; Kurtz, S.B.: The progression of vesico-ureteral reflux nephropathy. Ann. intern. Med. *92*: 776–784 (1980).

8 Aladjem, M.; Schoeneman, M.J.; Bennett, B.; Levitt, S.; Spitzer, A.; Greifer, I.: Focal segmental glomerulosclerosis with proteinuria and chronic interstitial nephritis. N.Y. St. J. Med. *March*: 579 (1978).

9 Bhathena, D.B.; Weiss, J.H.; Holland, N.H.; McMorrow, R.G.; Curtis, J.J.; Lucas, B.A.; Luke, R.G.: Focal and segmental glomerular sclerosis in reflux nephropathy (chronic pyelonephritis). Am. J. Med. *68*: 886 (1980).

10 Cotran, R.S.: Glomerulosclerosis in reflux nephropathy. Nephrology forum. Kidney int. *21*: 528–534 (1982).

11 Shimamura, T.; Morrison, A.B.: A progressive glomerulosclerosis occurring in partial five-sixths nephrectomized rats. Am. J. Pathol. *79*: 95–101 (1975).
12 Kiprov, D.D.; Colvin, R.B.; McCluskey, R.J.: Focal and segmental glomerulosclerosis and proteinuria associated with unilateral renal agenesis. Lab. Invest. *46*: 275–281 (1982).
13 Fairley, K.F.: Diagnosis in the difficult case. Kidney int. *8*: S12–S19 (1975).
14 Birch, D.F.; Fairley, K.F.; Pavillard, R.E.: Unconventional bacteria in urinary tract disease: *Ureaplasma urealyticum*. Kidney int. *19*: 58–64 (1981).
15 Fairley, K.F.; Birch, D.F.: Unconventional bacteria in urinary tract disease: *Gardnerella vaginalis*. Kidney int. (in press).

Prof. P. Kincaid-Smith, Director, Department of Nephrology,
The Royal Melbourne Hospital, Parkville, 3050, Victoria (Australia)

Contr. Nephrol., vol. 39, pp. 102–110 (Karger, Basel 1984)

9. End-Stage Reflux Nephropathy

Ross R. Bailey, Kelvin L. Lynn

Department of Nephrology, North Canterbury Hospital, Private Bag, Christchurch
New Zealand

Introduction

There is now considerable evidence that gross vesico-ureteric reflux (VUR) is the essential pathogenetic factor in the aetiology of the small, scarred, contracted kidney of non-obstructive, chronic atrophic pyelonephritis [1–4]. For this reason reflux nephropathy (RN) was suggested [1] as a more appropriate term for this entity.

This paper reports on the problem of end-stage RN in Australia and New Zealand and in our unit in Christchurch.

Australia and New Zealand

Over the past decade nephrologists have been recognizing RN as an important cause of end-stage chronic renal failure (ESCRF). The Australia and New Zealand Combined Dialysis and Transplant Registry now provides 6 monthly reports, and the recent data relating to RN are included in table I [5]. The corresponding data relating to children under the age of 16 years are summarized in table II.

Christchurch

Between 1 January 1970 and 1 July 1982, 207 patients entered the dialysis-transplant programme in Christchurch. In 25 (12%) of these patients RN was the cause of the ESCRF.

Table I. Patients presenting with end-stage RN as percentages of all cases with ESCRF

	New Zealand[1] (%)	Australia[2] (%)
1972–1973	–	19/297 (6)
1/1/75–31/10/80	31/463 (7)	192/2735 (7)[3]
1977–1978	8/72 (11)	27/450 (6)
1978–1979	4/88 (5)	29/463 (6)
1979–1980	8/93 (9)	43/539 (8)
1/11/80–31/10/81	11/109 (10)	53/558 (10)

[1] Present population approximately 3.21 million.
[2] Present population approximately 14.5 million.
[3] 94/192 (49%) were males.

Table II. Patients under the age of 16 years entering Australasian renal replacement programmes 1971 to 31/10/80

	Total number	Nephropathy	Reflux, %
Australia	158	54	34
New Zealand	32	6	19

Diagnosis of RN

RN was diagnosed at the time of presentation by 2 or more of the following features:

(1) High dose intravenous urography (IVU) (with or without tomography) showing the characteristic features described by *Hodson* [6, 7], namely calyceal clubbing, adjacent cortical scarring, arrest of renal growth. (2) Micturating cysto-urethrography (MCU) performed by radiologic [8, 9] or radionuclide techniques [10] showing VUR. (3) Cystoscopic evaluation of the ureteric orifices [11, 12].

In addition, 3 patients had nephrectomy of a small contracted kidney and 2 others had bilateral nephroureterectomy and removal of an ileal conduit prior to transplantation. All 7 kidneys showed the characteristic macroscopic and microscopic appearances of 'chronic diffuse pyelonephritis', i.e. RN [13, 14]. Patients with renal failure due to obstructive uropathy were excluded from the study.

Results

The clinical and investigatory details of the 11 male (age range at presentation = 3–41 years; mean age 19.3 years) and the 14 female (age range at presentation = 4–30 years; mean age 17.8 years) patients with ESCRF due to RN are included in tables III and IV. Of the 11 males only 2 had had a documented urinary tract infection (UTI). These were covert and detected at the time of presentation. 6 of the 14 females had suffered a proven UTI, while an additional girl had received one course of antibacterial treatment for a minor episode of frequency and dysuria.

19 patients had hypertension, which in 13 had not been detected prior to presentation. 4 patients presented with malignant hypertension. 8 of the 14 women presented during a pregnancy, 6 with severe or atypical "toxaemia of pregnancy".

39 healthy siblings, parents or offspring of 14 patients, had radiologic urinary tract investigations. Patient 2 had an affected brother and 3 of his 4 children were affected. 1 of the latter had severe but asymptomatic ESCRF leading to dialysis (patient 19). Patient 7 had a successful cadaveric renal transplant and gave birth to a son at 38 weeks gestation who was shown to have unilateral slight VUR at the age of 6 days. Patient 8 had a sister with bilateral gross VUR which was corrected surgically. She now has severe complicating hypertension and moderate renal insufficiency and has had a daughter with bilateral slight VUR. Patient 15 had a maternal cousin with known unilateral RN. Patient 25 has a sister and a daughter with RN. The latter has deteriorating renal function.

8 of the 11 male and 7 of the 14 female patients had severe renal failure at the time of presentation. All patients had proteinuria (mean 2.3 g/day; range 0.9–7.2 g) but none had the nephrotic syndrome (table IV).

The mean age of commencement of regular dialysis treatment was 25.1 years for the male and 27.2 years for the female patients. 3 have continued on home haemodialysis while 22 have received a total of 25 renal transplants. 14 of these 22 patients are at present well, with a functioning graft, 4 have returned to home haemodialysis and are awaiting a second graft, and 4 have died (table III). Of the latter, 1 committed suicide despite having normal renal function, and 3 died of uraemia following chronic rejection of their graft and no wish to return to regular dialysis treatment.

Of all patients reaching ESCRF in this unit there have been 12 who began dialysis aged less than 16 years. 6 of these 12 children had RN [15].

Table III. Clinical details

Patient No.	Sex	Presenting problem	Age at presentation years	History of UTIs	Hypertension (malignant*; age when noted, years)	Age when started dialysis years	Transplanted (failed*; dead†)
1	M	uraemic symptoms 4month	39	no	yes (39)	39	yes
2	M	asymptomatic proteinuria, gout	31	no	no	31	yes
3	M	proteinuria, gout, renal impairment, hypertension	26	no	yes (26)	36	yes*
4	M	enuresis, hypospadias, UTI, malignant hypertension	12	yes	yes (12)*	15	yes
5	M	enuresis, undescended testes, renal impairment, growth failure	6	no	no	8	yes
6	M	enuresis, undescended testes	7	no	yes (16)	18	yes†
7	F	growth failure, renal impairment	12	no	yes (20)	20	yes
8	F	UTI, hypertension	4	yes	yes (7)	21	yes
9	F	loin pain in 3rd pregnancy	30	no	no	41	yes
10	F	severe 'toxaemia' and renal impairment 32wk 2nd pregnancy	20	yes	yes (20)	22	yes†
11	F	severe 'toxaemia' and renal impairment 20weeks 1st pregnancy	27	no	yes (27)	30	yes
12	F	severe 'toxaemia' and renal impairment 24weeks 1st pregnancy	24	no	yes (24)	30	yes
13	F	enuresis, growth failure, uraemia, malignant hypertension	9	?yes (×1)	yes (9)*	9	yes
14	F	enuresis, severe 'toxaemia' at 20weeks 1st pregnancy, renal impairment, UTI	17	yes	yes (17)	25	yes
15	F	loin pain when bladder distended, renal impairment postpartum	17	no	no	23	yes
16	F	severe 'toxaemia' 12weeks 2nd pregnancy	21	no	yes (21)	39	no
17	F	severe 'toxaemia' 20weeks 1st pregnancy, UTI	26	yes	yes (26)	35	yes†
18	F	recurrent UTIs for 17 years	17	yes	yes (34)	49	yes†
19	M	family investigation	7	no	yes (11)	16	yes
20	M	recurrent UTIs	3	yes	no	17	yes*
21	M	uraemia	13	no	no	13	yes*
22	M	uraemia	27	no	yes (27)	37	no
23	F	recurrent UTIs	12	yes	yes (19)	23	yes
24	F	malignant hypertension, uraemia	13	no	yes (13)*	13	yes*
25	M	malignant hypertension	41	no	yes (41)*	45	no

Table IV. Investigations on patients

Patient No.	Renal function at presentation			24-hour urinary protein, g	Blood group	HLA antigens	
	plasma urea mg/100ml	plasma creatinine mg/100ml	GFR ml/min			A	B
1	221	12.4	6	1.2	B+	W32,–	5,7
2	240	7.0	15	4.0	0–	2,–	7,8
3	47	2.2	52	7.2	A+	1,3	12,40
4	55	1.9	20	1.0	A+	3,11	7,27
5	115	3.5	11	1.7	A+	9,–	12,W22
6	146	5.2	10	3.0	B–	1,2	8,12
7	50	–	–	2.0	A+	2,–	14,W40
8	43	–	–	2.0	A+	1,11	12,–
9	35	2.0	41	1.0	O+	3,–	7,W22
10	143	5.1	17	2.6	O+	9,11	12,W22
11	90	–	–	6,0	A+	2,–	8,12
12	61	2.0	39	4.5	AB+	1,9	7,–
13	188	6.6	5	0.5	A+	9,–	7,15
14	150	6.0	9	1.7	O+	2,9	27,–
15	115	3.3	20	1.8	O+	1,2	7,8
16	217	–	–	0.9	O+	3,9	–,–
17	40	–	–	1.9	B+	1,10	12,–
18	30	–	–	1.2	O+	–,–	7,–
19	80	1.5	30.8	0.2	O+	2,25	7,17
20	53	1.4	71.0	0.4	A+	2,9	8,15
21	252	8.9	4.8	0.9	O+	2,–	12,15
22	52	2.1	38.0	4.8	O+	9,30/31	12,14
23	30	0.8	66.0	3.1	A+	2,3	7,40
24	240	8.1	3.1	1.5	A+	3,–	7,35
25	161	4.1	30.0	2.3	O+	2,29	14,40

Discussion

VUR has long been recognized as a frequent association of the small scarred kidney in the adult and an almost invariable accompaniment in the infant and child. The observations that the severity of VUR and the presence of intrarenal reflux (IRR) are the most important determinants of renal damage or dysfunction have been major advances in the understanding of this renal lesion [3, 4, 16–18].

If VUR is bilateral and gross the patient may develop chronic renal failure which is usually preceded by hypertension. The latter may in turn lead to further renal damage. There are some patients, however, in whom VUR has ceased spontaneously or been surgically corrected, who have no complicating UTIs or hypertension, and yet their renal function continues to decline. *Zimmermann* et al. [19] and, more recently, *Kincaid-Smith* [14] have drawn attention to the associated glomerular lesion which may play an important role in the progression of the renal failure. The most important morphological lesion noted on light microscopic examination was focal and segmental hyalinosis with sclerosis or collapse of glomerular capillaries and thickening of their walls. *Kimmelstiel and Wilson* [20] described an "alternative glomerulitis" in one third of patients with "chronic atrophic pyelonephritis", while in the classic paper by *Weiss and Parker* [21] moderate to heavy proteinuria was a feature of many of the patients with "chronic pyelonephritis". Microscopically the glomeruli often showed concentric pericapsular fibrosis, with the glomerular tufts exhibiting varying degrees of sclerosis.

In the present study moderate to heavy proteinuria was a feature in the majority of patients. Renal biopsies were not obtained from any patients, but the characteristic glomerular lesions were seen in the 7 nephrectomy specimens. *Weiss* et al. [22] noted focal segmental glomerulosclerosis in the kidneys of all 23 patients examined, while in those kidneys studied by immunofluorescence microscopy, segmental or global deposits of C3 and IgM were invariably present. *Torres* et al. [23] made similar observations in 54 patients with RN. It appears highly likely that glomerular lesions play a major part in the progression of the renal failure in many patients with RN [19, 23, 24]. Figure 1 suggests the likely mechanisms by which RN may progress to ESCRF.

RN is a significant cause of ESCRF [25]. It is suspected that in some centres the condition is underdiagnosed. In Christchurch it is the commonest cause of chronic renal failure in children [15]. We have assessed

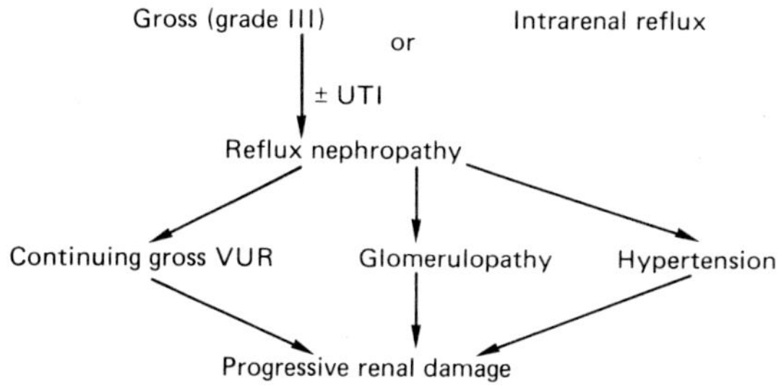

Fig. 1. Diagram suggesting the mechanisms by which RN may progress to ESCRF.

from the European Dialysis and Transplant Association Registry [26] that 0.3–0.4 children/million of the population/year under the age of 15 years will present with renal failure due to what is probably RN. However, this may well be an underestimate as it is known that some of the most severely affected children, particularly boys, may die from uraemia in early life and will not be considered for active treatment.

Of 965 patients referred to a Californian unit [27] for renal transplantation, 32 (3.3%) had bilateral primary, low pressure VUR. The mean age at the time of referral was 21.1 years (age range 5–38 years). 10 of the 32 patients had sterile VUR. The authors concluded that the severity of the VUR itself, rather than UTI, was the significant factor in the development of renal failure. 15 of 50 (30%) consecutive patients with ESCRF in the study of *Bakshandeh* et al. [28] were found to have VUR. The 7 males and 8 females ranged in age from 13 to 57 years (mean 30 years). 9 of the 15 patients had a positive history of UTIs. These authors indicated that their findings were at variance with the published causes of ESCRF and noted that VUR was not listed as an aetiology of renal failure in the Human Transplant Registry.

RN is an important cause of ESCRF which could potentially be eliminated by detecting gross VUR in infants or young children and having it corrected surgically. Some of these infants present with complicating UTIs as a marker of the condition, but this is frequently later in childhood or in early adult life, after renal damage has occurred.

A simple screening test to detect the potentially damaging degree of VUR in the new-born child is necessary.

In 1974 a *Lancet* editorial [29] appeared under the following heading: 'V.U.R. ± I.R.R. = C.P.N.?'

Soon after the Bermuda workshop, a variation was offered [30]:
'(V.U.R. ± I.R.R.) + U.T.I. = C.P.N.'

After another 4 years, a second formula is suggested:
RN (≡ CPN) ± UTI ± VUR | FGS ± BP = ESCRF,

where FGS = focal glomerulosclerosis; BP = blood pressure.

References

1 Bailey, R.R.: The relationship of vesico-ureteric reflux to urinary tract infection and chronic pyelonephritis – reflux nephropathy. Clin. Nephrol. *1*: 132 (1973).
2 Bailey, R.R.: An overview of reflux nephropathy; in Reflux nephropathy (Masson, New York 1979).
3 Rolleston, G.L.; Shannon, F.T.; Utley, W.L.F.: Follow-up of vesicoureteric reflux in the newborn. Kidney int. *8*: S59 (1975).
4. Aperia, A.; Brøberger, O.; Ericsson, N.O.; Wikstad, I.: Effect of vesicoureteral reflux on renal function in children with recurrent urinary tract infection. Kidney int. *9*: 418 (1976).
5 Disney, A.P.S. (ed.): Fifth report of Australia and New Zealand Combined Dialysis and Transplant Registry, Woodville (Australian Kidney Foundation, 1982).
6 Hodson, C.J.: The radiological diagnosis of pyelonephritis. Proc. R. Soc. Med. *52*: 669 (1969).
7 Hodson, C.J.: The effects of disturbance of flow on the kidney. J. infect. Dis. *120*: 54 (1969).
8 Rolleston, G.L.; Shannon, F.T.; Utley, W.L.F.: Relationship of infantile vesicoureteric reflux to renal damage. Br. med. J. *i*: 460 (1970).
9 Maling, T.M.J.; Rolleston, G.L.: Intra-renal reflux in children demonstrated by micturating cystography. Clin. Radiol. *25*: 81 (1974).
10 Bailey, R.R.; Stapleton, P.; Turner, J.G.; Brownlie, B.E.W.: Detection of vesicoureteric reflux using radionuclide micturating cystography. Aust. N.Z. J. Med. *6*: 542 (1976).
11 Lyon, R.P.; Marshall, S.; Tanagho, E.A.: The ureteral orifice: its configuration and competency. J. Urol. *102*: 504 (1969).
12 Vermillion, C.D.; Heale, W.F.: Position and configuration of the ureteral orifice and its relationship to renal scarring in adults. J. Urol. *109*: 579 (1973).
13 Heptinstall, R.H.: The enigma of chronic pyelonephritis. J. infect. Dis. *120*: 104 (1969).
14 Kincaid-Smith, P.: Glomerular lesions in atrophic pyelonephritis and reflux nephropathy. Kidney int. *8*: S81 (1975).
15 King, S.; Buttimore, A.; Lynn, K.L.; Bailey, R.R.: Active treatment of children with end-stage renal failure. N.Z. med. J. (in press).
16 Klare, B.; Amman, P.; Reinbold, F.; George, P.; Manz, F.; Möhring, K.; Schärer, K.: Kidney size and split renal function in reflux nephropathy. Abstr. Int. Symp. on Radionuclides in Nephrology, Boston 1978, p. 2.

17 Rolleston, G.L.; Maling, T.M.J.; Hodson, C.J.: Intrarenal reflux and the scarred kidney. Archs Dis. Childh. *49*: 531 (1974).
18 Ransley, P.G.; Risdon, R.A.: The renal papilla, intrarenal reflux, and chronic pyelonephritis; in Reflux nephropathy (Masson, New York 1979).
19 Zimmerman, S.W.; Uehling, D.T.; Burkholder, P.M.: Vesicoureteral reflux nephropathy. Evidence for immunologically mediated glomerular injury. Urology *2*: 534 (1973).
20 Kimmelstiel, P.; Wilson, C.: Inflammatory lesions in the glomeruli in pyelonephritis in relation to hypertension and renal insufficiency. Am J. Path. *12*: 99 (1936).
21 Weiss, S.; Parker, F.: Pyelonephritis: its relation to vascular lesions and to arterial hypertension. Medicine, Baltimore *18*: 221 (1939).
22 Weiss, J.; Bhathena, D.; Curtis, J.; Holland, N.; Lucas, B.; Luke, R.: Focal glomerulosclerosis associated with reflux nephropathy (RN): clinical features and results of transplantation. Nephrology 11th Annu. Meet., New Orleans 1978, p. 32A.
23 Torres, V.E.; Velosa, J.A.; Holley, K.E.; Kelalis, P.P.; Stickler, G.B.; Kurtz, S.B.: The progression of vesicoureteral reflux nephropathy. Ann. intern. Med. *92*: 776 (1980).
24 Cotran, R.S.: Glomerulosclerosis in reflux nephropathy. Kidney int. *21*: 528 (1982).
25 Bailey, R.R.: End-stage reflux nephropathy. Nephron *27*: 302 (1981).
26 Chantler, C.; Brunner, F.P.; Brynger, H.O.A.; Donckerwolcke, R.A.; Gurland, H.J.; Hathaway, R.A.; Jacobs, C.; Selwood, N.H.; Wing, A.J.: Combined report on regular dialysis and transplantation of children in Europe 1977. Proc. XVth Congr. EDTA, Istambul 1978.
27 Salvatierra, O.; Tanagho, E.A.: Reflux as a cause of end stage kidney disease: report of 32 cases. J. Urol. *117*: 441 (1977).
28 Bakshandeh, K.; Lynne, C.; Carrion, H.: Vesicoureteral reflux and end stage renal disease. J. Urol. *116*: 557 (1976).
29 Leading Article: V.U.R. ± I.R.R. = C.P.N.? Lancet *ii.*: 1120 (1974).
30 Leading Article: (V.U.R. ± I.R.R.) + U.T.I. = C.P.N. Lancet *ii*: 301 (1978).

Ross R. Bailey, MD, Department of Nephrology, Christchurch Hospital, Christchurch (New Zealand)

Contr. Nephrol., vol. 39, pp. 111–115 (Karger, Basel 1984)

10. Diffuse Parenchymal Lesions in Reflux Nephropathy and the Possibility of Making a Renal Biopsy Diagnosis in Reflux Nephropathy

Priscilla S. Kincaid-Smith

Department of Medicine, University of Melbourne, Victoria, Australia

In a series of studies of 197 patients with malignant hypertension 28 years ago, 6 showed what was described at that time as diffuse chronic pyelonephritis [1]. This was not a clear-cut entity at that time, nor indeed is it at the present time. The diffuse scarring in the renal parenchyma in the 6 patients was histologically similar to that seen in the coarsely scarred kidney of what was then called 'chronic atrophic pyelonephritis' and what we now refer to as 'reflux nephropathy' (RN).

There is additional evidence to suggest that diffuse parenchymal scarring, which cannot be detected on radiographs, may form part of the pattern of renal scarring seen in patients with vesico-ureteric reflux (VUR). Patients judged to have unilateral RN in whom the contralateral kidney is radiographically normal may show progressive deterioration due to disease in this same contralateral kidney [2, 3]. In these patients, glomerular lesions of hyalinosis and sclerosis are found in the radiographically 'normal' kidney. Accompanying this glomerular lesion there are often other features of parenchymal scarring. In the pig model of RN, fine diffuse parenchymal scarring is found in kidneys in which VUR has occurred over 6–18 months. This fine diffuse scarring may be present in kidneys in which no intrarenal reflux is documented and in which no coarse scars develop [4].

If diffuse parenchymal scarring occurs in apparent unilateral RN in radiographically normal kidneys, then why should not similar diffuse parenchymal lesions occur on both sides in patients in whom we do not currently make a diagnosis of RN because they lack coarse parenchymal scars? 6 adults have been described more recently in whom parenchymal scarring, detected on renal biopsy, resembled this diffuse reflux-related scarring. Further investigation of them revealed unsuspected VUR in 2 [5]. Since

Table I. Diagnosis of reflux nephropathy on biopsy

Glomerular features
Periglomerular fibrosis
Interstitial scarring around glomeruli
'Typical' focal and segmental hyalinosis and sclerosis
Granulated epithelial cells
Interstitial features
Inflammatory cellular infiltration
Diffuse cortical fibrosis
'Streaky' cortical fibrosis
Medullary fibrosis
Tubular features
Thyroid-like areas
Tamm-Horsfall casts
'Ischaemic' tubular atrophy
Vascular features
Interstitial scarring around arteries
'Typical' arterial and arteriolar changes
Other features
Dense collagen scars
Perirenal scars
Lymphatic dilatation

this second description of a possible diffuse form of RN, a further 127 biopsies in adult patients presenting with proteinuria but showing no coarse radiographic scars have suggested this same type of diffuse form of RN. They represent 8% of all biopsies (other than transplant cases) carried out over the same period. Thus, if diffuse cortical lesions do occur in RN they are not rare and comprise a significant proportion of adults being investigated for proteinuria. Only a small percentage of these patients show persisting VUR (10%). However, because it is calculated to cease spontaneously during childhood in 80% of cases, its absence in an adult does not exclude childhood VUR as a possible cause of the parenchymal lesion.

Fig. 1. Analysis of the features listed in table I in the two sets of biopsies. Analysis by Mann-Whitney rank sum method. F & SH = Focal and segmental hyalinosis and sclerosis.

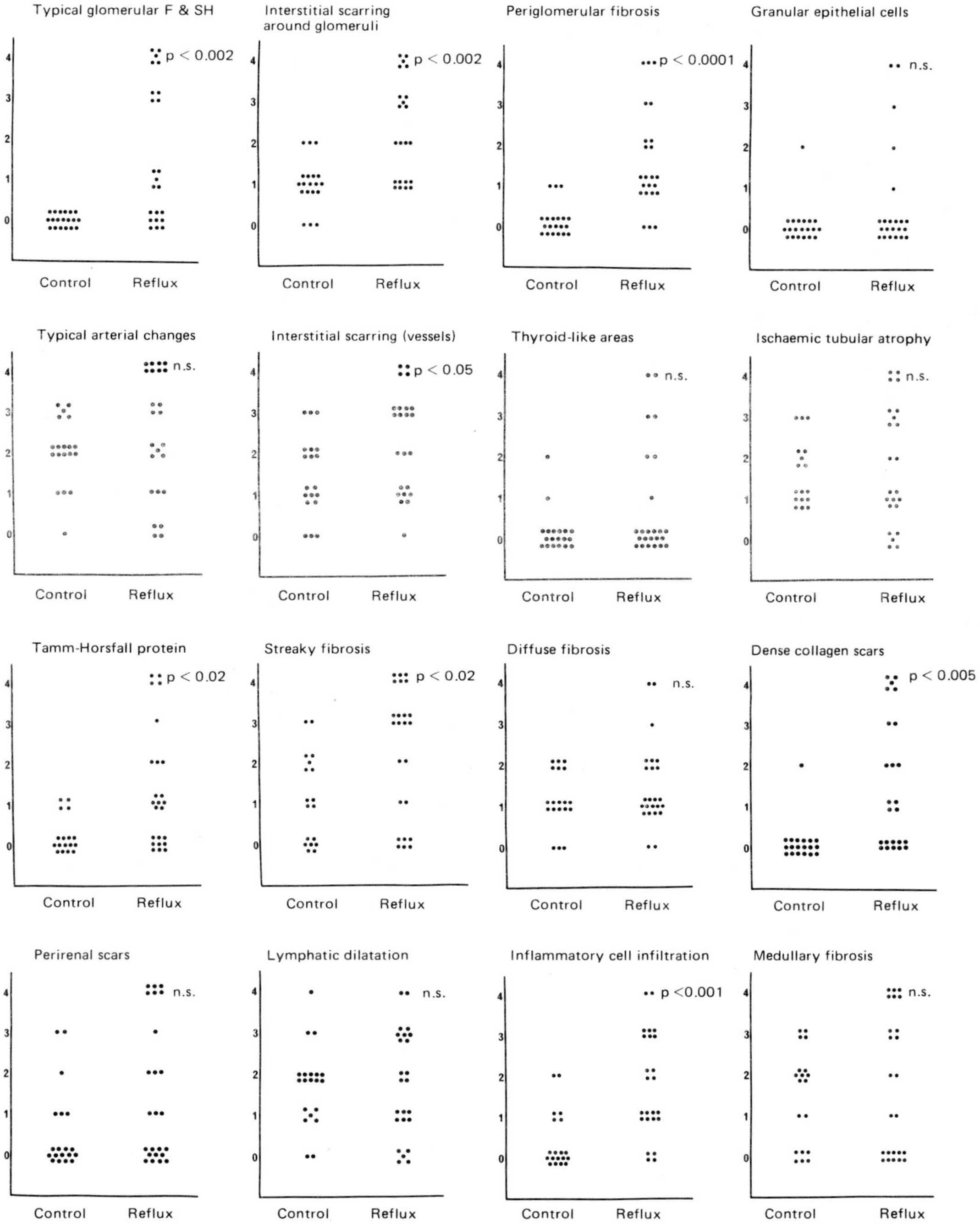
Typical glomerular F & SH
p < 0.002
Interstitial scarring around glomeruli
p < 0.002
Periglomerular fibrosis
p < 0.0001
Granular epithelial cells
n.s.
Typical arterial changes
n.s.
Interstitial scarring (vessels)
p < 0.05
Thyroid-like areas
n.s.
Ischaemic tubular atrophy
n.s.
Tamm-Horsfall protein
p < 0.02
Streaky fibrosis
p < 0.02
Diffuse fibrosis
n.s.
Dense collagen scars
p < 0.005
Perirenal scars
n.s.
Lymphatic dilatation
n.s.
Inflammatory cell infiltration
p <0.001
Medullary fibrosis
n.s.
Control
Reflux
0
1
2
3
4

Table II. Significant features derived from table I

	p
Periglomerular fibrosis	<0.0001
Inflammatory cell infiltration	<0.001
Interstitial scarring around glomeruli	<0.002
'Typical' glomerular focal and segmental hyalinosis and sclerosis	<0.002
Dense collagen scars	<0.005
'Streaky' cortical scars	<0.02
Tamm-Horsfall protein casts	<0.02
Interstitial scarring around vessels	<0.05

A study was set up to investigate whether the histological features of RN on a renal biopsy are sufficiently characteristic to allow differentiation of biopsies from patients with RN (biopsied because of proteinuria) from biopsies from other patients presenting with proteinuria. Accordingly, two series of renal biopsies were blinded and analysed histologically. The first group (24 biopsies) was from adults with known RN in whom a biopsy had been carried out because of proteinuria. A second group of age- and sex-matched biopsies from patients investigated for proteinuria were selected at random from the overall pool of biopsies carried out over the same time period. The findings in the two groups were compared.

Both groups were analysed for the features set out in table I, which were selected because they have been regarded as histological features seen in RN. The results of this analysis are shown in figure 1. As can be seen from these results, some of the features which were analysed appear to be of particular value in the renal biopsy diagnosis of RN and others appear relatively non-specific.

The most significant features in this analysis are listed in table II. The features in table II may therefore be important in detection of the diffuse form of RN. The proof that diffuse cortical scarring can result from VUR in man, as it can in the pig, may require long-term follow-up of children with VUR and a study of the renal lesions in kidneys which show no coarse scars.

References

1 Kincaid-Smith, P.; McMichael, J.; Murphy, E.A.: The clinical course and pathology of hypertension with papilleodema (malignant hypertension). Q. Jl Med. New Ser. *XXVII*: 117–153 (1958).

2 Kincaid-Smith, P.; Mathew, T.H.; Becker, E.L. (eds): Glomerulonephritis. Proc. Int. Symp. on Glomerulonephritis, Melbourne 1972 (Wiley & Sons, New York 1973).

3 Kincaid-Smith, P.: The prevention of renal failure. Proc. Vth Congr. Nephrol., Mexico 1972, vol. 3, pp. 100–118 (Karger, Basel 1974).

4 Hodson, J.; Kincaid-Smith, P. (eds): Reflux nephropathy, p. 197 (Masson, New York 1979).

5 Hodson, J.; Kincaid-Smith, P. (eds): Reflux nephropathy, p. 268 (Masson, New York 1979).

Prof. P. Kincaid-Smith, Director, Department of Nephrology,
Royal Melbourne Hospital, Parkville 3050, Victoria (Australia)

Contr. Nephrol., vol. 39, pp. 116–125 (Karger, Basel 1984)

11. Unilateral Reflux Nephropathy and Hypertension

Ross R. Bailey, Kelvin L. Lynn, Colin U. McRae

Departments of Nephrology and Urology, Christchurch Hospital, Christchurch, New Zealand

Introduction

Hypertension is a frequent late complication of reflux nephropathy (RN). And, although it may present in the malignant phase with rapidly declining renal funcion, it is much more likely to be 'benign' and relatively easy to manage. At the last symposium on this subject little attention was given to this important and frequent complication of RN. Perhaps this was because of our ignorance of its pathogenesis.

Hypertension in the context of unilateral RN raises the question of a possible surgical cure. Over the years many small scarred kidneys have been removed from hypertensive patients with varying reports of benefit. No prospective or controlled studies have been reported.

Review of Literature

Although *Ask-Upmark* [1] was the first to suggest a possible relationship between unilateral renal disease and hypertension, it was not until 8 years later in 1937 that *Butler* [2] reported that the removal of a small scarred kidney cured hypertension. The patient was a 10-year-old girl who was hospitalized with a urinary tract infection (UTI) and found to have a blood pressure of 190/120 mm Hg. After nephrectomy the blood pressure fell rapidly to 110/70 mm Hg and 3 months later was 92/60 mm Hg.

Over the next 20 years a vast literature was published on this subject, none of it controlled, and much of it anecdotal. *Smith* [3] attempted to introduce some order into the chaos of conflicting opinions concerning the prognosis of hypertension after unilateral nephrectomy. He reviewed the published literature between 1937 and 1956 of 575 patients who underwent unilateral nephrectomy for well-established hypertension. Of this number, 149 (26%) had a fall in blood pressure to 140/90 mm Hg or less for a period of at least 1 year. 62 (42%) of these 149 cured patients were diagnosed as having unilateral 'chronic pyelonephritis'. *Smith* [3] considered that many more failures than successes probably remained unreported. The following year *Thompson* [4] reviewed 3,000 patients who had undergone unilateral nephrectomy at the Mayo Clinic between 1940 and 1954. Of this group, 344 had hypertension and 7 were excluded from further study – of the remaining 337 (194 females) 100 had unilateral chronic pyelonephritis. 63 of these 100 patients had a normal blood pressure after 1 month. 64 of the patients with unilateral chronic pyelonephritis were followed for 1 year and 35 (55%) were still normotensive. *Yates-Bell* [5] detailed 66 patients with unilateral renal disease who underwent nephrectomy. 38% were cured (diastolic blood pressure of < 90 mm Hg at 1 year) and a few others were improved.

Kincaid-Smith [6] reviewed the literature for 1956 to 1961 and collated 326 patients with unilateral renal disease and hypertension. 57 of these had chronic pyelonephritis, of whom 23 were cured (< 140/90 at 1 year) and 33 showed substantial clinical benefit. *Luke* et al. [7] reported 34 patients with unilateral renal disease who underwent nephrectomy because of hypertension. 28 of these patients had unilateral chronic pyelonephritis and of these 11 were cured, 3 improved and 14 not helped. These authors concluded that the best results were in the young patients with a short history of hypertension and suggested that nephrectomy should be seriously considered if the unilateral kidney contributed less than 25% to the total glomerular filtration rate and the other kidney was completely normal. *Eliahou* et al. [8] reported 3 men and 4 women with unilateral atrophic pyelonephritis and severe hypertension. 3 of the patients were cured and 4 improved. *Haycock* [9] reported 2 girls, aged 7 and 10 years, with unilateral chronic pyelonephritis who were cured by nephrectomy. This author reviewed the published literature on the results of nephrectomy for unilateral renal disease and hypertension in children under the age of 15 years. Of 45 children (23 with unilateral chronic pyelonephritis) 34 were cured, 1 improved, 9 failed, and there was 1 postoperative death. *Haycock* [9] concluded that the results of surgery in childhood were better than those reported in adults.

This subject was most recently reviewed by *Pfau and Rosenmann* [10]. These authors, with little personal data, concluded, 'We believe that unilateral chronic pyelonephritis is rarely the cause of hypertension, and only occasionally will nephrectomy eliminate the associated hypertension in such a case.'

Is the Renin-Angiotensin System Involved?

Previous studies in our unit using renal vein renin (RVR) measurements [11, 12] showed no evidence that the renin-angiotensin-aldosterone system consistently played a role in the non-malignant hypertension of patients with strictly unilateral RN. The literature, moreover, has tended to support our findings [13–16], but not exclusively so [17].

Savage et al. [18] showed that the peripheral plasma renin activity was raised in 9 of 15 hypertensive children and, 8 of 100 normotensive children with either unilateral or bilateral RN. These authors suggested that an elevated plasma renin activity may indicate those patients at risk of developing hypertension.

A Prospective Trial

This long-term prospective trial was designed to study the hypertension of patients with unilateral RN [12]. Could prophylactic nephrectomy of the damaged kidney prevent hypertension developing in those patients whose blood pressure was still normal? Or would nephrectomy be beneficial to those patients already hypertensive?

This continuing study includes patients with well-documented unilateral RN (using diagnostic criteria detailed previously [11]) whose affected kidney has a glomerular filtration rate of $\leq$ 10 ml/min. In all patients the contralateral kidney was completely normal radiologically, showed compensatory hypertrophy and the total glomerular filtration rate (measured by ^{51}Cr EDTA clearance) was greater than 72 ml/min. Initially all patients in the series had differential renal function measured during ureteric catheterization. Recently unilateral renal function has been assessed using two non-invasive radionuclide techniques – ^{99m}Tc-dimercaptosuccinic acid

(DMSA) and ^{99m}Tc-diethylenetriaminepentaacetic acid (DTPA) studies. We have shown that both of these techniques correlated well with ureteric catheter studies [19]. Some of the patients had RVR concentrations measured. For patients to be classified as hypertensive a supine blood pressure > 140/90 mm Hg at 3 out-patient visits was required. No patient had malignant hypertension. The normotensive and hypertensive patients were then randomly allocated to either nephrectomy or conservative treatment.

Results

The clinical details of the patients in this continuing study are shown in tables I and II and summarized in table III. Radiological findings typical of the patients in the study are shown in figures 1 and 2.

In the normotensive group, 3 of 8 patients treated conservatively and 1 of 6 who underwent nephrectomy have become hypertensive during follow-up and have required continuing anti-hypertensive treatment (table I). Only one of the normotensive patients who became hypertensive had a RVR ratio suggesting that the damaged kidney may have been acting ischaemically.

Of the hypertensive group, all 5 treated conservatively have continued to require antihypertensive therapy. 3 of the 6 treated by nephrectomy have become normotensive (table II). The first of these was a 27-year-old grossly obese man who presented with acute pyelonephritis and was found to have unilateral RN, hypertension, and hypercalcaemia. 5 months later a parathyroid adenoma was removed without apparent effect on his blood pressure. 2 years later his blood pressure was 165/115 mm Hg and he weighed 127 kg. Over the next 9 months he dieted down to 100 kg and the blood pressure fell to 150/94 mm Hg. He then entered the study and underwent nephrectomy and his blood pressure has returned to normal. A 21-year-old girl's blood pressure fell from 145/100 to 124/84 mm Hg and has remained normal for 2 years. The blood pressure of a 12-year-old achondroplastic girl fell from 144/92 to 100/60 mm Hg after 1 year. The first 2 of the 3 patients whose hypertension was cured had the RVR ratio measured, and in the 21-year-old woman it was 2.12 suggesting that the damaged kidney was acting ischaemically. 1 hypertensive patient did not benefit from nephrectomy and has continued on antihypertensive therapy, while the 2 remaining patients required treatment for 4 years and 6 months, and at present are being observed without medication. It is possible that both of these patients benefited from the nephrectomy.

Table I. Clinical details of normotensive patients

No.	Sex	Age years	Clinical presentation	GFR of small kidney ml/min	PVR ratio	Initial mean blood pressure, mm Hg	Follow-up years	Recent blood pressure mm Hg	Clinical outcome
Normotensive-conservative									
1	F	50	loin pain	8.2	1.95	127/83	8	170/110	hypertensive after 3 months, Ca thyroid after 6 months, died Ca pancreas after 8 years, AHT
2	F	17	UTI in pregnancy	6.5	1.00	118/70	8	129/82	hypertensive on OC after 1 year (reversed), now N
3	F	46	UTI	8.0	0.30	140/80	6	160/90	hypertensive after 6 months, AHT
4	F	27	UTI, oedema	5.3	0.80	141/88	5	130/90	hypertensive after 5 years, AHT
5	F	7	Henoch-Schönlein purpura	4.7	ND	103/73	4	115/65	N
6	M	7	UTI	5.3	ND	100/65	2.5	95/65	N
7	F	24	UTI	6.0	ND	122/75	2.5	110/70	N
8	F	35	renal colic	3.8	ND	110/75	2	125/85	N
Normotensive-nephrectomy									
1	M	19	Ca bladder	7.2	0.97	115/73	8.5	120/75	N
2	F	20	UTI	9.7	1.26	128/73	8	120/70	N
3	M	26	loin pain	5.2	2.90	121/75	8	130/80	N
4	M	27	proteinuria	5.5	0.51	134/86	7	136/98	hypertensive after 10 months, AHT
5	F	20	UTI	2.0	1.05	130/80	6	122/82	N
6	M	23	UTI	6.0	ND	117/73	3	96/58	N

GFR = Glomerular filtration rate; AHT = antihypertensive therapy; N = normotensive; UTI = urinary tract infection; Ca = carcinoma;

OC = oral contraceptive; RVR = renal vein renin ($\frac{\text{abnormal}}{\text{normal}}$); ND = not done.

Table II. Clinical data of hypertensive patients

No.	Sex	Age years	Clinical presentation	GFR of small kidney ml/min	PVR ratio	Initial mean blood pressure, mm Hg	Follow-up years	Recent blood pressure mm Hg	Clinical outcome
Hypertensive-conservative									
1	F	26	pre-eclampsia	10.0	1.59	210/120	9	158/107	AHT
2	F	39	UTI	3.5	0.25	153/103	7	110/70	AHT
3	F	19	UTI	5.0	2.55	142/96	7	107/75	AHT
4	M	60	acute renal failure	4.0	ND	177/93	1	150/84	AHT
5	F	44	UTI, hypertension	10.0	ND	157/93	0.5	140/86	AHT
Hypertensive-nephrectomy									
1	F	39	hypertension	2.6	0.80	163/117	9	121/95	no benefit, AHT
2	F	19	loin pain	10.0	0.52	160/98	8	145/88	on AHT for first 4 years
3	M	27	UTI, hypertension	9.3	1.20	150/100	6	134/90	N
4	F	17	UTI	0.6	0.94	148/101	5	141/93	on AHT for first 6 months
5	F	21	UTI, hypertension	3.5	2.12	145/110	2	124/84	N
6	F	12	achondroplasia, UTI	2.2	ND	144/92	1	100/60	N

GFR = Glomerular filtration rate; AHT = antihypertensive therapy; N = normotensive; UTI = urinary tract infection;

RVR = renal vein renin ($\frac{\text{abnormal}}{\text{normal}}$); ND = not done.

Table III. Summary of outcome for all patients

Group and treatment	Number of patients	Number of hypertensive or on anti-hypertensive therapy during follow-up	Mean (range)	Follow-up period (years)
Normotensive	14	4	5.6	(2–8.5)
Conservative	8	3 (3 months, 6 months, 5 years later)	4.7	(2–8)
Nephrectomy	6	1 (10 months later)	6.8	(3–8.5)
Hypertensive	11	8	5.1	(0.5–9)
Conservative	5	5	4.9	(0.5–9)
Nephrectomy	6	3	5.2	(1–9)

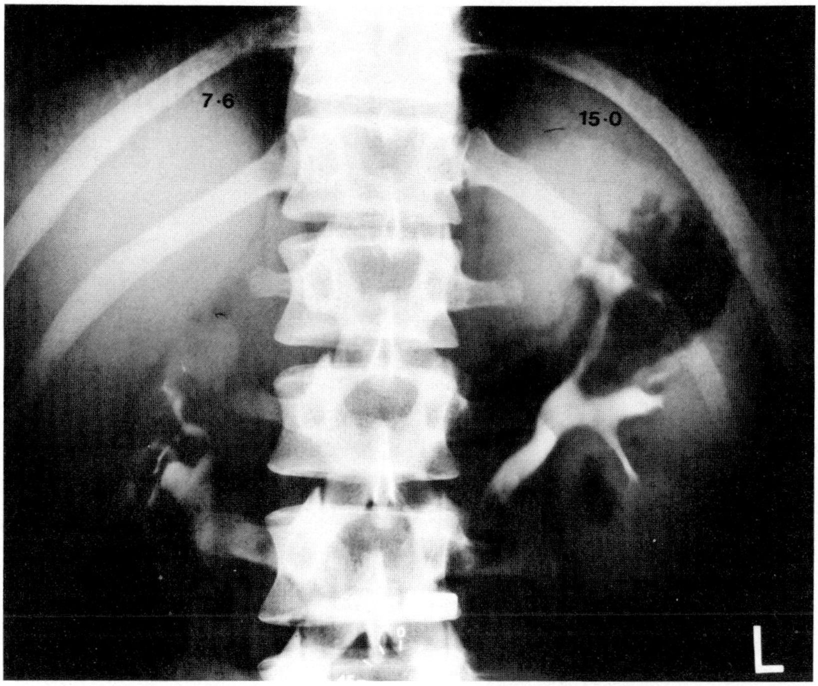

Fig. 1. The intravenous urogram of a 19-year-old man who was normotensive and underwent nephrectomy (table I).

Conclusion

The findings in this study are at present inconclusive. Such prospective studies are clearly important and will take many years to complete, not only because of the long natural history of the disease, but also because of the strict criteria for inclusion. The study does show that normotensive patients with unilateral RN are at risk of developing hypertension, but there is, as yet, no evidence to show that this can be prevented by prophylactic nephrectomy. There is evidence that some hypertensive patients may benefit from nephrectomy, but we have no reliable way of identifying them. It would appear as if nephrectomy is more likely to benefit younger patients with a recent onset of hypertension. We feel that nephrectomy should only be considered if the contralateral kidney is normal and the glomerular filtration rate of the damaged kidney is less than 10 ml/min. More than a quar-

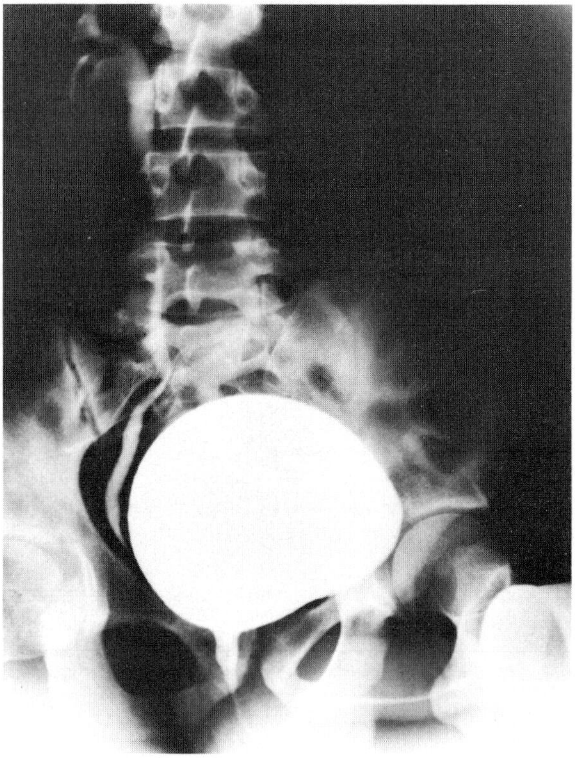

Fig. 2. The micturating cysto-urethrogram on the patient in figure 1.

ter of a century ago *Smith* [3] stated 'even in the presence of obvious unilateral renal disease, nephrectomy remains an experimental procedure and subject to experimental error'.

It is hoped that this long-term prospective study will enable further information to be gained on one of the major complications of RN – hypertension.

References

1 Ask-Upmark, E.: Über juvenile maligne Nephrosklerose und ihr Verhältnis zu Störungen in der Nierenentwicklung. Acta path. microbiol. scand. *6*: 383 (1929).

2 Butler, A.M.: Chronic pyelonephritis and arterial hypertension. J. clin. Invest. *16*: 889 (1937).

3 Smith, H.W.: Unilateral nephrectomy in hypertensive disease. J. Urol. *76*: 685 (1956).
4 Thompson, G.J.: Results of nephrectomy in hypertensive patients. J. Urol. *77*: 358 (1957).
5 Yates-Bell, J.G.: Nephrectomy in cases of hypertension. Br. med. J. *ii*: 1371 (1959).
6 Kincaid-Smith, P.: Renal ischaemia and hypertension: a review of the results of surgery. Australas. Ann. Med. *10*: 166 (1961).
7 Luke, R.G.; Kennedy, A.C.; Briggs, J.D.; Struthers, N.W.; Stirling, W.B.: Results of nephrectomy in hypertension associated with unilateral renal disease. Br. med. J. *iii*: 764 (1968).
8 Eliahou, H.E.; Boner, G.; Rakowczick, M.: Effect of nephrectomy on hypertension in unilateral non-vascular renal disease: report on 7 patients. J. Urol. *99*: 379 (1968).
9 Haycock, G.B.: Hypertension associated with unilateral renal disease in childhood. Report of 2 cases and review of the literature. Acta paediat. scand. *64*: 299 (1975).
10 Pfau, A.; Rosenmann, E.: Unilateral chronic pyelonephritis and hypertension: coincidental or causal relationship? Am. J. Med. *65*: 499 (1978).
11 Bailey, R.R.; McRae, C.U.; Maling, T.M.J.; Tisch, G.; Little, P.J.: Renal vein renin concentration in the hypertension of unilateral reflux nephropathy. J. Urol. *120*: 21 (1978).
12 Bailey, R.R.: Reflux nephropathy and hypertension; in Reflux nephropathy, pp. 263–267 (Masson, New York 1979).
13 Gunnels, J.C.; McGuiffin, W.L.; Johnsrude, I.; Robinson, R.R.: Peripheral and renal venous plasma renin activity in hypertension. Ann. intern. Med. *71*: 555 (1969).
14 Hollenberg, N.K.; Epstein, M.; Basch, R.I.; Merrill, J.P.; Hickler, R.B.: Renin secretion in the patient with hypertension: relationship to intrarenal blood flow distribution. Circulation Res. *24-25*: suppl. I, p. I-113 (1969).
15 Giese, J.; Aurell, M.; Munck, O.: Peripheral and renal venous plasma renin concentration in hypertensive patients with unilateral renal or renovascular disease. Scand. J. Urol. Nephrol. *6*: suppl. 15, p. 39 (1972).
16 Delin, K.; Aurell, M.; Granerus, G.: Renin-dependent hypertension in patients with unilateral kidney disease not caused by renal artery stenosis. Acta med. scand. *201*: 345 (1977).
17 Holland, N.: Reflux nephropathy and hypertension; in Reflux nephropathy, pp. 257–262 (Masson, New York 1979).
18 Savage, J.M.; Dillon, M.J.; Shah, V.; Barratt, T.M.; Williams, D.I.: Renin and blood-pressure in children with renal scarring and vesicoureteric reflux. Lancet *ii*: 441 (1978).
19 Bailey, R.R.; Reddy, J.; Boniface, G.R.; Turner, J.G.; McRae, C.U.: Estimating unilateral renal function with non-invasive methods. N.Z. med. J. (in press).

Ross. R. Bailey, MD, Departments of Nephrology and Urology,
Christchurch Hospital, Christchurch (New Zealand)

Contr. Nephrol., vol. 39, pp. 126–131 (Karger, Basel 1984)

12. Glomerular Lesions in the 'Normal' Kidney in Patients with Unilateral Reflux Nephropathy

Ross R. Bailey, Charles P. Swainson, Kelvin L. Lynn, Alastair F. Burry

Departments of Nephrology and Pathology, Christchurch Hospital, Christchurch, New Zealand

Introduction

There is now convincing evidence [1–8] that an associated glomerulopathy (focal and segmental sclerosis and hyalinosis) plays an important role in the deterioration of renal function in patients with reflux nephropathy (RN). The pathogenesis of this lesion is uncertain, but an immunologic mechanism appears likely. The lesion has been demonstrated in kidneys showing RN, but there is little evidence available as to whether the glomerulopathy affects the radiologically 'normal' kidney of patients with strictly unilateral RN. However, *Kincaid-Smith* [2] in a review of 105 patients briefly alluded to 4 patients with unilateral RN who had focal and segmental hyalinosis in the contralateral non-scarred kidney. We report 2 more such patients.

Case Reports

Patient 1. A 24-year-old man was found to have proteinuria. He had no history of renal disease, but had suffered gout 1 year previously. On examination he was well, with a blood pressure of 110/60 mm Hg. Urinalysis showed 2+ protein and a negative reaction for blood while, on microscopy, there were 60 white cells/mm^3 and no red cells. The specimen was sterile on culture. Urine fibrin degradation products were slightly increased at 0.2 mg/dl. Plasma creatinine 1.8 mg/dl, Cr^{51}-ethylenediaminetetraacetic acid (EDTA) clearance 66 ml/min, maximum urinary concentrating ability (following intranasal desmopressin) 515 mmol/kg and 24 h urinary protein excretion 2.2 g. Antinuclear antibodies, streptococcal antibodies and hepatitis B surface antigen were negative, and serum complement (C3 and C4), serum protein electrophoresis and serum immunoglobulins were all normal. Blood group 0 positive and tissue type HLA A1, –; B8, 14.

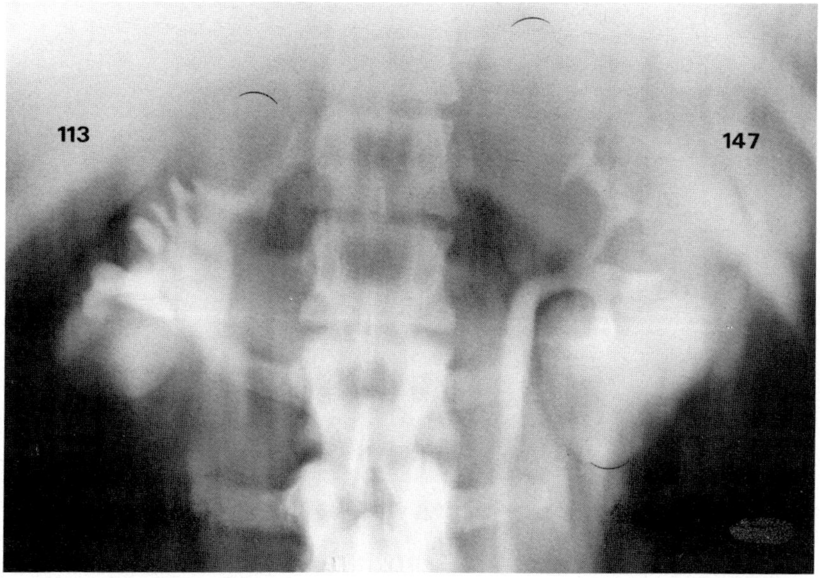

Fig. 1. Intravenous urogram on patient 1.

An intravenous urography (IVU) showed the left kidney to measure 14.7 cm in length and to be structurally normal. The right kidney was 11.3 cm in length and showed the characteristic features of RN (fig. 1). A ^{99m}Tc-dimercaptosuccinic acid (DMSA) scan showed 29% of the isotope uptake in the right kidney. Voiding cysto-urethrography (VCU) showed gross vesico-ureteral reflux (VUR) on the right side (fig. 2). A renal biopsy was obtained from the 'normal' left kidney. On immunofluorescence there was segmental, fine, granular glomerular basement membrane and mesangial deposition of IgM, while on light microscopy all 7 glomeruli showed varying degrees of focal segmental sclerosis and hyalinosis. There was patchy interstitial fibrosis, tubular atrophy and a chronic inflammatory cell infiltrate, together with moderate hyaline thickening of the arterioles. The electron microscopic sections showed some increase in mesangial matrix and some basement membrane thickening, but no deposits were demonstrated and the appearances were considered to be non-specific. The overall biopsy appearances were those of focal glomerulosclerosis.

Patient 2. A 46-year-old Samoan man presented with intermittent left loin pain. 2 years earlier he had suffered pneumonitis following accidental petrol inhalation. He was on no medications. Urinalysis showed 3+ proteinuria and on microscopy there were <100 red cell/mm^3. Urine specimens were sterile on culture. Plasma urea 54 mg/dl; plasma creatinine 1.7 mg/dl; creatinine clearance 84 ml/min; maximal urinary concentrating ability 551 mmol/kg, and 42 h urinary protein excretion = 4.5 g. Antinuclear antibodies and streptococcal antibodies were negative and the serum complement (C3 and C4) normal. Hepatitis B surface antigen was positive and the antibody negative. Liver function tests normal. Serum total pro-

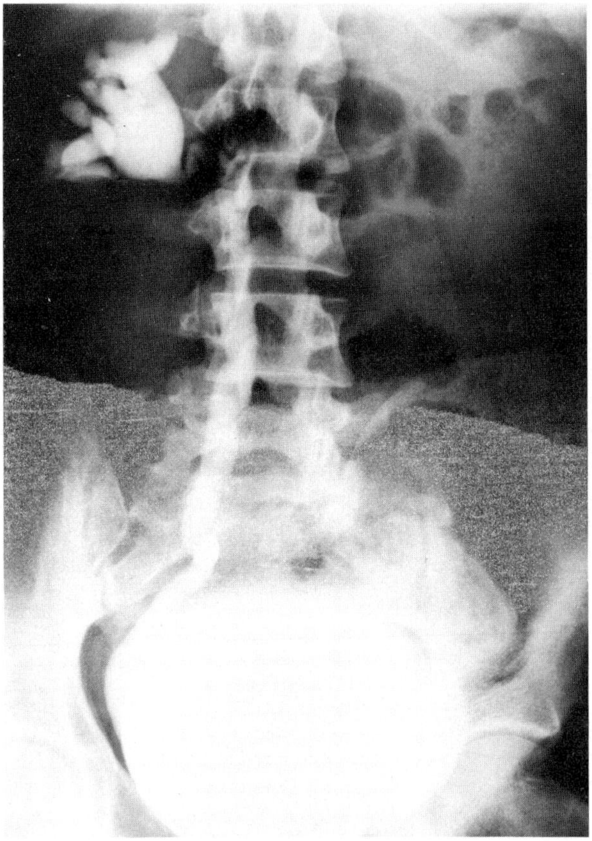

Fig. 2. Micturating cysto-urethrogram on patient 1.

teins 67, with 38 g/l of albumin. Serum lipid studies showed changes consistent with a type V hyperlipidaemia. Blood group 0 positive and tissue type HLA A2, –; B12, W22.

An IVU showed the left kidney to measure 15 cm in length and to be radiologically normal, while the right kidney measured 12 cm in length, was a little low in position, slightly rotated and showed the characteristic features of RN. A renal biopsy of the radiologically 'normal' left kidney showed light microscopic features of a severe focal and segmental sclerosis and hyalinosis.

When seen 3 years later in this department his blood pressure was 130/80 mm Hg and he was taking digoxin 0.0625 mg daily, frusemide 40 mg daily and dyazide (25 mg hydrochlorothiazide – 50 mg triamterene) 1 tablet daily because of paroxysmal atrial fibrillation and complicating cardiac failure. 12 months earlier he had developed gout. The diuretic was discontinued and allopurinol commenced. Urinalysis showed 3+ proteinuria and a negative reaction for blood while, on microscopy, there were no cells or casts and the specimen was

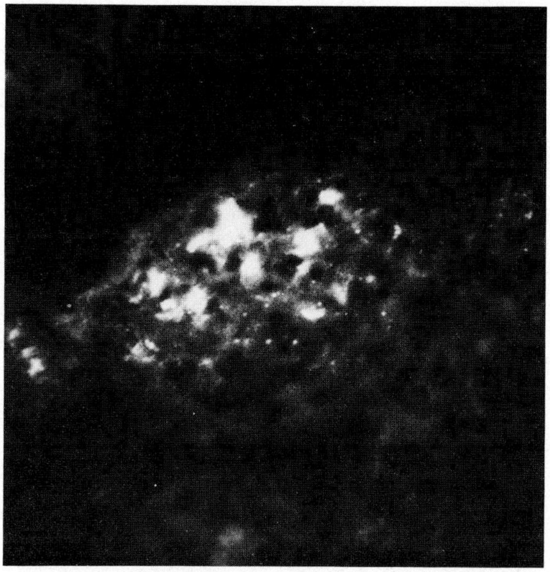

Fig. 3. Glomerulus showing patchy mesangial deposition of IgM.

sterile on culture. Urine fibrin degradation products increased at 0.4 mg/dl. Plasma urea 65 mg/dl; plasma creatinine 2.4 mg/dl; creatinine clearance 45 ml/min; ^{51}-Cr EDTA clearance 60 ml/min; maximal urinary concentrating ability 480 mmol/kg, and 24 h urinary protein excretion 4 g. Hepatitis B surface antigen (e antigen negative) and antibody positive. Liver function tests normal. Type V hyperlipidaemia was confirmed.

A repeat IVU showed no change. A VCU showed no VUR. A repeat renal biopsy on the 'normal' left kidney showed, on immunofluorescence, patchy mesangial deposition of IgM (fig. 3), while on light microscopy (fig. 4) 10 of the 15 glomeruli were totally sclerotic and the remaining 5 were hypertrophied and showed varying degrees of segmental sclerosis with increased mesangial matrix, capsular adhesions and insudation of hyaline material into mesangial areas. Foam cells were also present in some mesangial areas. There was extensive tubular atrophy, interstitial fibrosis and chronic inflammatory cell infiltration. The intact tubules were hypertrophied and the arterioles showed moderate mural thickening and mild arteriosclerosis. Electron microscopic examination showed extensive fusion of epithelial cell foot processes and marked expansion of mesangial areas with increased matrix and occasional large electron-dense aggregates in the paramesangial regions beneath the endothelium and within the mesangium. These features were those of an advanced focal and segmental glomerulosclerosis.

Discussion

Both of these men had unilateral RN with the contralateral kidney showing compensatory hypertrophy and being radiologically normal. Both

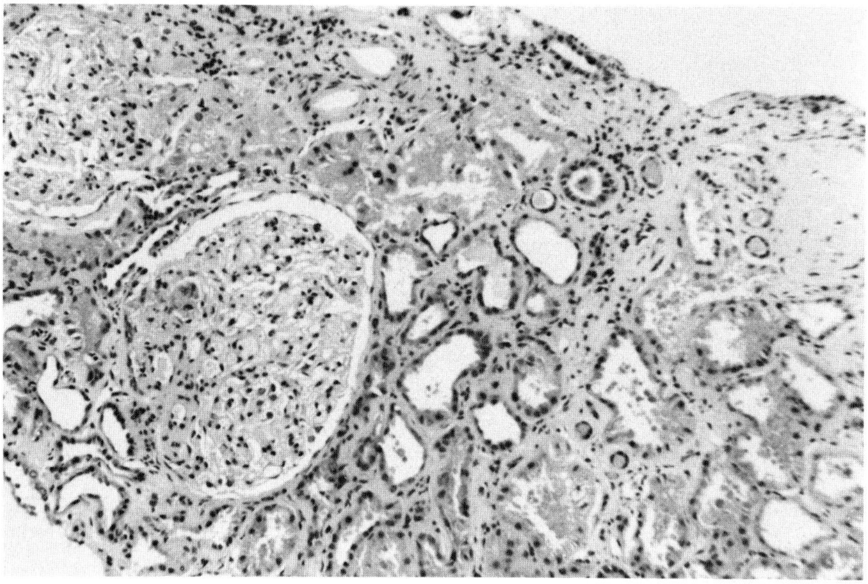

Fig. 4. Section of kidney showing a hypertrophied glomerulus with segmental sclerosis towards the stalk, a hyalinized glomerulus, and an essentially normal glomerulus. HE. × 210.

patients, however, had significant proteinuria, impaired glomerular and tubular function and histological evidence of focal glomerulosclerosis in the 'normal' kidney. In both cases the lesion appears to be progressive.

The pathogenesis of this glomerular lesion remains uncertain, but there is now considerable evidence [1–8] to show that it contributes in a major way to the deterioration of renal function that may occur in some patients with RN.

References

1 Zimmerman, S.W.; Uehling, D.T.; Burkholder, P.N.: Vesicoureteral reflux nephropathy. Evidence for immunologically mediated glomerular injury. Urology *2*: 534 (1973).

2 Kincaid-Smith, P.: Glomerular lesions in atrophic pyelonephritis and reflux nephropathy. Kidney int. *8*: suppl. 4, S81 (1975).

3 Aladjen, M.; Schoeneman, M.J.; Bennett, B.; Levitt, S.; Spitzer, A.; Greifer, I.: Focal segmental glomerulosclerosis: with proteinuria and chronic interstitial nephritis. N.Y. St. J. Med. *March*: 579 (1978).

4 Senekjian, H.O.; Stinebaugh, B.J.; Mattiolo, C.A.; Suki, W.N.: Irreversible renal failure following vesicoureteral reflux. J. Am. med. Ass. *241*: 160 (1979).
5 Bhathena, D.B.; Weiss, J.H.; Holland, N.H.; McMorrow, R.G.; Curtis, J.J.; Lucas, B.A.; Luke, R.G.: Focal and segmental glomerular sclerosis in reflux nephropathy. Am. J. Med. *68*: 886 (1980).
6 Torres, V.E.; Velosa, J.A.; Holley, K.E.; Kelalis, P.P.; Stickler, G.B.; Kurtz, S.B.: The progression of vesicoureteral reflux nephropathy. Ann. intern. Med. *92*: 776 (1980).
7 Cotran, R.S.: Pathogenetic mechanisms in the progression of reflux nephropathy, the roles of glomerulosclerosis and extravasation of Tamm-Horsfall protein. Proc. 8th Int. Congr. Nephrol., Athens 1981, p. 374.
8 Cotran, R.S.: Glomerulosclerosis in reflux nephropathy. Kidney int. *21*: 528 (1982).

Ross R. Bailey, MD, Departments of Nephrology and Pathology,
Christchurch Hospital, Christchurch (New Zealand)

Contr. Nephrol., vol. 39, pp. 132–145 (Karger, Basel 1984)

Discussion on Chapters 4–12

Dr. *P. Kincaid-Smith*: Dr. *Bailey*, in some of the families you showed you implied that you were making a diagnosis of reflux nephropathy (RN) in patients with end-stage renal failure. We found quite a mixture of types of glomerulonephritis in patients with vesicoureteric reflux (VUR). In one group that I analyzed, we found 3 IgA nephropathies among 24 refluxers. I'm just wondering if there might have been other diseases which caused the end-stage renal failure in your series, or if you confirmed RN by some objective means in those families.

My second question is: Should one really be looking for an HLA association in a disease that is not, or probably not, an immunologically related disease?

Dr. *R. Bailey*: The families that we investigated with end-stage renal failure had end-stage RN. They had bilateral gross VUR, and small, scarred kidneys. Most had been followed for a period of time, and had abnormal ureteral orifices.

Dr. *P. Kincaid-Smith*: Those were all in the family units?

Dr. *R. Bailey*: They were in the 18 individuals who entered the renal replacement program with end-stage RN. With regard to the question of markers, I'm not a geneticist and it is possible that HLA may be the wrong marker on chromosome 6. But it could be something else that is very close.

Dr. *R. Heptinstall*: Well, if you know nothing about it, who then advised you to trace the HLA types?

Dr. *R. Bailey*: Initially, because we had good evidence it was congenital and was occurring in families, we looked at genetic markers and, like many other people, looked for them using the HLA system. I still think that there is a distinct possibility that there is some such link. HLA may be a marker to the real marker. That's why I suggested measuring other things on chromosome 6 such as 21-hydroxylase.

Dr. *J. Winberg*: Dr. *Bailey*, could you make clear to us what you actually studied?

Dr. *R. Bailey*: Well, in a large number of the 68 families the propositi who had normal renal function were mothers who had RN, and their newborn infants were then investigated at birth; a micturating cystogram (MCU) was performed as soon after birth as possible. We were clearly not looking for RN in this group, but for VUR. In some children who were older, we may have missed some cases because VUR may, by then, have disappeared. Later we concentrated on RN. So in the very young, we looked for VUR. In the older ones, we looked for kidney scarring.

Dr. *J. Winberg*: The weak point then is that you don't know whether in such a protocol there is VUR in newborns whose mothers don't have RN. You assume that it is so, but you don't know.

Dr. *R. Bailey*: You mean that the prevalence of VUR in newborn infants with normal mothers is a study that cannot be performed on ethical grounds?

Dr. *Abbott*, in our department, has gone part of the way towards it. In 50 children whose bag-collected specimens were infected, suprapubic aspiration was performed. 5 again had a positive culture and 45 were sterile. In all some contrast material was infused at the time of bladder needling and in 10% of the 45 sterile cases VUR was demonstrated, which suggests that there may be an appreciable population of refluxers in otherwise healthy normal infants.

Dr. *J. Winberg*: As Dr. *Asscher* also pointed out earlier, we don't know this normal incidence. We have done some MCUs in newborns with renal masses which eventually turned out to be suprarenal lesions. Some had VUR, although they had no renal disease, so I think that it may not be so uncommon, unless it is a procedural artifact.

Dr. *J. Hodson*: Once again, I would like to warn against the value that can be placed on one MCU.

Dr. *N. Goldraich*: We also performed a study to establish the incidence of abnormalities in the urinary tract among relatives of children with VUR. The index cases were 26 children (6 males and 20 females) with primary VUR, without duplex kidneys. 51 parents and 43 siblings were investigated. We found abnormalities in 8% of the fathers, in 26.9% of the mothers and in 39.5% of the siblings. Among the 51 parents we found VUR in 4, RN in 2, a duplex kidney in 1, a caliceal diverticulum in 1 and pelviureteral junction (PUJ) obstruction in 1. Among the siblings, we found VUR in 6, VUR plus RN in 4, PUJ obstruction in 2, duplex kidneys in 2 and urethral valves in 1.

The prevalence of VUR and/or RN was 17% in the overall sample, 23.3% among the siblings, and 11.8% among the parents. We also did not manage to establish the pattern of genetic inheritance of these anomalies. We recommend the systematic and early investigation of siblings and children of patients with VUR.

Dr. *R. Bailey*: Dr. *Goldraich*, you said that none of your patients had surgery and possessed all grades of VUR. I think your work also emphasizes how early in life renal damage occurs, with many patients who already have scars under the age of 2 years. I think that further confirms that we have to be looking at birth and the first few months of life for a way of diagnosing and preventing the baby at risk. But I don't know if you can really conclude, for the reasons we have just been discussing, that the fact that no more scars developed was because of your prophylactic antibacterial regimen. I think the same might happen whether you treated them or not, providing they remained symptomless.

Dr. *N. Goldraich*: We can conclude that if they are treated at the time of the first urinary tract infection (UTI) fewer kidneys become scarred than if treatment is delayed.

Dr. *W. Asscher*: Was there a control group?

Dr. *N. Goldraich*: This is an ongoing study, and the control group will be those who were infants when we began to treat them. 2 years later they will be pre-school children. The numbers are not yet big enough to make comparisons between the results of the treated and untreated groups. We have to wait for these. If we eventually prevent scars in all pre-school children there will be a difference between the treated and untreated, as at present we already have more scars in the pre-school age than in the infants.

Dr. *J. Winberg*: The existence of RN is denied among most pediatricians – at least among those I meet at home. If so, its absence simply results from the widespread use of antimicrobials for all fevers in babies. Dr. *Goldraich*, however, is experiencing the situation existing in our countries 30 or 40 years ago.

Dr. *J. Hodson*: Dr. *Goldraich*, I gather your practice comprises what you might call two completely different socioeconomic groups.

Dr. *N. Goldraich*: Yes.

Dr. *J. Hodson*: Is there any difference between them in the incidence and severity of RN?

Dr. *N. Goldraich*: No, there is no difference.

Dr. *P. Kincaid-Smith*: I'm interested in the apparent prevalence of RN in the Brazilian population. *Kunin* in the USA found very little VUR among his black girls with UTI. My own experience in South Africa is that RN is a pretty rare condition in Black Africans, if it is present at all. I would like to know if there is any difference between the different racial groups in Brazil.

Dr. *N. Goldraich*: No, we have found no difference between the black and white populations. But we don't have a large black population in the south of Brazil. Usually in South Brazil the races mix a lot so we do not see the same situation that obtains in the USA.

Dr. *J. Duckett*: I'd like to make a comment about perineal hygiene. In our country we have a very low incidence of UTI in black children. I think this results from a genetic trait and has nothing to do with hygiene.

Dr. *R. White*: On the same theme, one thing that occurs to me is that in the black families there may be fewer hangups about toilet training in the child, and it is possible this may have something to do with the non-development of unstable detrusor contractions or delay in voiding control and so on. There may be a genetic difference in the tendency to VUR, but as far as the UTI is concerned it may be environmental.

Dr. *J. Conway*: How do you explain Dr. *Svenson*'s thesis then that the basic fact is the migration of bacteria from the perineum, if everyone denies that perineal hygiene has nothing to do with it?

Dr. *S. Svenson*: That's not what we're saying. What we *are* saying is that individuals differ as regards their natural defences against bacteria and, if you are in the unfortunate position of possessing an inadequate host defence mechanism in the urethral area, you will be prone to UTI, and there is probably no way to wipe off attached bacteria. I don't think it is a matter of hygiene.

Dr. *J. Hodson*: To start with a statement of fact: when I first started diagnosing RN radiographically in 1956 I rarely came across a female patient with coarsely scarred kidneys over the age of 40 years. The use of antibiotics first spread widely just after the war, in 1950. Thus, all adult women at that time would have spent their childhood in the pre-antibiotic era. And without antibiotics RN is just as much a killing disease as is pneumonia, although it may take a little longer. What we see now are either what might be called antibiotic breakthroughs, or they have never been infected, or their early UTIs went undiagnosed and untreated.

Dr. *W. Asscher*: I was going to say something about the theory of hyperfiltration as a predisposition for glomerulopathy and proteinuria. I agree with Dr. *Kincaid-Smith* that there doesn't seem to be enough in the way of diminution of renal parenchyma in many of these patients, or even those who deteriorate, for hyperfiltration of remaining glomeruli to be a relevant issue.

Dr. *Dillon*, how many of Dr. *Smellie*'s patients with high renin levels were taking oral contraceptives – as this would greatly affect their renin levels? Also, did you relate the renin levels to their level of sodium excretion?

Dr. *M. Dillon*: The patients that I reported were those in whom we had eliminated interfering factors. The 'pill' wasn't actually a difficult issue because several patients of whom it was entirely unsuspected were, in fact, surreptitiously 'taking the pill' during the time many of the specimens were obtained. So we eliminated them. We also eliminated the odd pregnancy which seemed to have slipped in. So none of those patients were subject to this type of interfering medication so far as we could elicit.

As for the sodium balance, when we first set up our renin assay we were very impressed by *John Laragh*'s beautiful curves [*Brenner* et al.: Essential hypertension: renin, aldosterone, heart attack and stroke. New Engl. J. Med. *286*: 441–449, 1972], and I thought that we ought to relate all our renin results to the sodium balance by some means or another. We discovered, however, that those curves were founded on very low sodium intakes at one end of the spectrum and some extremely high ones at the other. In the middle of the curves, there really isn't much correlation. And we found that most of our children on standard ward diets or standard home diet were, in fact, in the middle, with no sufficient data to justify using sodium as a factor. The same result obtained with the hypertensive patients.

Dr. *W. Asscher*: Would you also assure us then that those with high renin levels didn't have high sodium levels, which occasionally happens in RN.

Dr. *M. Dillon*: There was no evidence to suggest that they were wasting sodium.

Dr. *R. White*: I would like to refer back to the present grading of VUR because, for good or ill, this is what three important ongoing studies are based on, and I would like Dr. *Duckett* to speak on this matter.

Dr. *J. Duckett*: It was *Parkkulainen* in Finland in 1966 who first came up with a 1–5 classification of VUR [*Heikel and Parkkulainen*, Ann. Radiol. *9*: 37, 1966]. It clearly defines both what is happening at the forniceal and caliceal levels and the amount of dilatation that occurs at various places of the upper tract. Clearly what we have been calling 2B was his grade 3. So it is easy now to bring these two classifications together.

We would like to bring them together all over the world so that we are all talking about the same thing. To define it accurately, grade 1 is partly up the ureter; 2 to the kidney without any dilatation at all; 3 is with dilatation and minimal, if any, blunting of the fornix; 4 is blunting of the fornix but with maintenance of the papillary impression, and 5 is where you've got clubbing, and clearly no papillary impressions at all. We have found this classification to be eminently practical and it is not too different from that put forward by the British Medical Research Council, and by the two International ongoing trials.

Dr. *J. Hodson*: I agree this classification, which has been adopted by the European Study with only minor modifications, is a realistic way of grading what is seen during voiding cystourethrography (VCU). But I must stress again that *what* is seen depends very much on the details of the technique used, and differs with the age of the child, the urine flow at the time and probably the time since the last UTI. This is an examination which has never been subjected to a properly conducted trial of its reproducibility. I do not believe it is realistic, therefore, to base a decision on one study.

Dr. *J. Duckett*: Well, let me make another point, I'm sorry Dr. *Conway* is not here to defend the idea of standardizing the volume that is refluxed. I think that this may be totally irrelevant, because of the very variable volumes of the renal pelves and ureters that are found, except perhaps in the case of repeated examinations in the same patient. I don't believe that radionuclide cystography is ever going to produce a realistic grading of VUR.

And the other point is that if the infusion is carried out at a pressure of 60 cm of contrast, all bladders are filled to the same pressure level and voiding is commenced after that level is reached. In this way maximal filling may be achieved and standardized. If the patient voids before a pressure of 60 cm is reached then maximum filling may be assumed.

Dr. *S. Koff*: I can't let that go by in Dr. *Conway*'s absence. In fact there have been studies done which show precisely the opposite, that the height of the fluid column during the cystogram bears absolutely no relationship to the pressure in the bladder until the latter fills to capacity and stops filling. Only then does the bladder pressure commence to rise. But during the inflow there is no rise in bladder pressure.

Dr. *J. Duckett*: I agree. That's what I thought I was saying. We determine maximum filling by no more flow coming from the bottle at 60 cm of water.

Dr. *P. Kincaid-Smith*: I think it essential to get accurate figures on what percentage of infants with severe VUR have RN. I think I'm right in saying that in the original Christchurch series, which is the biggest one I know of, that it was only 22%. And yet today we hear talk about an incidence of renal damage of 80% or more in infants with gross VUR.

Dr. *R. Bailey*: I think that in the Christchurch infants with gross VUR at the time of presentation, the figure was about 70%. But only 70% of them presented with UTI.

Dr. *P. Kincaid-Smith*: Dr. *Winberg*, the incidence of gross VUR in your infants was much less, wasn't it?

Dr. *J. Winberg*: Yes. Disregarding those with obvious dysplasia we only had 1 or 2 with RN and gross VUR at their first UTI.

Dr. *P. Kincaid-Smith*: I was wondering why there appeared to be such a different incidence in the two series.

Dr. *M. Taylor*: Obviously there is a big problem with regard to how one compromises in the collection of patients for a study like this. One ought to make a statistical statement to look at how big 'n' must be to beget 'p'; the percentage difference in the outcome. Of course, we met the same problem. Before I came away I asked our statistician, if we are looking for a 10% difference in a parameter, how big 'n' had to be in each group. The answer was 'n' has to be 380 in each limb! So that some doubts are likely to be cast on any conclusions based on a study with only a few patients in each limb.

Dr. *J. Hodson*: Some time back Dr. *Weiss* remarked that many of their cases show intrarenal reflux (IRR). If one thinks about this, does it really mean that IRR occurs every time the child micturates and, if so, is this happening without the formation of scars? Or is it a procedural artifact from the MCU?

Dr. *R. Weiss*: Of those that did have IRR above the age of 6, a few, if I recall correctly, do not have any scarring, which suggests that it is artifactual.

Dr. *J. Hodson*: Which brings us back to the infusion pressure used during MCU. Our pig work has shown us that there is a very critical pressure above which IRR occurs, and this may vary from day to day governed by such physiologic parameters as blood pressure, glomerular filtration rate (GFR), etc.

I believe that this can happen in normal kidneys. In the middle of the night if a child is bladder-trained, his bladder fills up to a capacity rarely reached during the day. And there is evidence that the bladder doesn't then simply remain inert but occasionally contracts, how forcefully one simply doesn't know. Is that not so, Dr. *van Gool*?

Dr. *J. van Gool*: It does contract.

Dr. *J. Hodson*: So if VUR is also present, then, varying according to certain factors the urine will be propelled up to, and perhaps *into*, the kidney and ebb out again when the contraction wave recedes. A process which, if it occurs at all, is likely to be repeated at intervals, presumably without causing damage. Also, very occasionally one sees in cystograms of children with VUR up slightly or severely dilated ureters, a generalized form of IRR and, unless this is completely a procedural artifact, it may represent a repetitive phenomenon. And if this persists, one might well expect a diffuse effect on the kidneys. Time will show.

Dr. *R. Weiss*: If it turns out that most of the children that have had IRR all come from one center and one radiologist then we'll have an answer. But if they come from multiple centers and involve children of different ages, some with and some without RN in the 5- and 10-year follow-ups, we also may have an answer.

Dr. *P. Ransley*: We must be very cautious here, between the occurrence of IRR and our ability to visualize it. I consider the cystogram has to be carried to very unphysiological limits to force enough contrast into the parenchyma for it to be visible on poor quality radiographs.

Dr. *J. Winberg*: Dr. *Ransley*, you once presented to us a scheme as to which cases of VUR to operate and which not to. You avoided those below 1 year of age. Have you now changed your mind?

Dr. *P. Ransley*: All that I've seen in the last few years has confirmed that opinion. I think that dilated ureters associated with thin bladder walls in infants are a contraindication to surgery.

Dr. *W. Asscher*: It seems to me that every time we hear a surgeon talk about Dr. *Stephen*'s ideas on congenital malformation, and VUR not being related to the kidney disorder, we tend to avoid this issue. I would like to ask, do we really feel that VUR is in fact responsible for these gross changes in the neonate or does it occur in utero? Over the years we have seen the age at which we are trying to prevent the problem becoming younger and younger and still no one seems very successful in doing so. We now hear that even under the age of 1, we're not doing any good. Has anybody seen this disease in utero?

Dr. *J. Duckett*: I'd like to ask Dr. *Bailey* whether, because there is an equal sex distribution of RN in infants, UTI can be incriminated as the cause of end-stage disease in children, as it may well be in the 30-year-old female after several pregnancies. Of your patients under 16, I maintain that some of those were born with 'dysplastic' kidneys.

Dr. *R. Bailey*: It is a difficult problem. Dr. *Winberg* has documented some infants with VUR among whom already at birth some had severe renal damage. And this was excluding those with posterior urethral valves in which many have congenital damage. But kidneys commence excretion at about the 10–12th week of fetal life, and no one has any idea what may happen to them after that in utero. And, so far, I am not aware of any intrauterine study carried out in a family, say with a strong family history.

Dr. *J. Hodson*: In our hospital 2 cases of urethral obstruction with upper tract dilatation have been diagnosed in utero by means of ultrasound, and this was shown to be correct postpartum.

Dr. *R. Bailey*: But as regards the question of UTI, the young male under the age of 1 year, and particularly under the age of 3 months, is at especial risk. UTI has an equal prevalence in both sexes in this age group and my impression is that they usually have some congenital abnormality, often VUR.

Dr. *P. Kincaid-Smith*: I'd like to comment on Dr. *Stephen*'s theory. I understand that his whole concept of the development of the dysplastic upper urinary tract is totally theoretical and really has very little basis in fact. This was pointed out by Dr. *Friedland* in Bermuda 4 years ago and admitted by Dr. *Stephens* himself. I have looked at some of his original kidneys and the argument that they were dysplastic was based on the presence of abnormal tissues, such as cartilage or even bone. But you can find the same thing in papillae in women of 40 or 50 with analgesic nephropathy. So I have never accepted the argument that those kidneys were truly dysplastic simply because of the unusual tissue present in them. I think it is probable that a neonatal kidney subject to any injurious effect is much more likely to contain abnormal tissue than a woman who has analgesic nephropathy.

Dr. *T. Risdon*: Dr. *Kincaid-Smith*, the diagnosis of dysplasia is considerably more complicated than the mere histologic presence of cartilage, etc.

Dr. *P. Kincaid-Smith*: Of course. I'm just saying that Dr. *Stephen*'s work was theoretical, and I am not saying there aren't dysplastic kidneys. I'm saying that some of the kidneys that I looked at from the Melbourne Children's Hospital could well have resulted from VUR but were labelled 'dysplastic' because of abnormal tissue in them.

Dr. *R. Risdon*: The mere presence of a bit of bone in a kidney obviously doesn't mean anything at all. The distribution is quite different in analgesic nephropathy anyway.

Dr. *P. Kincaid-Smith*: That's exactly the point I'm making. I have no doubt that there are some congenital abnormalities that occur in kidney development, but probably not those in that particular group of kidneys.

Dr. *R. White*: Do you accept, Dr. *Risdon*, that it is possible that intrauterine VUR can lead to some of these abnormalities that one sees in neonates?

Dr. *R.Risdon*: I'm very glad that this subject has been brought up because I think it is a very realistic theory. There is not an awful lot of factual evidence in its support, but it does help to explain some of the more puzzling aspects of these very young children with 'bad' kidneys and 'bad' ureters. The mere fact that there is VUR as well as bad kidneys doesn't necessarily mean to say they are related. They may both be reflections of a malformed urinary tract.

I think it is very important that we try to distinguish those cases where the kidney may be congenitally abnormal from those born with a normal kidney and who acquire disease later.

Dr.*J. Winberg*: Is not one acceptable method of distinguishing between congenital and acquired disease to count the number of papillae (renal lobes) present? If they are well below average, this may indicate a congenital abnormality.

Dr. *J. Duckett*: In the case of very severe kidneys, yes. They are deformed, and it is difficult to identify them. But what I'm trying to postulate is that there may be gradations between congenitally 'bad' kidneys and those resulting from VUR and UTI, or just high pressure VUR with obstruction. I like neither to use the term 'dysplasia', which I regard as extreme, nor 'hypoplasia' which is another nebulous term. I am rather intrigued as to what a series of carefully conducted biopsies might reveal.

Dr. *J. Hodson*: We had all this out in Bermuda at our last meeting, when Dr. *Stephens* himself was present. It is all theory and we are no further on, because these small kidneys are not being accurately categorized.

Dr. *J. Winberg*: I think many of Dr. *Stephen*'s kidneys were very tiny from the beginning and there was no question that these were congenitally defective. But we are now suggesting there may be another group – less damaged – and of secondary, rather than primary etiology.

This would support what Dr. *Bailey* said, that males with early UTI have a very high rate of functional or structural malformation. I think that shows that too few neonates with UTI are being diagnosed, as our experience is the opposite, namely that neonates with UTI have a very low rate of malformation.

Dr. *R. Bailey*: But in Dr. *Abbott*'s study in which he screened 1,460 neonates within the first week of life, he found a 1% prevalence of UTI and 8 out of those 14 infants had VUR.

Dr.*J. Winberg*: Yes. If you say that VUR is a malformation, okay. But if we discount VUR, there are very few malformations.

Dr. *M. Dillon*: I want to support the prospect of prenatal ultrasound as a means of identifying those foetuses that have VUR or urethral obstruction. I have diagnosed at least 1 child in whom both VUR and a dilated urinary tract were identified in the absence of organic obstruction. I think that there may well be important opportunities of solving some of our problems here so long as the children are referred early after delivery for the next stage of review.

Dr. *S. Koff*: We are shortly presenting a paper describing 9 cases of fetal hydronephrosis. The majority of these were non-obstructive and were refluxing and, because of the tremendous dilatation in the urinary tract, they were easily picked up in utero by ultrasound. I also think we may learn a lot if this becomes a routine antenatal procedure.

Dr. *J. Hodson*: Is your ultrasound good enough to pick up the thickness of the bladder wall?

Dr. *S. Koff*: Yes.

Dr. *J. Hodson*: That is another thing which ought to be looked for in an antenatal study.

Dr. *J. Hodson*: We now come to an important matter with wide clinical implications, Dr. *Kincaid-Smith*'s claim that a diagnosis of chronic diffuse RN can be made from renal biopsy.

Dr. *P. Kincaid-Smith*: One must realize that by the time adulthood is reached, only 10% of refluxers still reflux, so this is only acceptable as a criterion when positive What I'm proposing is that there are sometimes diffuse acute lesions, in what is normally assumed to be uninvolved parenchyma, which occur simultaneously with the large acute lesions that give rise to the coarse scars. In other words, if a refluxing kidney has coarse scars and a biopsy is taken from non-scarred tissue there are diffuse specific changes present by which the etiology can be identified.

Dr. *W. Asscher*: Did your patients have normal kidney function? Because I'd be very surprised to get an abnormal biopsy from non-scarred tissue if the function was normal.

Dr. *P. Kincaid-Smith*: They had normal kidney function. The mean renal function between the two groups was no different. The serum creatinine levels were about the 0.12 level. They were marginally elevated but not different from the other group.

Dr. *R. Heptinstall*: I am reluctant to join this discussion because I do not believe that chronic pyelonephritis is a diffuse disease. It is a focal disease.

There were a few things I didn't understand about Dr. *Kincaid-Smith*'s study. She had 24 adults in whom she had made the diagnosis of RN, chronic pyelonephritis, whatever you like to call it. That is group number one. Two was an age-matched group of 24 patients who had proteinuria. What was group number three again?

Dr. *P. Kincaid-Smith*: Group three was made up of patients with proteinuria whom I suspected, on the biopsy appearances, also had RN. They were from 127 out of 1,500 biopsies in whom I diagnosed RN on the histological appearance that was demonstrated in Bermuda [*Kincaid-Smith and Hodson* (eds): Reflux nephropathy, Chapter 26, Masson, New York, 1979].

In none of these kidneys was coarse scarring present but they all had proteinuria. If all the histological features I described are grouped, there is a highly statistical significant difference between the two: those with proteinuria alone, and those with proteinuria plus the peculiar histological changes.

Dr. *R. Heptinstall*: But why did you choose a group of 24 patients with proteinuria?

Dr. *P. Kincaid-Smith*: They were all biopsied because of proteinuria.

Dr. *R. Heptinstall*: So all the patients with RN in this series have proteinuria. And now, what was the age spread of these patients?

Dr. *P. Kincaid-Smith*: If I remember correctly, between 18 and 26 years.

Dr. *R. Heptinstall*: Do you know the blood pressures of the two groups? You have not got them listed? I ask you this because I think it is important, as some of the changes you are describing could be due to ischemia on the basis of vascular lesions.

Dr. *P. Kincaid-Smith*: I have not got them with me. I think it was very much the same in the two groups.

Dr. *Heptinstall* went on to describe a method of 'ranking' histologic findings which has been used by *Boitnott* of the Pathology Department at Johns Hopkins [Boitnott, J.R.: The use of ranking in the statistical assessment of morphologic data. Solez and Whelton (eds.) Acute renal failure: correlations between morphology and function, p. 13. Marcel Dekker, New York 1984]. He considered Dr. *Kincaid-Smith*'s data eminently suitable to be analyzed in this way.

Dr. *J. Hodson*: There is some recently published work which bears on this problem and on Dr. *Kincaid-Smith*'s talk. We found in rabbits, repeatedly inoculated intravenously with rabbit urine, that a localized interstitial fibrocellular reaction occurred around those cells of the tubule in which Tamm-Horsfall protein (THP) is found. This occurred in 100% animals after 48 weeks. If THP-depleted urine was used as the inoculating agent, no reaction occurred. But if pure rabbit THP was inoculated, a 100% positive result was obtained, only local segments of the tubules again being affected [*Mayrer* et al.: Tubulointerstitial nephritis and immunologic responses to Tamm-Horsfall protein in rabbits challenged with homologous urine or Tamm-Horsfall protein. J. Immun. *128*: 2634–2642, 1982]. So that a section of most tubules was affected, but only a section. Is this a focal disease? As I understand it, Dr. *Kincaid-Smith* is talking about a diffuse yet focal condition rather like this.

The second experimental data referred to by Dr. *Kincaid-Smith* were the lesions found in the 3- to 4-year survivors of our previous pig series, all of whom had severe hypertension. They had severe coarse scarring on one side, and in both the 'spared' portions of this, and throughout the opposite kidney, multiple tiny 'pit' scars, very like the 'pores' found in an orange skin, were found. It was in relation to these 'pit' scars that the findings described by Dr. *Kincaid-Smith* in her talk were first identified [*Kincaid-Smith and Hodson*: Lesions in the pig kidney with chronic reflux nephropathy; in Hodson, Kincaid-Smith, Reflux nephropathy, chap. 20, Masson, New York 1979].

Dr. *J. Winberg*: Today we have had an insight into the natural history of this disease and, as a pediatrician, this is a very valuable experience. Dr. *Bailey* mentioned that there were almost as many adult males as females with end-stage RN. I think this fact has been used to support the idea that UTI does not play a major role in its causation.

Figures from our epidemiological study in infants showed a male:female ratio of UTI was 154:440. On follow-up, we found that of the 154 boys, 18 had scars, and of the 440 girls, 20 had scars. So the ratio in infected cases was about 1:1 with regard to scarring. So the incidence of RN in adults correlates with these figures.

With regard to the problem of missing UTI in infancy, I must recall that one third of our males – about 50 – had their first UTI during the first 30 days of life. It was their first, and usually their only documented UTI during this period. It was symptomatic and was treated. Of the females, about 20 (5%) had their first symptomatic UTI at this age. As Dr. *White* said, many could easily have been missed as UTIs and their fevers treated symptomatically.

The other matter about which I would like to hear opinions is that when we made a survey in Sweden of chronic renal failure in children below the age of 14, defined as 2 mg/100 ml of creatinine or more lasting at least 6 months, we found 77 cases in a 4-year period and none of them could be identified as RN.

Looking at the figures published by *Chantler* [Archs Dis. Childh. *55*: 435–445, 1980], in which 16% of children with end-stage renal disease were considered to have RN, these are very different figures. I wonder whether someone will comment on this.

Dr. *P. Kincaid-Smith*: You obviously cured them all! You cured their UTIs as infants so they didn't progress!

Dr. *J. Winberg*: I don't know whether that is the explanation, or whether we have failed to identify them in the older age groups.

Dr. *R. Bailey*: If one considers end-stage renal disease in children – and the European Dialysis and Transplant figures for children are probably the best – they confirm the figures that I showed, namely that one third of the group with end-stage renal failure had RN.

So, I think that the population that we're seeing with end-stage renal failure is different to that which you are seeing with UTIs in infants. But this does not explain why no child goes into end-stage renal disease in Sweden due to RN.

Dr. *J. Winberg*: There were 77 children in Sweden during 4 years with chronic renal insufficiency; a creatinine about 2 for at least 6 months.

Dr. *R. Bailey*: And they all had MCUs and no VUR?

Dr. *J. Winberg*: They had an intravenous urogram (IVU) if their disease was not obvious glomerular nephritis.

Dr. *R. Bailey*: Well, maybe that's where you have been misled, because those with RN will have renal impairment, proteinuria and, as Dr. *Kincaid-Smith* showed, microscopic hematuria as well. So from the evidence of urine sediment and biochemistry, one would diagnose them as glomerulonephritis.

Dr. J. Winberg: Those with glomerulonephritis were biopsied, almost all of them. They usually showed inflammatory reactions and there were none,or very few, with focal segmental sclerosis. Some of them were rapidly progressive nephritis. They fell into the usual classification of glomerular nephritis. Would you think this sufficient diagnostic evidence?

Dr. *P. Kincaid-Smith*: Well, I'm sure we'd find a completely different distribution of our diseases if we looked at all our adult patients with raised serum creatinine levels, and it is difficult to compare different groups like this, because they follow different courses. For example, we have very many patients with analgesic nephropathy with a creatinine level of 3, but only 8 or 9% of our end-stage renal population are due to this disease. But I certainly would confess that until I tumbled to the significance of this glomerular lesion, we had previously diagnosed quite a few of our patients with RN as glomerular nephritis. And it was only when we looked at their kidneys that I perceived our mistake. We then found that what we thought was glomerular nephritis was, in fact, RN. You can certainly mistake RN for glomerular nephritis on a biopsy.

Dr. *J. Winberg*: So what you are intimating is that with any child with chronic renal insufficiency one has to perform an IVU and MCU to be quite sure that it is not RN, whatever kind of symptomatology the child shows.

Dr. *P. Kincaid-Smith*: I can only say that in an adult we would always do that to pinpoint the diagnosis as clearly as we can. If the function is too bad to show up in the IVU, we even carried out arteriography with some patients to find out what is wrong with them.

Dr. *R. Weiss*: Does anyone know what the positions and configuration of ureteric orifices are in adults that you think have, or have had, VUR? In other words, in patients who present with renal failure and bilateral scarred kidneys in the 20- to 30-year age group, and in whom a MCU is negative for VUR, is it worth looking at the ureteral orifices in order to get further evidence as to etiology?

Dr. *R. Bailey*: Yes. *Heale*, when he was in Christchurch, and Vermillion studied this very point in a large series of adult patients (about 170) which they published in the *Journal of Urology* [*109*: 571, 1973]. The abnormal appearances of the ureteric orifice remained throughout adult life. Even though the VUR may have stopped, the configuration and abnormality were still there. The study showed excellent correlation with the renal damage.

Dr. *P. Kincaid-Smith*: In a much smaller study we have not been able to confirm these results nearly as clearly.

Dr. *R. White*: To go back to the aetiology of chronic renal failure in childhood, certainly RN figures fairly prominently in our own series of chronic renal failures. I also agree that one can be easily misled into believing that the child has some sort of glomerular nephritis. Unless one follows the patient from an identifiable acute nephritic illness in the beginning into chronic renal failure one cannot be certain. And so I consider that a MCU must be an essential investigative procedure in all cases of chronic renal failure in children.

Dr. *J. Winberg*: Unless you have a biopsy which identifies it as a well-known type of glomerular nephritis.

Dr. *R. White*: I remember at least 2 children in whom we saw what we called focal glomerular sclerosis on biopsy, but in whom we found VUR as well.

Dr. *W. Asscher*: One slight note of caution. In order to assess whether or not the cause of kidney failure in a patient already on a dialysis program might have been RN, one must take into account the observations of *Torres* et al. [The progression of vesicoureteral reflux nephropathy. Ann. intern. Med. *92*: 776–784] who showed that some patients who entered the dialysis program with undoubted glomerular nephritis later were shown to reflux on MCU. This was brought up in the Bermuda meeting; it may occur, it is said, in any condition in which the urine flow rate is greatly diminished, as is the case in many dialysis patients, and has nothing to do with the etiology of the end-stage renal failure.

Dr. *W. Asscher*: Dr. *Kincaid-Smith* made a great point about the functional deterioration in pregnancy. Is this any worse than for glomerular nephritis?

Dr. *P. Kincaid-Smith*: No. I think it relates to the initial degree of impairment of renal function. As you know, by no means everyone agrees with us about this. *Katz* et al. published a series of 150 patients and, although in fact 3 or 4 of their patients with initially impaired renal function did deteriorate, during pregnancy, they really made a big point about the good prognosis of the remainder [*Katz* et al.: Pregnancy in women with kidney disease. Kidney int. *18*: 192–206, 1980].

But it has been our invariable experience with patients who have impaired renal function – be it from glomerulonephritis, or RN, or analgesic disease – that they all deteriorate during pregnancy. They commonly have tiny little kidneys.

Dr. *P. Ransley*: The data that we have heard this morning are entirely consistent with the aetiology of the renal disease being either renal dysplasia; an unrecognized 'big bang' early in infancy; continuing sterile VUR damage, or continuing asymptomatic bacteriuric damage. There has been nothing which points to any one single pattern in the pathogenesis; perhaps they are in fact several different patterns.

I personally believe that the nephron hyperperfusion story does play a big part in many of these children at puberty. And of course Dr. *Kincaid-Smith*'s finding of disease, in what pyelographically appears an almost normal kidney on one side, is a very worrying one. I'd like to hear from her what part hypertension played in the lesions in these 'good' kidneys, and the possible contribution untreated hypertension toward the production of the glomerular appearances she were describing.

Dr. *P. Kincaid-Smith*: We could certainly exclude hypertension as a significant causative factor in this diffuse type of damage. Malignant hypertension can cause a segmental glomerular lesion. I would say fairly categorically that it doesn't produce anything that in any way resembles the series of changes I described earlier.

Dr. *R.Risdon*: I would agree. As to how much loss of renal mass is required before glomerulopathy commences, there was a paper in *Laboratory Investigation* [*Kiprov* et al.: Focal and segmental glomerulosclerosis and proteinuria associated with unilateral renal agenesis. Lab. Invest. *46*: 275, 1982] where there was a long follow-up of people with unilateral renal agenesis to see what their long-term prognosis was. A very small proportion of them developed renal failure.

Dr. *W.Asscher*: On the same theme, in *Kidney International* [Nephrology, suppl. 2, 528–534, 1982] there was also a follow-up of kidney donors and people who have had nephrectomies, from about 1 to 18 years of age and not a single instance of this glomerular lesion was encountered.

Dr. *K. Verrier-Jones*: If one looks at proteinuria in schoolgirls with covert UTI, it tends to be elevated in those with RN, whether the RN is unilateral or bilateral. The degree of proteinuria is not great, perhaps about 300 mg a day would be the mean. But this is definitely higher than in the controls, who never had UTI. I would like to ask Dr. *Kincaid-Smith* whether she thinks these girls have a bad prognosis? It amounts to a very small amount of proteinuria, but is definitely elevated above the normal.

Dr. *P. Kincaid-Smith*: You certainly can't say all cases with proteinuria are at risk. But one can say that it is very unlikely for anybody to have a bad prognosis who has not got proteinuria. As you saw from my graphs, the higher the proteinuria the worse the prognosis. Certainly there may be a worse prognosis in your cases. There is about a 50% risk of a bad one in those with proteinuria.

Dr. *R. Bailey*: I would say that about 25–30% of cases have a significant proteinuria and a bad prognosis, whether one or both kidneys are affected. As regards hypertension, there is nothing to be done for those whose renal state is deteriorating, other than to treat the hypertension aggressively, when there may even be some improvement in renal function.

Another facet is the question of oral contraceptives and their well-known association with severe hypertension in such cases. I advise against this form of contraception. I don't forbid them, but the patients go to the family planning clinic and get vigorous contraceptive advice. We have had some 30 cases who have become severely hypertensive 'on the pill', although this state can usually be reversed.

As regards saralasin, we have found its response to be non-specific, whereas captopril appears to have a greater effect on cases of RN than in other forms of hypertension.

Dr. *M. Dillon*: Our own conclusion so far is that a dramatic response to captopril is of some significance with regard to the choice of treatment.

Dr. *K. Verrier-Jones*: The contraceptive pill is obviously a very relevant issue to most young women these days. I consider that if one denies it to the young woman who has VUR and some renal scarring, there will be an increase in the number of unwanted pregnancies, which can have such a seriously deleterious effect in this disease. In my group of patients, some 20 or 30 girls have been taking oral contraceptives for 3 years or so. So far none has deteriorated medically.

Dr. *R. Weiss*: Dr. *Bailey*, were your patients matched in terms of duration of hypertension prior to randomization for conservative therapy versus nephrectomy.

Dr. *R. Bailey*: No.

Dr. *R. Weiss*: Then do you have any data regarding the duration of their hypertension?

Dr. *R. Bailey*: I have it, but not here. They were all in good health and most of them were found to be hypertensive on clinical examination. So they had a very short, if any, history. They were mainly fresh patients coming to us.

Dr. *R. Weiss*: And did you have any biopsy or material from the contralateral, supposedly normal, kidney to see if there were any arteriolar lesions in it?

Dr. *R. Bailey*: No biopsies were done on the normal side. One thing I didn't mention was that one of the essential things in the protocol was a total GFR of over 70 ml/min.

Dr. *M. Dillon*: The failure of nephrectomy to relieve hypertension associated with unilateral RN focuses attention on the means of excluding disease in the 'good' kidney. I would have thought that a case might then be made for renal segmental vein renin sampling in order not to miss a localized origin of renin production. Also, did radionuclide scans show up any abnormalities at the time of the initial workup or later?

Dr. *R. Bailey*: Following our earlier study published in the *Journal of Urology* [*Bailey* et al.: Renal vein renin concentration in the hypertension of reflux nephropathy. J. Urol. *120*: 21, 1978], we lost some enthusiasm for renal vein renin estimations. In our adult population, it didn't seem to be helping us at all. One of the main problems was sampling the tiny scarred opposite kidney and at the moment we have given up this approach. The radiologic studies I mentioned were mainly radionuclide micturating cystograms. We do dimercaptosuccinic acid (DMSA) scans, but not routinely on entry into the protocol, as we have very good radiology.

Dr. *P. Kincaid-Smith*: What did you actually measure? Was it concentration of renin in the veins?

Dr. *R. Bailey*: Originally just the standard test, renal vein renin estimations from each side.

Dr. *P. Kincaid-Smith*: But it was the actual renin concentration that you measured.

Dr. *R. Bailey*: Plus renin activity measured by generated angiotensin I. The thing we do is to measure the renin secretion rate, not the concentration, because renal blood flow is so low.

Dr. *W. Asscher*: That is when you are talking about kidneys with GFRs of less than 10%.

Dr. *R. Bailey*: Quite right.

Dr. *M. Dillon*: The point I'm making is that the critical thing in your study is what the other kidney is doing, and what you are looking for is some pathology on the side where you've got good blood flow. So I think segmental renal vein sampling and a DMSA scan on that side are the things you ought to do.

Dr. *R. Bailey*: The good kidney showed suppression by the criteria that you use. Deep down, my personal opinion is that the renin-angiotensin system has absolutely nothing to do with the hypertension of RN. We have spent a decade wasting our time. That's what I think.

Dr. *M. Dillon*: If that is your argument for the case you are making, I don't think that it is an acceptable one.

Dr. *J. Hodson*: Some of our pigs with sterile scarring are hypertensive, and they are responding dramatically to captopril. Unfortunately the control pigs also show a small, much less dramatic response. We also have supporting evidence of a rise in peripheral renin levels in these pigs as the hypertension develops. The study is not yet finished, and we have not yet published our results. Another observation we have made is that over periods of months the pressure levels vary without treatment and on a regular diet. I wonder if this mimics the clinical picture.

Dr. *M. Dillon*: I think that we will see hypertension from scarred zones in kidneys seemingly resolving by itself, and that after some treatment children can be taken off therapy.

Dr. *W. Asscher:* I don't think you can conclude just because the high pressure responds to captopril that it is a renin-originated hypertension.

Dr. *P. Kincaid-Smith*: I agree. I think as yet this question is unresolved. There is no doubt on the histological side that you can see big positive granules in the sorts of cells that should be making renin in these pigs, whether or not you can measure it in veins. But the final answer is something that is going to need more refined techniques.

Contr. Nephrol., vol. 39, pp. 146–151 (Karger, Basel 1984)

13. Long-Term Follow-Up of Infants with Gross Vesico-Ureteric Reflux

Ross R. Bailey

Head of the Department of Nephrology, Christchurch Hospital, Christchurch, New Zealand

Introduction

Early reports from this institution demonstrated that the majority of those infants who presented under the age of 1 year with gross vesico-ureteric reflux (VUR) already had renal damage at the time of presentation, or were observed to develop renal scarring (reflux nephropathy, RN) during the first few years of life [1–4].

This study reports the long-term follow-up of 31 infants with gross VUR. These 31 infants were diagnosed in the paediatric unit between 1952 and 1970. Prior to 1970 infants with VUR were treated with prophylactic antibacterial therapy and were rarely subjected to ureteric reimplantation unless there was radiologic evidence of renal damage. Analysis of this early experience formulated the more recent urologic practice of reimplanting all ureters with gross VUR at the time of diagnosis [5].

The patients have been subdivided into 3 groups as follows: 1. Those still under regular supervision. 2. Those now lost to regular follow-up. 3. Those who have died.

Results

31 infants (16 boys; 15 girls) with a total of 44 grossly refluxing ureters (18 unilateral; 13 bilateral) were included in the study (table I). 9 of the 18 infants with unilateral gross VUR had moderate (7) or slight (2) VUR on the other side. Infants with obstructive uropathy were excluded. The mean age at presentation was 15.3 weeks (boys 11.3 weeks; girls 19.5 weeks). 24

of the 31 infants had a urinary tract infection (UTI) at the time of presentation. Many were ill at the time of presentation and had failed to thrive. In 12 of the 26 in whom RN was eventually documented, it was already present when they were first investigated at 4–48 weeks of life (mean 20.2 weeks).

5 infants died within the first year of life – in 3 this was due to sepsis following reconstructive surgery, 1 had only a single kidney which was severely damaged and the other multiple congenital abnormalities. Of the remaining 26 infants, 7 were followed for varying periods before they left the area and were lost to follow-up. The remaining 19 have been under regular follow-up in this department of 12–30.5 years (mean 16.9 years). Of these 19 patients, 4 appear to have normal kidneys. 5 developed bilateral RN, and 2 of these have a glomerular filtration rate (GFR) of <70 ml/min. The remaining 10 patients have unilateral RN, with a mildly elevated blood pressure for their age; 2 a GFR of <70 ml/min; 1 proteinuria alone, and 1 mild hypertension, proteinuria and a GFR of 67 ml/min (table I). 12 of these 19 patients subsequently had reconstructive surgery, and in 11 of these 12 it was undertaken after RN had been demonstrated radiologically.

Conclusion

This study has demonstrated that almost one half of those infants diagnosed as having gross VUR in their first year of life already had RN at the time of presentation. Of the 14 patients who later developed RN all did so within 5 years and usually within 3 years of birth. Clearly the damage resulting from gross VUR develops very early in life. In addition, those children with advanced disease may not survive the infantile period, as was demonstrated in this study. With the improved paediatric intensive care facilities which are now available 3 of these 5 children might have survived.

After gross VUR has been surgically corrected the major risks to the patient are the development of hypertension or complicating glomerulopathy. The marker for the latter is proteinuria, which is now present in 2 of the 19 patients still under follow-up. There are 4 patients whose blood pressure is now elevated for their age. 2 of these are women who will almost certainly have a sharp rise in blood pressure when they become pregnant. The 6 patients with a GFR of <70 ml/min reflect an overall reduction in functioning renal mass. None has yet developed a progressive reduc-

Table I. Clinical and radiologic data and current status of all patients

No.	Sex	Age at presentation weeks	Clinical presentation	Side of gross VUR	Age when definite renal damage first first noted	Age of surgery	Duration of follow-up, years	Current status
A								
1	F	35	UTI, vomiting	R + L	24 months	8 years	30.5	L > R RN, GFR 105 ml/min
2	F	10	F	R + L	41 months	14 months	22.5	L > R RN, GFR 70 ml/min
3	M	21	UTI	R + L	17 months	6, 29 months	22.5	L > R RN, ileal conduit, GFR 51 ml/min
4	M	6	vomiting	L	normal	NS	19	normal IVU, GFR 134 ml/min
5	M	6	UTI, F	L	25 months	NS	18.5	L RN, GFR 99 ml/min, 120/85
6	F	10 days	Single umbilical artery	L	60 months	NS	18	L RN, GFR 109 ml/min
7	M	3	UTI, F	R	14 months	NS	17.5	R RN, 144/96, GFR 96 ml/min
8	F	18	UTI, vomiting	L	11 months	13 months, 5 years	16.5	L RN, GFR 67 ml/min, proteinuria, 125/80
9	F	17	UTI, vomiting	L	4 months	9 months	16	L RN, enuretic, GFR 60 ml/min
10	F	7	UTI, F	L	28 months	NS	15.5	L RN, GFR 97 ml/min
11	F	12	UTI, F	R + L	42 months	4 years	15.5	L RN, proteinuria, GFR 102 ml/min
12	F	43	UTI	R	21 months	22 months	14.5	R RN, GFR 110 ml/min, 125/80
13	M	3	F	R + L	13 weeks	1 years	14.5	L > R RN, GFR 45 ml/min
14	M	7	UTI, F	R + L	7 weeks	11 weeks, 30 months	14.5	R > L RN, GFR 79 ml/min
15	M	4	UTI, F	L	20 months	3.5, 12 years	14	L RN (single kidney), GFR 59 ml/min
16	M	41	UTI, F	L	10 months	10, 34 months	13.5	L RN, GFR 137 ml/min
17	F	26	UTI	L	normal	1 years	13	normal IVU, GFR 130 ml/min
18	M	4	UTI, F	R + L	normal	NS	12.5	normal IVU, GFR 117 ml/min
19	M	6 days	UTI, vomiting	R	normal	NS	12	normal IVU, GFR 126 ml/min

B								
20	M	23	UTI	R + L	5 months	8 months	10.75	L Nx, R hemi-Nx, lost to follow-up when GFR 69 ml/min
21	F	20	F	R	29 months	30 months	10	R RN, lost to follow-up
22	M	11	UTI, F	L	19 months	26 months	9	L RN, GFR 60 ml/min
23	M	7	UTI, diarrhoea	L	7 weeks	11 weeks, 25 months	2.5	L RN, lost to follow-up
24	F	4	UTI, F	R	4 weeks	1 month, 1 years	1	R Nx, lost to follow-up
25	F	42	UTI	R + L	42 weeks	NS	42 weeks	R > L RN, lost to follow-up
26	F	1 day	control	R + L	normal	NS	5 days	lost to follow-up
C								
27	F	48	UTI, F	R + L	11 months	11 months	11 months	died aged 11 months after ileal loop
28	F	9	D-trisomy	R	9 weeks	NS	8 months	died aged 8 months
29	M	23	UTI	R + L	5 months	6 months	6 months	died 4 days after bilateral re implantation
30	M	17	UTI, F	R	4 months	NS	4 months	died aged 4 months, absent L kidney, R RN
31	M	4	UTI, F	R + L	4 weeks	9 weeks	9 weeks	died 6 days after ileal loop aged 9 weeks, L > R RN

F = Failure to thrive; NS = no surgery; Nx = nephrectomy; GFR = glomerular filtration rate either measured by ^{51}Cr-EDTA clearance or assessed by Cockcroft and Gault formula [6]; IVU = intravenous urogram.

Table II. Clinical details on children (< 16 years) presenting with end-stage reflux nephropathy

No.	Sex	Age at presentation	Clinical presentation	Time from diagnosis of renal disease to dialysis; months
1	M	13	hospitalized following an accident and found to have renal failure	19
2	F	9	hypertensive encephalopathy, renal failure	1
3	M	6	measles, failure to thrive	26
4	F	12	malignant hypertension, renal failure	2
5	M	7	family investigation	89
6	M	13	anemia, uraemic symptoms	<1

tion in GFR. There are no more than 1 or 2 of the 19 patients still under follow-up who appear likely to develop chronic renal failure.

As a comparison, 6 children under the age of 16 years have reached end-stage RN and entered our dialysis-transplant programme during the last 8 years of this follow-up period (table II) [7]. None of these 6 children presented in the infantile period, presumably they were not fortunate enough to develop a complicating UTI to bring them to clinical attention.

Although 12 of the 19 patients still under follow-up underwent ureteric reimplantation, this was not done in 11 of them until RN had been detected. It is impossible to conclude whether this late surgery has been in any way beneficial to the growing kidneys and prevented progressive RN.

It can be concluded that infants who present within the first year of life with UTI as a marker of gross VUR will ultimately do well, as long as there has not been severe RN by the time of presentation. The problem with end-stage RN is that these patients do not come to clinical attention until irreversible RN has already occurred. If this important cause of hypertension and chronic renal failure is going to be eliminated, then gross VUR must be detected very soon after birth and corrected surgically.

References

1 Rolleston, G.L.; Shannon, F.T.; Utley, W.L.F.: Relationship of infantile vesicoureteric reflux to renal damage. Br. med. J. *i*: 460 (1970).

2 Rolleston, G.L.; Shannon, F.T.; Utley, W.L.F.: Follow-up of vesico-ureteric reflux in the newborn. Kidney int. *8*: S59(1975).
3 Rolleston, G.L.; Maling, T.M.J.; Hodson, C.J.: Intrarenal reflux and the scarred kidney. Archs Dis. Childh. *49*: 531 (1974).
4 Bailey, R.R.: The relationship of vesico-ureteric reflux to urinary tract infection and chronic pyelonephritis – reflux nephropathy. Clin. Nephrol. *1*: 132 (1973).
5 McRae, C.U.; Shannon, F.T.; Utley, W.L.F.: Effect on renal growth of reimplantation of refluxing ureters. Lancet *i*: 1310 (1974).
6 Charleson, H.; Bailey, R.R.; Stewart, A.: Quick prediction of creatinine clearance without the necessity of urine collection. N.Z. med. J. *92*: 425 (1980).
7 King, S.Y.; Buttimore, A.; Lynn, K.L.; Bailey, R.R.: Active treatment of children with end-stage renal failure. N.Z. med. J. *95 (719)*: 763–766 (1982).

Ross R. Bailey, MD, Department of Nephrology, Christchurch Hospital, Christchurch (New Zealand)

Contr. Nephrol., vol. 39, pp. 152–163 (Karger, Basel 1984)

14. Renal Functional Changes in Schoolgirls with Covert Asymptomatic Bacteriuria

Kate Verrier Jones, William Asscher, Roger Verrier Jones, Kevin Mattholie, Kenneth Leach, Mair Thompson

Departments of Renal Medicine, Child Health and Medical Physics at the Royal Infirmary and University Hospital of Wales, Cardiff, Wales

Introduction

'Chronic pyelonephritis' (reflux nephropathy, RN) is an important cause of end-stage kidney failure in children [8, 17], and its close association with vesico-ureteric reflux (VUR) has been observed repeatedly [4, 10, 12, 14, 16, 18]. Not surprisingly considerable time and effort has been expended on eradicating urinary tract infection (UTI) and correcting VUR in an attempt to prevent the associated kidney damage. Most of this damage develops before the age of 4 years [1]; in prospective studies of schoolgirls over 4 RN rarely occurs in kidneys which are normal at the outset, even when VUR is present and UTI is left untreated [6, 15]. This suggests that treatment may not be necessary in girls over 4 in whom the kidneys are radiologically normal.

Little is known about the effect of VUR and UTI on renal function and before a policy of non-treatment is advocated it seems prudent to evaluate their effects on the glomerular filtration rate (GFR). We report such a study.

Subjects and Methods – Part 1

Study Population, Follow-Up, and Treatment

In 1971, 89.3% of all schoolgirls between the ages of 4 and 11 years (n = 13,369) in the City of Cardiff, Wales, were screened for UTI by means of a mobile laboratory [3]. In 207 girls (1.7%) covert UTI was identified. All 207 were allocated at random to a treatment or control group. The treatment group received short (mostly 7-day) courses of antimicrobial agents whenever colony counts exceeded 10^8 colony-forming units (CFU)/l. Treatment was

Table I. Distribution of RN and VUR in 96 kidneys from 48 girls with covert UTI (grade of VUR given in parentheses)

Radiological Findings	VUR	No VUR	Total
Scarred kidneys	(1) 2 11 (2) 3 (3) 6	9	20
Normal kidneys	(1) 5 24 (2) 13 (3) 6	52	76
Total	(1) 7 35 (2) 16 (3) 12	61	96

selected on the basis of multi-disk sensitivity of the urinary isolates. During the initial 4-year follow-up, each girl was seen 4–6 times a year, and subsequently they attended the clinic at least once a year.

Radiological Investigations

When first seen, during 1971 and 1972, excretion urography (intravenous urography, IVU) and micturating cysto-urography (MCU) were carried out on all 207 girls. These investigations were repeated in 1975 and 1976 after a follow-up period of 4 years [5]. In 1979, 120 of the 207 girls, then aged 12–19, were still attending the clinic. Consent to measure GFR was obtained from 60, and in 48 this was done. Table I gives the original radiological findings in these 48 girls; 18 had RN, and in 2 the condition was bilateral. VUR was detected in 25 individuals, among whom 35 kidneys were drained by refluxing ureters; in 11 cases VUR was associated with RN. VUR was graded 1–3 as recommended by the British Medical Research Council Bacteriuria Committee [13]. Where the two original investigations had shown different grades of VUR the more severe one was used for analysis.

Measurement of Glomerular Filtration Rate

Girls were asked to keep to a normal fluid intake on the morning of the investigation and were given a 300-ml drink shortly before the study. They were then positioned over the gamma camera so that both kidneys could be visualized, and technetium-labelled stannous DTPA (^{99m}TC-DPTA) was administered by rapid intravenous injection. The dose was adjusted according to the weight of the subject [10 MBq (0.27 mCi) plus 1.5 MBq (0.04 mCi)/kg], and the study continued for 30 min from the time of injection. Blood samples were taken 2, 3 and 4 minutes after injection for estimation of GFR [9]. The percentage contribution from each kidney was assessed from the relative uptake over the first 3 min of the study [11]. All values obtained were corrected for surface area and expressed per 1.73 m^2.

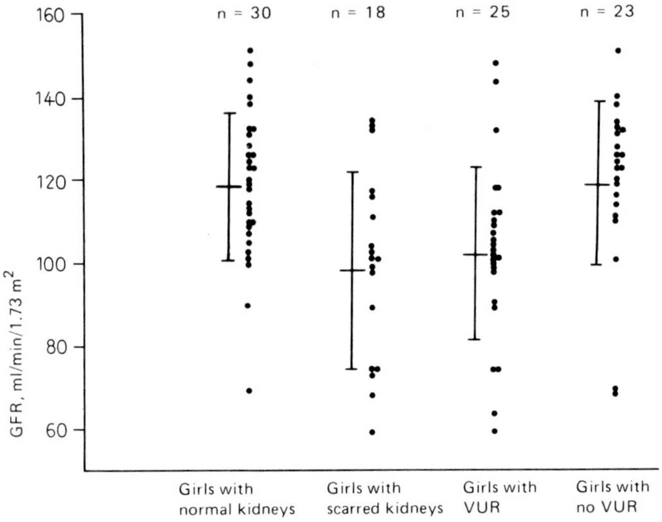

Fig. 1. GFRs in 48 girls with covert UTI. Bars denote mean ± SD.

Bacteriological Methods

At each clinic visit a midstream urine specimen was collected after perineal washing with green soap solution and cultured on dipslides. Identification of organisms was carried out by standard techniques [7], and the sensitivity of the isolates to antimicrobials was determined by the disc-diffusion method. All subjects were also sent dipslides for further urine culture at 2-month intervals. Of the 48 girls studied, 22 returned these slides regularly, 12 returned them occasionally, and 14 never returned them. Bacteriuria was regarded as significant if there was a pure growth of $> 10^8$ CFU/l. If the specimen showed a mixed growth, a further dipslide was sent and significant bacteriuria considered to be present only if that dipslide showed a pure growth of $> 10^8$ CFU/l. The mean number of cultures obtained from each girl over the 7 years of follow-up was 30 (range 16–50). The amount of UTI experienced by each girl was calculated from the number of infected specimens divided by the total number, and this was expressed as a percentage. Statistical analyses were performed with Student's t-test, p value of < 0.05 being regarded as significant.

Results in Part 1

GFRs are expressed in ml/min/1.73 m^2. Mean values are expressed ± SD. The mean GFR for the whole group was 112 ± 22. Figure 1 shows the rates in girls with normal and those with scarred kidneys, and in those with refluxing and non-refluxing ureters. The mean rate in girls with scarred kidneys (99 ± 24) was significantly reduced ($0.005 > p > 0.002$) compared with those with normal kidneys (119 ± 18). In the 25 girls with VUR the

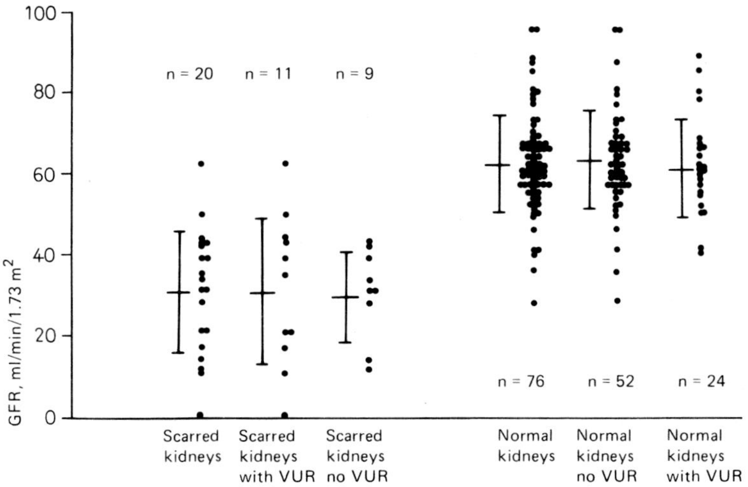

Fig. 2. GFRs from 96 single kidneys of 48 girls with covert UTI. Bars denote mean ± SD.

mean GFR (103 ± 21) was reduced compared with the 23 in whom no VUR was present (120 ± 20); this difference was significant ($0.01 > p > 0.005$). Only 1 of the subjects with normal kidneys had a GFR of less than 90, compared with 5 of the 23 girls with renal scarring.

Figure 2 gives the GFR of individual kidneys. The mean in scarred kidneys was 31 ± 15 as compared with 62 ± 12 in normal ones; this difference was highly significant ($0.001 > p > 0.0005$). The presence of VUR did not influence the GFR in either scarred or unscarred kidneys. The mean in 11 scarred kidneys with VUR was 31 ± 18 and in 9 scarred kidneys without VUR 30 ± 11. Likewise, the GFR of normal kidneys with VUR (61 ± 12) was not significantly different from those with no VUR (63 ± 12). Figure 3 shows the GFR of normal kidneys related to the grades of VUR present. Kidneys drained by ureters with grade 1 VUR had a mean GFR of 59 ± 5, and this was not significantly different from those with grade 2 (63 ± 15) or grade 3 VUR (58 ± 8). In 8 girls with normal kidneys and unilateral VUR the mean GFR was 57 ± 8 on the side with, and 56 ± 12 on the one without, VUR.

Tables II and III summarize the effect of duration of UTI over the 7 years of follow-up. GFR was not significantly affected by either the duration of UTI, or the presence or absence of VUR in either normal or scarred kidneys.

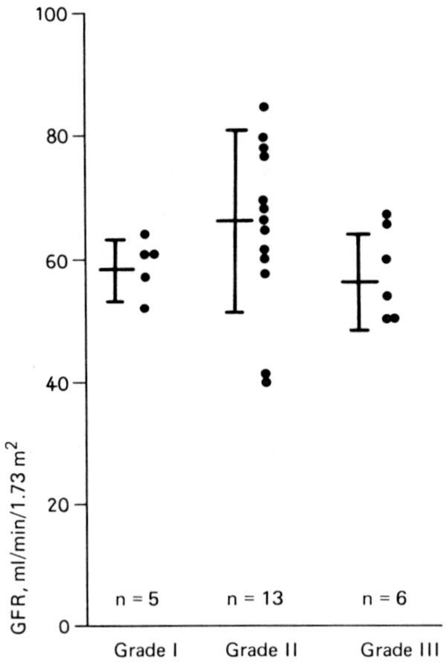

Fig. 3. Effect of grade of VUR on GFR in 24 unscarred kidneys of girls with covert UTI. Bars denote mean ± SD.

Table II. Effect of percentage of infected urine samples and VUR on GFR in 76 radiologically normal kidneys

% infected specimens during 7-year follow-up period	Normal kidneys with VUR: GFR, ml/min/1.73 m^2		Normal kidneys with no VUR: GFR, ml/min/1.73 m^2	
	mean (± SD)	number	mean (± SD)	number
0–20	52	1	57 (± 17)	10
21–40	72 (± 19)	3	64 (± 5)	12
41–60	58 (± 18)	6	60 (± 6)	11
61–80	58 (± 5)	7	65 (± 16)	10
81–100	66 (± 7)	7	67 (± 14)	9

Table III. Effect of percentage of infected urine samples and VUR on GFR in 20 kidneys with radiological scarring

% infected specimens during 7-year follow-up period	Scarred kidneys with VUR: GFR, ml/min/1.73 m^2		Scarred kidneys with no VUR: GFR, ml/min/1.73 m^2	
	mean (± SD)	number	mean (± SD)	number
0–20	–	0	39	1
21–40	31 (± 16)	3	13	2
41–60	33 (± 19)	3	37	2
61–80	30 (± 27)	4	34	1
81–100	35	1	34 (± 8)	3

Table IV shows the GFR in the treated and untreated groups of girls. Treatment reduced the duration of covert UTI but had no effect on GFR. The mean GFR of 'normal' kidneys opposite scarred ones (72 ± 15) in 16 girls with unilateral RN (fig. 4) was significantly greater than that of individual kidneys in girls without RN (60 ± 12), thus confirming that compensatory hypertrophy of 'opposite' kidneys had occurred ($0.01 > p > 0.005$). 8 of these 'opposite' kidneys had been exposed to VUR and the mean GFR (71 ± 12) was not significantly lower than that of the opposite kidneys which had not been so exposed (74 ± 18). Similarly the duration of UTI did not influence the GFR of these opposite kidneys.

5 girls with RN had abnormally low GFRs (below 80). 2, both with a total GFR of 74, had bilateral RN. The 3 others (total GFRs 59, 63 and 68) had unilateral RN; the GFRs in their 'opposite' kidneys were 52, 56 and 59 (i.e. all well below the mean for all opposite kidneys); 1 of which was drained by a refluxing ureter. 2 of them were in the treatment group and had a high proportion of infected urine samples (56 and 64%). The third, who was in the control group, had UTI in 34% of samples, but no documented UTI during the 3 years before estimation of her GFR. 2 also had proteinuria exceeding 300 mg/24 h; all 3 were normotensive.

Table IV. Effect of treatment on GFR in 48 girls with covert UTI

	Control group			Treatment group		
	GFR ml/min/1.73 m^2	% infected urine samples		GFR ml/min/1.73 m^2	% infected urine samples	
	mean (± SD)	mean (± SD)	number	mean (± SD)	mean (± SD)	number
All girls (n = 48)	113 (± 21)	69 (± 22)	21	109 (± 24)	41 (± 22)	27
Girls with scarring (n = 18)	104 (± 19)	75 (± 18)	9	93 (± 28) 99 (± 30)	42 (± 15) 42 (± 16)	9 7
Girls with normal kidneys (n = 30)	123 (± 18)	66 (± 24)	12	116 (± 17)	40 (± 25)	18

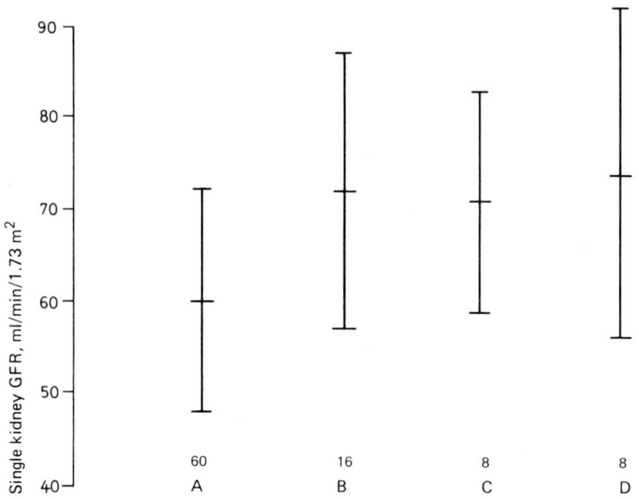

Fig. 4. GFRs in individual normal kidneys. A = Opposite other normal kidneys. B = Opposite scarred kidneys. C = Opposite scarred kidneys with VUR. D = Opposite scarred kidneys without VUR. Numbers indicate size of group. Bars denote mean ± SD.

Table V. Radiological findings in 44 kidneys from 22 girls who underwent second DTPA study

Radiological Findings	VUR	No VUR	Total
Scarred kidneys	1 (0) 5–2 (2) 3 (3)	3	8
Normal kidneys	12	24	36
Total	17	27	44

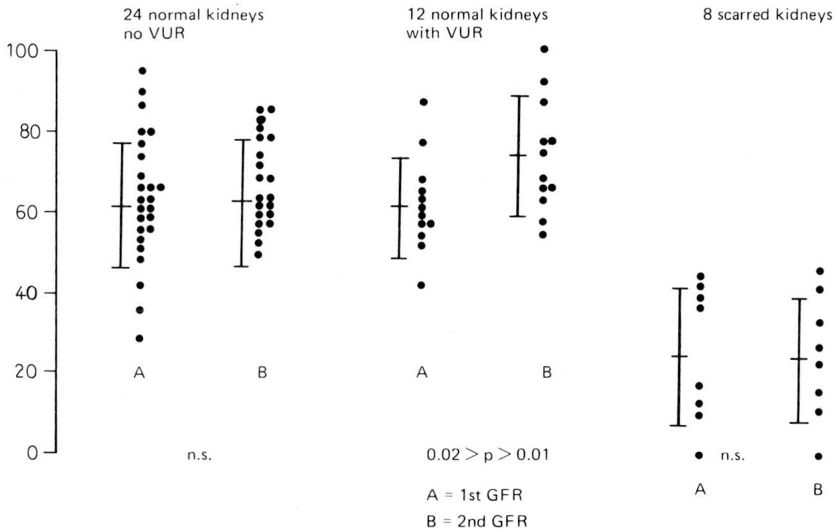

Fig. 5. GFR in 36 normal and 8 scarred kidneys before and after 2-year follow-up period.

Subjects and Methods – Part 2

22 girls underwent a second GFR estimation using the same technique. The mean time interval between the first and second studies was 26 months (range 22–29). 8 had unilateral RN; the remainder had normal kidneys. 12 of the latter and 3 of those with RN were associated with VUR (table V).

Results in Part 2

There was no change in the mean GFR for the 24 normal kidneys not associated with VUR (fig. 5). The mean GFR for 12 radiologically normal kidneys associated with VUR increased from 62 ± 12 to 72 ± 14 ml/min/

1.73 m^2. This was significant at the 2% level ($0.02 > p > 0.01$). The mean GFR for 8 scarred kidneys did not alter during the follow-up period (first GFR: 28 ± 15 ml/min/1.73 m^2, second GFR: 27 ± 17 ml/min/1.73 m^2).

Discussion

During the past decade there has been considerable interest in screening for covert UTI with a view to preventing kidney failure from RN. Although there is a clear association between UTI, VUR and RN, the role of the former two factors in producing kidney damage at different ages and in different clinical situations is not clear. While no one would argue the need to treat children with symptoms, the wisdom and practicality of providing effective long-term or intermittent treatment for symptomless, and usually less motivated, children and parents, are far from clear. It is therefore mandatory to define the relative importance of UTI and VUR in the pathogenesis of RN.

By measuring the clearance of ^{99m}Tc-DPTA, we have assessed the effects of UTI, VUR, and RN on the GFR both separately and in combination in these children. Whereas the total GFR for girls with scarred kidneys was reduced compared with those with normal kidneys, there was considerable overlap between the two groups. The GFR in individual kidneys with RN was reduced to about 50% of the normal mean. This emphasizes the serious effect of RN on renal function. However, when the total GFR of each pair of kidneys was considered, this effect was partially masked by compensatory hypertrophy of the contralateral kidney.

In this study MCU had been carried out 3–4 years before the determination of GFR, and in the intervening period VUR may have cleared spontaneously in some subjects. Nevertheless, our findings show that: (1) VUR of at least 4 years' duration did not influence the GFR in either scarred or normal kidneys; (2) that half of those showing compensatory hypertrophy had been subject to VUR for the same period; (3) that in normal kidneys exposed to grade 3 VUR (MRC grading, which is unlikely to disappear spontaneously), there was no reduction in GFR, and (4) that in cases where unilateral VUR was present in the absence of scarring there was no difference in GFR between the two sides.

Hence, VUR alone does not appear to influence GFR. The reduction in total GFR in individuals with VUR is therefore accounted for by the presence of RN in this group rather than the effects of VUR. If we assume that kidney function and growth are interrelated, our findings accord with the observations of *Smellie* et al. [19] who showed that kidney growth in children with symptomatic UTI treated by continuous antibiotic therapy was also not influenced by the presence or severity of VUR.

Aperia et al. [2] determined GFR in children with UTI using the clearance of inulin as a measure, and studying individual kidney function by using unilateral external ureteric compression to obtain urine samples from one side at a time. They found a reduced GFR in kidneys drained by grade 3 refluxing ureters, which became more marked with age. They did not, however, analyse the data with respect to renal scarring, which may well account for the discrepancy between their findings and ours. *Wikstad* et al. [20] described a reduction in the area of the renal parenchyma in kidneys drained by grade 3 refluxing ureters in children aged 4 months to 13 years. 5 of their 8 children developed scarring during the 4 years of observation, and in 2 others a relative decrease in kidney size was thought to be due to a failure of kidney growth. The high incidence of progressive scarring in that study may have been related to the younger age of their patients compared with ours for UTI and VUR in combination are known to be most damaging to the kidneys before the age of 4.

In our study prolonged UTI was not associated with a reduction of GFR in girls after age 4 and no benefit from intermittent antibiotic treatment was shown. In those with scarred kidneys, who might have been expected to show progressive renal damage, there was no difference in function between kidneys exposed to severe VUR or prolonged UTI or both, and those not so exposed. Since we found no relation between the duration of UTI and GFR, it is not surprising that our treatment did not benefit kidney function. These results differ from those of *Smellie* et al. [19] who showed, in uncontrolled studies, that long-term prophylaxis of symptomatic UTIs benefitted kidney growth: This difference may be due to the fact that their children, unlike ours, had symptomatic UTIs, which are presumably caused by more virulent pathogens than those encountered in the asymptomatic variety. It is also possible that their continuous long-term treatment achieved better eradication of bacteria than the short courses we employed. It should be borne in mind, however, that long-term antibacterial prophylaxis of symptomless UTIs is unlikely to succeed since asymptomatic patients are usually less compliant with treatment than those with symptoms.

From our findings, therefore, it appears that treatment of covert UTI, whether for short or long periods, is unlikely to be beneficial, and that the incidence of end-stage kidney failure will be uninfluenced by screening for covert bacteriuria after the age of 5 years.

Acknowledgements

This study was supported by a project grant from the Medical Research Council to K.V.J., A.W.A., and E.R.V.J. We thank Mrs. *Lynne Court* and Mrs. *Ruth Mackenzie* for their help and Mrs. *Gaynor Jones* for secretarial work. Part of this article has been reproduced by kind permission of the editor of the *British Medical Journal.*

References

1 Anonymous: Covert bacteriuria – peril or partnership. Br. med. J. *i*: 1649–1650 (1978).
2 Aperia, A.; Broberger, O.; Ericsson, N.O.; Wikstad, I.: Effect of vesicoureteric reflux on renal function in children with recurrent urinary tract infection. Kidney int. *9*: 418–423 (1976).
3 Asscher, A.W.; McLachlan, M.S.F.; Verrier Jones, R.; Meller, S.; Sussman, M.; Harrison, S.; Johnston, H.H.; Sleight, G.; Fletcher, E.W.: Screening for asymptomatic bacteriuria. Lancet *ii*: 1–4 (1973).
4 Bailey, R.R.: The relationship of vesicoureteric reflux to urinary tract infection and chronic pyelonephritis – reflux nephropathy. Clin. Nephrol. *1*: 132–141 (1963).
5 Cardiff Oxford Bacteriuria Study Group: Sequelae of covert bacteriuria in schoolgirls. A four-year follow-up study. Lancet *i*: 889–894 (1978).
6 Cardiff Oxford Bacteriuria Study Group: Long-term effects of bacteriuria on the urinary tract in schoolgirls. Radiology *132*: 343–350 (1979).
7 Cowan, S.T.; Steel, K.J.: Manual for the identification of medical bacteria (Cambridge University Press, London 1965).
8 Habib, R.; Broyer, M.; Benmaiz, H.: Chronic renal failure in children. Causes, rate of deterioration and survival data. Nephron *11*: 209–220 (1973).
9 Hilson, A.J.W.; Mistry, R.D.; Maisey, M.N.: ^{99m}Tc-DTPA for the measurement of glomerular filtration rate. Br. J. Radiol. *49*: 794–796 (1976).
10 Hodson, C.J.: Natural history of chronic pyelonephritic scarring. Br. med. J. *ii*: 191–194 (1965).
11 Kainer, G.; McIlveen, B.; Hoschl, R.; Rosenberg, A.R.: Assessment of individual renal function in children using ^{99m}Tc-DTPA. Archs Dis. Childh. *54*: 931–936 (1979).
12 McLachlan, M.S.F.; Meller, S.T.; Verrier Jones, E.R.; Asscher, A.W.; Fletcher, E.W.; Mayon White, R.T.; Ledingham, J.G.G.; Smith, J.C.; Johnston, H.H.: Urinary tract in schoolgirls with covert bacteriuria. Archs Dis. Childh. *50*: 253–258 (1975).
13 British Medical Research Council Bacteriuria Committee: Recommended terminology of urinary tract infection. Br. med. J. *ii*: 717–719 (1979).
14 Newcastle Asymptomatic Bacteriuria Research Group: Asymptomatic bacteriuria in school children in Newcastle upon Tyne. Newcastle asymptomatic bacteriuria investigation. First report 1975. Archs Dis. Childh. *50*: 90–102 (1975).

15 Newcastle Covert Bacteriuria Research Group: Covert bacteriuria in schoolgirls in Newcastle upon Tyne. A five-year follow-up. Archs Dis. Childh. *56*: 585–592 (1981).
16 Savage, D.C.L.; Wilson, M.D.; Ross, E.M.; Fee, W.M.: Asymptomatic bacteriuria in girl entrants to Dundee primary schools. Br. med. J. *iii*: 75–80 (1969).
17 Scharer, K.; Brunner, F.P.; Dehn, H. van: Combined report on regular dialysis and transplantation in children in Europe. Proc. Eur. Dial. Transpl. Ass. *9*: LXII (1972).
18 Smellie, J.M.; Hodson, C.J.; Edwards, D.; Normand, I.C.S.: Radiological features of urinary infection in childhood. Br. med. J. *ii*: 1222–1226 (1964).
19 Smellie, J.M.; Edwards, D.; Normand, I.C.S.; Prescod, N.: Effects of vesicoureteral reflux on renal growth in children with urinary tract infection. Archs Dis. Childh. *56*: 593–600 (1981).
20 Wikstad, I.; Aperia, A.; Broberger, O.; Ekengren, K.: Vesicoureteral reflux and pyelonephritis. Long time effect on area of renal parenchyma. Acta radiol. (Diag.) *20*: 252–260 (1979).

Kate Verrier Jones, Departments of Renal Medicine, Child Health and Medical Physics at the Royal Infirmary and University Hospital of Wales, GB-Cardiff CF2 ISZ (Wales)

Contr. Nephrol., vol. 39, pp. 164–168 (Karger, Basel 1984)

Discussion on Chapters 13 and 14

Dr. *Richard White*: Dr. *Bailey*'s long-term follow-up is a marvellous study and shows us some important information. His figures show that about 50% of his total cases already had reflux nephropathy (RN) by the time he first saw them. This gets back again to the need to find a way of picking up vesicoureteric reflux (VUR) before the first urinary tract infection (UTI).

But I would like him to explain why 3 of the 10 patients that were followed for 30 years with unilateral RN, had a declining glomerular filtration rate (GFR)?

Dr. *R. Bailey*: 2 of them have a GFR of below 70 ml/min. They weren't declining. They were just lower. I can't explain that. We've been following them serially and there has been no change. The other kidney seems to be structurally normal. But both have a very small kidney on the side that is damaged. Neither have proteinuria. They are the residual from the group originally described by *Rolleston* et al. [Follow-up of vesico-ureteral reflux in the newborn. Kidney int. *8*: S59–S64, 1975]. They are the ones with gross VUR, though gross VUR detected in the first year of life by means of associated UTI is still a relatively uncommon condition, which explains why the registration for these trials is so slow. It is perhaps unfortunate that those who end up with end-stage renal failure are not from that group at all.

Dr. *M. Taylor*: Dr. *Bailey*, you have put a lot of emphasis on the possibility of sterile VUR giving rise to significant nephropathy, you say that 24 of the 31 patients had UTI at presentation. That leaves 7, some of whom you said had generalized illness, with jaundice and other symptoms compatible with acute pyelonephritis. I'm not quite clear about the exclusion of UTI in this remainder.

Dr. *R. Bailey*: It was excluded by suprapubic bladder aspiration for cultures – our hospital was the place where this technique was virtually invented. Dr. *Chatham* was doing it before anyone else, so far as I can ascertain, and certainly it was published very early on. So that they did suprapubic aspiration on these infants almost routinely and that's why so many patients with asymptomatic UTI's were detected. And that experience was followed by the prospective studies of suprapubic bladder aspiration on all neonates. So I think there was good evidence that UTI was being excluded, as 'bag' urine or voided urine specimens were never used.

Dr. *M. Taylor*: I'm not quite clear why you carried out the IVUs and cystograms if you hadn't diagnosed a UTI.

Dr. *R. Bailey*: I think if you go back to the original papers, you will find that 79% had UTI. The other 21% were investigated for a number of reasons. Family involvement, single umbilical arteries and other congenital anomalies.

Dr. *R. Weiss*: To return to the point that Dr. *White* mentioned about the 2 patients with the low GFRs. It is well known that when nephrons are lost early in life almost complete compensatory hypertrophy follows so that only one surviving kidney can act as two normal-sized ones, function-wise. I don't think that 60 or 70 ml/min represents adequate compensatory hypertrophy, considering that these babies had what was virtually a total loss of one kidney very early in life. I think that this might possibly be explained by the dysplasia theory, namely that the contralateral kidney, although it may appear normal, in fact does not have a complete complement of nephrons, and that there may be areas of dysplasia within it.

Dr. *P. Kincaid-Smith*: You could equally hypothesize that they had lost nephrons due to their gross VUR in infancy in the 'good' kidney in the absence of focal scarring, and that they are examples of the diffuse form of RN that I described earlier.

Dr. *R. Bailey*: Indeed, some of the infants with gross VUR on one side had slight or moderate degrees of it on the other. That I didn't discuss.

Dr. *P. Ransley*: Further to follow Dr. *White's* argument; Dr. *Bailey*, you first said that 50% of these babies already had RN at the outset. Then you made your case for progressive RN and suggested that the pyelographic changes represented progressive RN in response to continuing VUR and UTI. I would not accept that at all. I think that we are all agreed that the difficulties of defining renal parenchyma by intravenous urogram (IVU) in babies makes it very difficult to make any comment on the radiographs you showed us; the ones at 0 and 2 years. This is just the situation in which we hope the dimercaptosuccinic acid (DMSA) scan will prove to be more accurate, in spite of the problems of movement in babies we discussed earlier. I therefore don't believe that your case for progressive RN is substantiated, and that the incidence of RN at the beginning was probably much higher.

Dr. *P. Kincaid-Smith*: Dr. *Ransley*, I am not clear as to your present policy with regard to the surgery of VUR. You seemed to imply that if they still have VUR when they enter teenage that you may do surgery at that time. I would say, however, that most people who see a lot of teenagers and adults with VUR would consider there is no indication for surgery at that stage.

Dr. *P. Ransley*: I wrote in 1978 that I believed no child should leave childhood still refluxing. But I don't hold that view anymore, whether their kidneys are scarred or not, provided they can be kept free from UTI.

Dr. *R. Bailey*: What then are your criteria for surgery on VUR at any age.

Dr. *P. Ransley*: Mostly symptoms; I consider the persistence of symptoms is my prime reason for surgery.

Dr. *R. Bailey*: What symptoms?

Dr. *P. Ransley*: Either breakthrough UTI, or UTI occurring in spite of prophylaxis. I accept that the incidence of UTI is commonly unaltered by surgery. But the symptoms associated with those UTIs are not the same before and after surgery.

Dr. *P. Kincaid-Smith*: There was a controlled trial from the Stamford group a few years ago in which it was shown quite clearly that, although the rate of UTIs was the same in both groups, the rate of renal involvement as they defined it, which I am pretty sure was on symptoms, was higher in the non-operated group. I think that's the best data I know on this question, and my own experience in a few cases is similar.

Dr. *R. Bailey*: But providing the patient is, or can be, subjected to regular supervision UTI is now so easy to control that very few must come into the breakthrough group. I would never make UTI an indication for surgery in any patient at any age.

Dr. *R. White*: Our surgeons keep saying that the ones that are operated on lose their symptoms more quickly. In fact, as the follow-up is largely in the hands of non-surgeons now, this can only be an impression, and one I don't share.

Dr. *P. Kincaid-Smith*: Let's hope the present long-term studies will provide that answer. The most fascinating thing to me about this and other studies in schoolgirls with asymptomatic UTI is how benign the prognosis is when they are followed up in this sort of way. It gets away from the idea we have had for many years, namely that all the 'action' in this matter of RN is in childhood. I am not quite clear whether one or both groups were being treated during the follow-up period.

Dr. *K. Verrier Jones*: The control groups was completely untreated in the first 4 years of the follow-up. The only indications for giving the treatment were if they had fever and loin pain. I think I'm right in saying only 1 patient was so treated.

After the first 4 years of follow-up, when I first became involved, I tried to carry on with the short courses of antibiotics, since that was the type of treatment these girls expected. So they still fell into two groups. But a small number of girls in the control group have subsequently developed backaches, or dysuria; problems of that nature, and when they have asked me for treatment I haven't withheld it.

Dr. *W. Asscher*: But the control group were kept off treatment as far as possible, isn't that right?

Dr. *K. Verrier Jones*: Yes. Except for the few that developed symptoms, but this really amounted to very inadequate treatment.

Dr. *P. Kincaid-Smith*: And the other group was on continuous prophylaxis?

Dr. *K. Verrier Jones*: No, no one was on continuous prophylaxis.

Dr. *W. Asscher*: The contrast between the two groups is, in fact, not very distinct. Initially it wasn't very distinct, and it is even less so now. As you noticed from the figure, 70% of the control group had UTI, the same for 40% of the group that was treated. So although there are differences in the sum of the days during which they were exposed to UTI these were not absolutely clear-cut.

Dr. *P. Kincaid-Smith*: Nonetheless, they obviously behave in a very benign manner with only short courses of treatment.

Dr. *W. Asscher*: Oh, yes.

Dr. *R. Bailey*: This is also our experience in Christchurch. Since January 1967, we have been screening women, children, and anybody else for UTI, asymptomatic UTI. And among our positives a proportion has been shown to have RN. And we have yet to see a single patient from that population develop a progressive condition with proteinuria and hypertension and deteriorating renal function. The patients with end-stage RN are not from that group. They come from elsewhere.

Dr. *W. Asscher*: I would like to ask this meeting, has anybody ever recorded the actual onset of proteinuria in a case of RN?

Dr. *P. Ransley*: Not with normal kidney function.

Dr. *W. Asscher*: When I looked back on the records of these patients that go on to kidney failure, I found that they had proteinuria at the time of their first visit. I have never caught one in the act of developing it.

Dr. *P. Kincaid-Smith*: If you define proteinuria as less than 100 mg/day, I'm pretty sure we've got 2 patients from our original pregnancy bacteriuria screening program that have gone on to develop progressive renal failure who certainly didn't have proteinuria at the start. But I'd have to look back in the records to see whether they were symptomatic in pregnancy. That is a 15-year follow-up.

Dr. *R. Bailey*: It is a rare happening.

Dr. *J. Winberg*: Yes. But it commences rather early on in the picture when it does occur.

Dr. *J. Duckett*: These patients are only treated intermittently by short courses of antibiotics. The two groups are comparable. Even though you treat one group periodically, the results are the same at the end. That is essentially what you are saying.

Dr. *K. Verrier Jones*: Yes. That's right.

Dr. *J. Duckett*: Then let me ask you this. If you had those patients on prophylactic antibiotics continuously, as Dr. *Smellie* does, the incidence of their UTIs would be nil?

Dr. *K. Verrier Jones*: Yes.

Dr. *W. Asscher*: Forgive me interrupting, but we wouldn't get the necessary compliance. I mean these girls are asymptomatic. Even in Germany where one excepts more cooperation among the lay population than in the UK, only 30% compliance was obtained in similar circumstances.

Dr. *J. Duckett*: The point I am trying to make is that these are select groups of benign patients. They are discovered because of covert UTI. They are quite different from those who come to me as a urologist with an attack of symptomatic pyelonephritis in whom VUR is demonstrated, and whom we then place on prophylactic antibiotics. Because if *they* do not comply, or forget their medicine, a large percentage come back with other attacks of pyelonephritis. This is our clinical experience, and one cannot deny that this is a different type of patient to those whom you are following. You can't compare apples and oranges.

Dr. *J. Winberg*: I think what Dr. *Duckett* has just said is very important, namely that we have to separate our patients into different clinical groups. We have studied one cohort of patients, our infants with first UTI. Those of Dr. *Verrier Jones* were symptomless schoolgirls picked up by a screening exercise. These are not the same necessarily as the symptomatic children who are referred to a urologist.

Dr. *W. Asscher*: Our study was designed to answer a public health problem.

Dr. *J. Duckett*: And so it may not be directly extrapolated to the clinical field. We are supposed to be considering VUR right now. Introducing your schoolgirls seems to imply that they are reflux patients and that these as a group are benign. I don't think you can make that claim.

Dr. *W. Asscher*: Children identified with covert UTI in general pursue a very benign course. That is very important to know if one has to advise health authorities on what to do about preventing kidney failure because one simply does not identify the right type of case by screening for symptomless UTI. That is what this study is beginning to say. Dr. *Verrier Jones* is fortunately young enough still to carry on for 20 more years. And perhaps then she'll come back with the proof that this conclusion as it stands today is wrong.

Dr. *K. Verrier Jones*: I agree that we are seeing the other end of the spectrum from the patients who present symptomatically to pediatricians or urologists. But I also think there is quite a lot of overlap between these groups. And one factor that must always be taken into account is that, once a child has been diagnosed as having UTI and somebody has found a scar on a kidney, there is a very considerable difference in the way the family reacts than if they think the child has only had a UTI. While I'm sure some of our children have fever and loin pain ans so on, it's not something I very often meet. I do a clinic with a urologist, and he asks the children whether they have had any further UTI. Sometimes they say no; other times they say yes. They haven't been ill enough to come to the hospital, so we don't see them with these attacks; and I often wonder what these attacks are really like. I doubt if they are really as sick as the patients Dr. *Winberg* has just described.

Dr. *R. White*: Can the technique of diethylenetriaminepentaacetic acid (DTPA) measurement of split renal function be adapted to the very young children, or will we have to use DMSA?

Dr. *K. Verrier Jones*: We don't find the technique difficult, but I cannot vouch for the accuracy of the method.

Dr. *P. Ransley*: We have had very successful individual kidney GFR measurements in babies. A big dilemma for the urologist is the 8-year-old patient still with VUR – less than it was 5 years ago – whose kidneys are growing and who, when you take her off chemoprophylaxis, remains asymptomatic but has repeatedly positive urine cultures. Does one treat her or not? I think such a case may fit into Dr. *Verrier Jones* group, and perhaps we can take courage from her work and not treat such a case. One last question: What was the lowest total corrected GFR for her group?

Dr. *K. Verrier Jones*: I think it was 59 ml/min.

Dr. *P. Ransley*: I would like to predict that none of your patients will ever end up with renal failure. Our strong impression being that the bad ones get worse and the good ones get better. In other words, children with corrected GFRs below 40 are very likely to develop proteinuria and progressive renal failure later on, say in early adult life; above 40 the prognosis appears to be much better.

Dr. *P. Kincaid-Smith*: In relation to that last point, we have certainly seen adults with RN and normal renal function, certainly with GFR way above 40, pass into renal failure. Something else I would like to suggest is that the prognosis of any group, particularly the slightly older children who present with a symptomatic UTI, will depend on whether or not they are kept under medical supervision in the first place, and how effective this supervision is in the second. I think the proof can be illustrated by comparing Dr. *Smellie*'s immaculate series with others in which medical care has been sporadic. I don't think one can prognose in general from just how the child first presents.

Dr. *J. Winberg*: We can confirm Dr. *Verrier Jones'* observations from our own experience in patients who presented with asymptomatic UTI. But I would also say that they were taken care of as small children and this might be the critical factor.

Dr. *J. Conway*: As someone who has catheterized some 12,000 young girls over the last 15 years, I can say that their perineal region is usually extremely unsavory, and one marvels how infrequently this seems to lead to UTI.

Dr. *J. Winberg*: We can't go into detail about that now. But we already know that there is a very well-balanced bacterial situation between aerobes and anaerobes in this area. Little girls up to the age of 2–3 years are heavily colonized, but only 1% of them get UTI. After the age of 4 years virtually no Gram-negative organisms are found except in those who have recurrent UTIs, and that is not because of bad hygiene.

Section IV: Prospective Trial of Surgery versus Conservative Treatment

Contr. Nephrol., vol. 39, pp. 169–185 (Karger, Basel 1984)

15. A Prospective Trial of Operative versus Non-Operative Treatment of Severe Vesico-Ureteric Reflux: 2 Years' Observation in 96 Children[1]

The Birmingham Reflux Study Group[2]

The Children's Hospital, Birmingham, England

Introduction

The relationship between vesico-ureteric reflux (VUR) and coarse renal scarring is now firmly established [1–4], the term 'reflux nephropathy' (RN) [5] being widely accepted as an alternative to 'chronic pyelonephritis'. There is substantial evidence that intrarenal reflux (IRR) plays a role in its aetiology [6]; in pigs made to reflux experimentally, infected urine produced scars which were related anatomically to compound, refluxing papillae [7]. Although there is some experimental evidence that scarring may be initiated by IRR with sterile urine [8], there is little to suggest that RN occurs in humans in the absence of urinary tract infection (UTI).

The prevention of recurrent UTI in children with VUR by means of regular chemoprophylaxis [9] might therefore appear a logical way of minimizing RN. Using impaired renal growth as an indication of progressive RN, however, the Cardiff-Oxford Bacteriuria Group [10, 11] was unable to demonstrate any difference between *symptomless* bacteriuric schoolgirls who received chemoprophylaxis and those who did not. Furthermore, they did not observe new scars developing in previously unscarred kidneys despite the persistence of VUR, in many instances with UTI. These findings strongly suggest that the scarring process is initiated early

[1] This paper was drafted by R.H.R.W. and C.M.T.

[2] Members of Group: *R.H.R. White* and *M.H. Winterborn*, Paediatric Nephrologists; *C.M. Taylor* and *R.C. Clark*, Senior Paediatric Registrars; *R. Astley* and *K.J. Shah*, Paediatric Radiologists; *J.J. Corkery* and *P. Gornall*, Paediatric Surgeons.

in childhood and imply that medical intervention after the fifth birthday may be ineffective.

An alternative means of preventing infected urine reaching the renal parenchyma is the abolition of VUR by surgical reimplantation of the affected ureter. *McRae* et al. [12] reported improved renal growth following reimplantation of severely refluxing ureters, but made no comparison with matched patients managed with chemoprophylaxis alone. By eliminating the substantial bladder residue which results from the return of urine from a severely dilated, refluxing ureter, surgical reimplantation might be expected to hasten the disappearance of symptoms due to both UTI and bladder instability. In fact *McRae* et al. [12] could detect no difference in the incidence of UTI postoperatively, although *Scott* [13] noted slight improvement. The possible benefits of reimplantation must be weighed against the continuing tendency towards spontaneous resolution of VUR observed over a long period of time [1, 3, 14].

These questions have preoccupied workers in this field for a number of years, and led us to the conclusion that a prospective study in which suitable patients were randomly allocated to operative treatment or to chemoprophylaxis alone was the only satisfactory way of providing answers. The study which we describe in this paper incorporates clinical, functional and radiological assessment at entry, and again 2 and 5 years after allocation. We now report our findings in 96 children who complied with the protocol and from whom adequate data were obtained during their first 2 years' observation.

Patients and Methods

Grading of VUR

The severity of VUR was graded on the evidence of a single cysto-urethrogram (voiding cysto-urethrography, VCU) as follows: *Grade I.* VUR of contrast medium, on filling or micturition, which fails to reach the renal pelvis. *Grade II*: Contrast medium reaching the renal pelvis but not causing distension or any disturbance of the normal acute forniceal angles of the calyces. *Grade III*: Contrast medium distending the pelvicalyceal system and widening the forniceal angles.

Patients

Children suitable for entry into the study were drawn from two sources. 60% were refered by consultant paediatricians in the West Midlands Health Region, the diagnosis of VUR

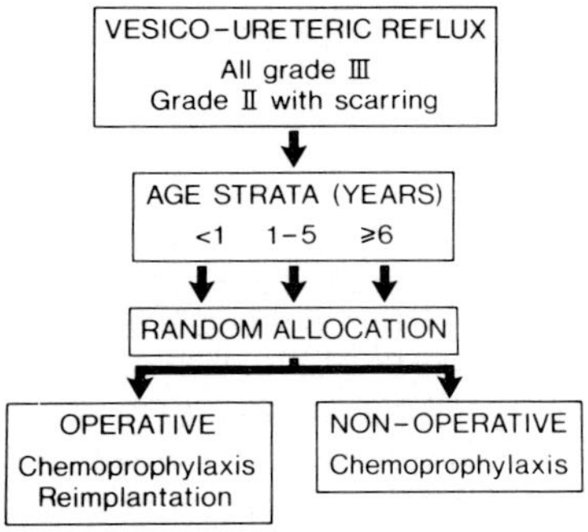

Fig. 1. Flow-diagram illustrating the allocation procedure.

already having been established as a result of investigating symptomatic UTI. The remainder were referred by their general practitioners, or attended the Accident and Emergency Department of the Hospital, with a diagnosis of UTI.

The following criteria were required for entry into the study: (1) Age of patient less than 15 years at time of allocation; (2) VUR diagnosed in the absence of active UTI, less than 6 months previously; and (3) VUR grade III, with or without RN, or grade II associated with RN. One or both ureters could be allocated in accordance with these criteria; grade I VUR in one ureter did not preclude allocation of an eligible contralateral ureter.

Exclusions

Any of the following abnormalities excluded entry: (1) A refluxing ureter draining a poorly or non-functioning kidney, as judged by excretion of radio-opaque contrast material on intravenous urography (IVU). However, VUR of sufficient grade in a contralateral ureter draining an adequately functioning kidney did not exclude entry. (2) A completely duplicated ureter. (3) Ureterocele. (4) Obstructive uropathy. (5) Neuropathic bladder. (6) Urinary calculus. (7) Previous surgery to the lower ureter or near the bladder base and considered likely to prejudice the reimplantation operation. (8) VUR up a ureter draining an ectopic or horseshoe kidney.

Allocation Procedure

Eligible patients were stratified and separately randomized in three age groups: (1) <1; (2) 1–5; (3) ≥ 6 years old at allocation (fig. 1). Within these age strata no distinction was made between unilateral and bilateral VUR, or between grade III VUR and grade II VUR with RN, in the allocation to either treatment group.

Allocation was made by opening the next of a batch of sealed envelopes. Each batch consisted of 8 envelopes, containing 4 operative and 4 non-operative allocations, which were prepared by a secretary and placed in random order, the envelopes being numbered consecutively and labelled with the appropriate age group.

Initially it was intended to obtain informed consent from the parents of eligible children. However, early experience indicated that a substantial proportion of parents withheld consent when faced with the choice of operation or no operation. The Research Ethical Committee of Central Birmingham Health District gave its unanimous approval to our proceeding without informed consent after interviewing representatives of the Study Group and accepting that, with existing knowledge, there was no agreement regarding the ideal choice of management.

Treatment

All patients received prophylaxis with a suitable antibiotic in appropriate single nightly dosage [15, 16] for an initial period of 2 years, after which clinical, functional and radiological reassessment took place. The alternative of omitting prophylaxis in the operative group was rejected because it was considered that short courses of antibiotics would probably be administered haphazardly for UTI or other infections and thus introduce an uncontrolled variable. The trial was therefore designed to assess whether ureteric reimplantation conferred any benefits additional to those of conventional medical management.

Children who drew operative management underwent reimplantation of their affected ureters within 6 months of diagnosis of VUR. A shorter interval,although desirable, was found impracticable, allowing for the time required for initial referral of the patient, assessment in our clinic, arrangement of baseline investigations, and the surgical waiting list. Operations were performed by one of two surgical teams, using either a modified Leadbetter-Politano method (J.J.C.) or the Cohen technique (P.G.).

Monitoring Progress

On allocation each child was assessed clinically by one of us, and the height, weight and blood pressure (BP) recorded. A mid-stream urine (MSU) sample was cultured. Renal excretory function was assessed by determination of the plasma creatinine, using an automated reaction-rate method, and by slope clearance of ^{51}Cr-edetic acid (C_{EDTA}) as described by *Chantler and Barratt* [17]. The maximum renal concentrating capacity was assessed by measuring the osmolality of a timed overnight urine collection (ONU) made during fluid deprivation [18]. In the operative group the tests were generally carried out during the hospital admission for surgery, immediately pre-operatively. In non-operative patients living at a distance from the hospital, and in all infants, the tests were performed during an overnight stay; older children living nearby collected the ONU sample at home, following written instructions, and attended as day cases for the clearance studies.

Radiographs of the IVU were reviewed by the radiologists who, at the time of allocation, noted the presence or absence of calyceal distortion and parenchymal loss. Renal length measurement was deferred until the results of the trial were analysed. The degree of VUR was graded on the VCU films.

Regular hospital attendance, at either The Children's Hospital or the referring regional Hospital, was requested every 3 months, and parents were instructed to report sooner if symptoms of UTI developed. The height, weight, and BP were recorded at each visit. In the Renal Clinic patients were screened for UTI by microscopy of uncentrifuged urine [19] obtained by clean-catch or by Hollister U-bag, and culture was carried out when bacteriuria, or an excess of leucocytes, were seen. In other clinics urine culture was routinely undertaken.

All patients underwent reassessment of renal function together with repeat IVU and VCU 2 years after allocation. Children treated surgically required an additional IVU and VCU 6 months postoperatively, in order to eliminate the possibility of ureteric obstruction and ensure that VUR had been abolished, but these films were not included in the radiological analysis.

Table I. Patients withdrawn from the study

Reason for withdrawal	Number of patients	
	Op.	Non-op.
Unacceptable radiographs	2	3
Operative delay ≥6 months	3	0
Previous ureteric surgery	0	1
VCU during UTI	0	1
Parental objection	0	1
Unrelated death	1	1
Total	6	7

Analysis of Results

The IVU films were returned to the radiologists following obliteration of identification labels, allowing renal length measurements and the documentation of RN to be recorded without knowledge of the mode of treatment. Renal length was related to the intervertebral distance L1–L3 and expressed as a standard deviation (SD). The formula:

$$SD = \frac{\text{Renal length} - [2.6 + 0.98\,(L1-L3)]}{0.72}$$

was derived from the nomogram of *Eklöf and Ringertz* [20].

Preliminary tests showed that the method of measuring renal length was reproducible for both radiologists, and yielded negligible observer error between them. The radiological work-load was accordingly shared. Because more than half of the examinations were performed at the referring hospitals, there were sometimes difficulties, mostly owing to inadequate bowel preparation. When these arose, measurements were made by both radiologists; and when, despite this, there was still any difficulty in interpretation, a joint discussion was held between the two radiologists together with RCC, to resolve discrepancies. This led to a small number of children being withdrawn from the trial (table I). In all cases showing the

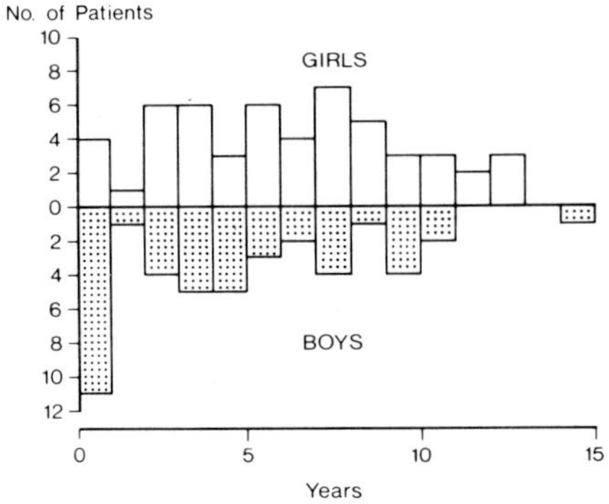

Fig. 2. Sex and age at allocation of the 96 children in the study.

development of a new scar, or progression of an existing one, and in all infants both radiologists made independent assessments.

The clinical, laboratory and radiological data were transferred to computer cards and stored in an ICL 1906A computer (Department of Social Medicine, University of Birmingham). The computer was programmed to compare the observations recorded at entry, 2 and 5 years, and to evaluate differences statistically, using Student's t-test, Fisher's exact test and Yates' corrected χ^2 test where appropriate. The present analysis is confined to the first 2-year observation, since sufficient data on the 5-year follow-up are not yet available. Although all the data were separately analysed for each age stratum, as well as for all ages together, only singificant results for individual age strata will be presented, for the sake of brevity.

Results

Clinical Data

During the period July 1975 to December 1981, 109 children completed 2 years' observation; however, 13 were withdrawn for failing to comply with the study protocol (table I), leaving 96 for analysis. Figure 2 shows the age and sex distribution at entry. The predominance of males in infancy and of females in later childhood reflects changes in the sex incidence of UTI with increasing age.

The randomization of patients and the resulting allocation of ureters to the two treatment groups are given in table II. This also shows that similar proportions of patients in each treatment limb were allocated for unilat-

Table II. Randomization of patients and ureters

		Operative	Non-operative
Patients			
Total		49	47
One ureter allocated		29	28
Both ureters allocated		20	19
Ureters			
VUR grade:	III	65	65
	II	4	1
Age, years:	<1	10	13
	1–5	33	26
	≥6	26	27
Total		69	66

eral or bilateral VUR. The ratio of unilateral to bilateral VUR was broadly similar in the three age strata. Grade III VUR was present in 130 and grade II VUR in 5 ureters. All 5 grade II ureters were associated with contralateral grade III VUR and, by chance, 4 were allocated to operative and only one to non-operative treatment.

Height

Body height was analysed for each age stratum as the mean height SD score [21], which enables comparisons to be made between children of different ages. There was no significant difference at any time in the mean scores between operative and non-operative groups in any age stratum. However, the growth rate during the 2-year period for 1- to 5-year-old children was slightly greater in the operative group (change in mean height SD: operative +0.41, non-operative −0.001; $t = 2.114$, $p < 0.05$). This was not seen in other age strata, neither was a difference in growth rate observed when all ages were analysed together.

Blood Pressure

Hypertension was defined according to the criteria of the National Heart, Lung and Blood Institute [22]. No child developed hypertension during the 2-year observation period, but 1 girl aged 12 with bilateral grade

Table III. Number of patients with breakthrough UTI

Age years	Operative		Non-operative	
	UTI	total	UTI	total
<1	1	7	3	8
1–5	3	22	4	19
≥6	8	20	4	20
Total	12	49	11	47

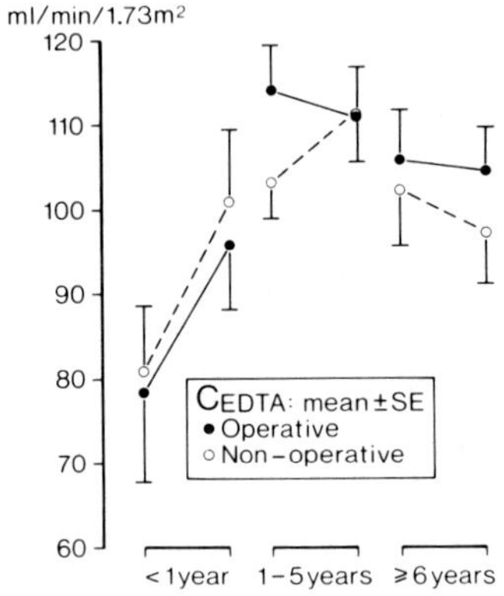

Fig. 3. Clearance of C_{EDTA} for each age stratum, at allocation and after 2 years' observation.

III VUR, RN and reduced glomerular filtration rate (GFR) was already on treatment for hypertension at allocation.

Urinary Tract Infection

24% of all patients were observed to have one or more episodes of breakthrough UTI. The incidence of UTI in both treatment groups was similar for each age stratum as shown in table III.

Renal Function

GFR showed no significant difference between treatment modalities at any age, whether assessment by plasma creatinine or C_{EDTA} (fig. 3). The rise in C_{EDTA} clearance observed in the <1 year age group reflects the normal physiological increase in GFR [23].

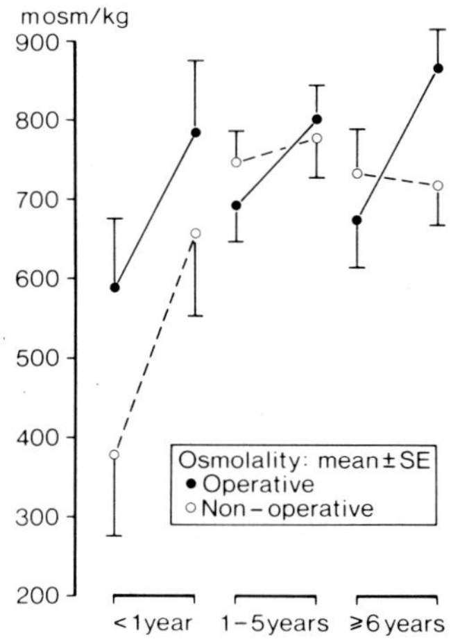

Fig. 4. Overnight urine osmolality (displayed as in fig. 3).

Changes in ONU concentration are similarly displayed in figure 4. There was no significant difference in osmolality between treatment groups in any age stratum at entry; however, there was a significantly higher mean osmolality at 2 years in the operative group of children aged ≥6 years (operative: 865 ± 48 mosm/kg; non-operative: 715 ± 49 mosm/kg; t = 2.17, $p < 0.05$). The change in osmolality observed over the 2-year period was also significant (operative +175, SD 60; non-operative −7, SD 42; t = 2.47, $p < 0.05$). However, it must be stated that, of the 20 children ≥6 years old undergoing operative treatment, ONU collection was inadvertently omitted in 8 at entry, and in 4 at 2 years, leaving only 10 with complete data. To ensure that the decreased ONU concentration in patients managed non-operatively was not an artefact created by residual dilute urine secreted the previous evening, 13 children recently shown to have persisting gross VUR were asked to perform two ONU concentration tests at home, once with, and once without double voiding at bedtime. Both tests yielded similar results (mean osmolality without double voiding 679 ± 49 osm/kg; with double voiding 690 ± 63; t = 0.1378).

Radiological Data

The 96 patients yielded 135 kidneys drained by severely refluxing ureters, now referred to as the 'allocated' kidneys. Table IV shows the effect of patient randomization on the distribution of scarred and small kidneys (length < −2SD) at allocation. In the age stratum < 1 year there were more scarred kidneys in the non-operative (10/13) than in the operative group

Table IV. Radiological data at allocation and after 2 years' observation

	Operative	Non-operative
At allocation		
Number of ureters	69	66
Existing scarring	34	39
Renal length < -2.0 SD	12	18
At 2 years		
Progression of scarring	7	11
Renal length decrease ≥ 1.0 SD	22	20
New scars	2	2

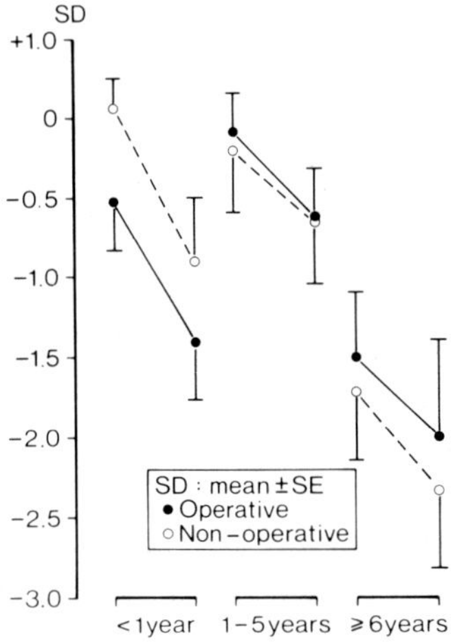

Fig. 5. Renal length standard deviations (displayed as in fig. 3).

(3/10). Although just significant ($p < 0.05$), we consider that this discrepancy is a chance finding which will disappear when more patients of this age have been recruited. At other ages, and for the data as a whole, there were no significant differences in the proportions of small or scarred kidneys between operative and non-operative groups at allocation.

Table IV also shows that, after 2 years' follow-up, there were no significant differences between the two treatment groups in the proportion of kidneys which showed either fresh or progressive scarring or impaired growth (which we defined as a decrease of renal length ≥ 1.0 SD). Changes in mean renal growth over the period of observation are further illustrated in figure 5, divided according to the three age strata and the two treatment

Table V. Comparison of radiological data at entry and after 2 years' follow-up, in allocated and unallocated kidneys

	Allocated	Unallocated	p
At entry			
Number of ureters	135	55	
Existing scarring	73	5	<0.0005
Renal length SD	−0.74 ± 0.16	0.47 ± 0.13	<0.001
At 2 years			
Progression of scarring	18	2	n.s.
Renal length SD change	−0.57 ± 0.08	−0.27 ± 0.09	<0.01
Renal length decrease ≥1.0 SD	42	5	<0.01
New scars	4	1	n.s.

Table VI. Radiological changes in kidneys exposed to breakthrough UTI, related to mode of treatment, and compared with unexposed kidneys

	Exposed to UTI			Not exposed to UTI
	operative	non-operative	all	
Total	17	18	35	100
Scarred at allocation	8	11	19	54
Progression of scarring	2	2	4	14
Renal length decrease ≥1.0 SD	8	5	13	28
New scars	0	1	1	3

modes. No significant differences were demonstrable. Growth was retarded at all ages.

In table V the radiographic changes in allocated kidneys are compared with those of the 55 contralateral kidneys where the criteria for inclusion in the study were not met. As might be expected, these unallocated kidneys were of greater mean length, showed less existing scarring, and grew significantly larger. However, the proportions of kidneys showing new or progressive scars did not differ from those of the allocated kidneys.

Table VII. Details of patients developing new scars

Management	Operative		Non-operative		
Age, years/months	2/4	7/2	3/8	6/9	3/6
Sex	F	M	F	F	M
UTI episodes	0	0	0	4	1
VUR grade	III	III	III	III	nil[1]
Previous scarring	no	yes	no	yes	no
Renal length SD					
At entry	0.88	−0.99	0.81	−0.36	3.57
At 2 years	−0.92	−2.21	−0.91	−0.14	1.44

[1] Unallocated kidney, contralateral to grade III VUR.

35 of the allocated kidneys were exposed to breakthrough UTI during the observation period. The radiological findings in these kidneys are detailed in table VI; no differences were found between treatment groups. When allocated kidneys exposed to UTI were compared with unexposed ones (table VI) there was no difference in the proportion demonstrating new or progressive scars. New scarring occurred in 5 kidneys, details of which appear in table VII; breakthrough UTI was demonstrated in only 2 instances, 1 being an unallocated kidney with a non-refluxing ureter.

Surgery was successful in abolishing VUR in 67 our of 69 ureters (97%). The 2 failures continued to have significant VUR; there were no cases of postoperative ureteric obstruction. On the other hand, 48 (74%) of the 65 grade III ureters managed non-operatively still demonstrated grades II–III VUR after 2 years.

Discussion

This study was designed in the mid-1970s and employs conventional methods of imaging and assessing renal function. The 2-year observation period can only be regarded as brief, in the light of the natural history of VUR and RN. Therefore, conclusions must be drawn cautiously; it would be premature to construe our findings as condemning reimplantation as a mode of treatment, and the results of 5 and 10 years' follow-up will be of greater importance.

We were unable to demonstrate any differences in renal excretory function between the two treatment groups; however, C_{EDTA} measures total renal function and is incapable of identifying subtle changes in individual kidney function which may have occurred even in this short observation period. By means of ^{99m}Tc-DTPA renograms, *Verrier Jones* et al. [24] have confirmed that impaired renal function is directly related to the presence of RN and is not affected by the persistence of either VUR or UTI.

The finding of impaired ONU concentration in older children managed non-operatively was unexpected. Artefactual dilution by residual urine in the presence of persistent VUR has been discounted. The ONU does not measure the maximum renal concentrating ability but tests the osmolality after approximately 14 h fluid deprivation, and is dependent upon the patient's compliance. Nevertheless, we assumed that the degree of error would be evenly distributed between the two treatment groups. Possibly the small number of operative patients in the 6-year-old stratum who completed this investigation may have introduced a sampling error.

Savage et al. [25] demonstrated impaired renal concentrating ability in bacteriuric 5-year-old girls who had VUR, in contrast to those without VUR and healthy controls. However, the authors commented that: 'This disability of the kidneys to concentrate the urine adequately is maximal when there is radiological evidence of parenchymal disease . . .'. *Uehling* [26] also demonstrated impaired ONU osmolality in children with recurrent UTI but showed a greater reduction in those with RN, the VUR itself having no apparent influence. Since the incidence of RN in our operative and non-operative older children was similar, the difference observed in ONU osmolality is puzzling, and requires further evaluation.

Improved renal growth has been reported following ureteric reimplantation [12]; however, these observations were uncontrolled and we cannot confirm them. New scars and progression of existing ones were seen equally among operative, non-operative, and unallocated kidneys and bore no apparent relationship to either persistent VUR or breakthrough UTI. This accords with the findings of the Cardiff-Oxford Bacteriuria Study Group [11] in schoolgirls. *Smellie and Normand* [27] noted that most of the few fresh scars reported in the literature had developed before the age of 5 years. Nevertheless, this study confirms, as we [4] and others [27] have done previously, that fresh scars may rarely develop, or appear to do so, at a later age. Interpretation of the significance of new scars demands an appreciation that the radiologically apparent scar probably represents the late result of fibrous contraction [28]; thus, the possibility that the scarring process in our patients had been initiated 2 years previously could not confidently be ruled out with the techniques employed. Alternative imaging techniques such as ^{99m}Tc-DMSA scanning may be capable of overcoming this difficulty [29].

Breakthrough UTI occurred in a 24% of our patients. However, we made no special endeavour to monitor compliance with medication, nor did we consider it reasonable to expect those children who were asymptomatic to attend the clinic, often at great personal inconvenience, at intervals of less than 3 months. The rate of UTI was similar in operative and non-operative patients, confirming previous observations [12] and lending no support to the theory that the predisposition of a refluxing urinary tract to UTI is caused by incomplete hydrodynamic washout of bladder bacteria [30].

We emphasize the interim nature of this report. Whereas VUR was abolished in 97% of ureters subjected to surgery, 74% of grade III ureters managed non-operatively for 2 years still demonstrated grades II–III VUR. In the children studied over much longer periods by *Smellie* et al. [3] and *Edwards* et al. [14], a continuing tendency to resolution of VUR was observed, which was not attributed to the control of UTI by means of long-term chemoprophylaxis. Nevertheless, only 41% of grossly refluxing ureters had undergone resolution, and this will make an interesting comparison with our own patients, analysed after 5 years' conservative management.

Although RN is recognized as an important cause of end-stage renal failure [31], only a small fraction of all children with VUR will develop the extensive bilateral parenchymal scarring which is necessary to cause such functional impairment. Nevertheless, patients with even focal, unilateral renal scarring are at increased risk of developing hypertension [32], so the prevention of RN must continue to be the main aim in the management of VUR.

Controlled trials in this field are new [33] and have an important contribution to make, but it is already apparent from our preliminary results that neither chemotherapy nor surgical intervention are likely to exert a profoundly beneficial influence on the course of the parenchymal scarring process, once initiated. This is illustrated graphically by figure 5, which suggests that poor renal growth is a continuing feature of RN throughout

Table VIII. Prevalence of existing renal scarring related to age of patient at allocation

Age group	Number of kidneys	
	scarred	unscarred
<1 year	13	10
≥1 year	60	52

childhood, irrespective of treatment, so that a substantial proportion of kidneys in older children have become reduced to less than −2 SD in length, the limit below which normal growth may never be resumed [34].

Were the acquisition of RN a continuing process caused by persistent VUR and UTI, we could expect to find a higher incidence in older children than in infants. It can be seen from table VIII that this is not the case. Its occurrence so early in life perhaps parallels the rapid development of segmental inflammation and fibrosis demonstrated experimentally in pigs when infected urine is refluxed into compound papillae – the 'big bang' theory [35]. On the other hand, the term 'reflux nephropathy' may also embrace examples of congenital malformation associated with VUR, in addition to lesions acquired postnatally, and these could not be expected to benefit from either chemoprophylaxis or ureteric reimplantation.

Table IV shows that more than 50% of kidneys were already scarred at the time of allocation, and controlled trials with such unsatisfactory ingredients will inevitably require large numbers of patients if significant differences between treatments are to be demonstrated. It may already be too late to influence subsequent events once the child has presented clinically and, if the acquired form of RN is to be prevented, a more rational approach would be to screen infants for VUR before their first episode of UTI. Although justified in the at-risk younger siblings of known cases of VUR [36], the conventional VCU method is unfortunately too invasive to employ in preventative screening of infant populations, and future progress will depend on the elaboration of a more suitable technique.

Acknowledgements

We thank the many colleagues who referred patients and helped with their care. We particularly wish to acknowledge the contribution of Dr. *Harley R. Powell* (Department of

Nephrology, The Royal Children's Hospital, Melbourne) to the trial design, while in Birmingham in 1974. We are also grateful to Prof. *E.G. Knox* (Department of Social Medicine, University of Birmingham) for his help with the planning and analysis, to Mr. *R. Lancashire* for the computer handling of data and to Miss *Valerie A. Bailey* for her part in the organization as well as typing the manuscript. The figures were kindly prepared by the Medical Illustration Department; figures 1, 3, and 5 are reproduced by courtesy of the *British Medical Journal*.

References

1 MacGregor, M.E.; Freeman, P.: Childhood urinary infection associated with vesico-ureteric reflux. Q. Jl. Med. *44*: 481–489 (1975).

2 McLachlan, M.S.F.; Meller, S.T.; Verrier Jones, E.R.; Asscher, A.W.; Fletcher, E.W.L.; Mayon-White, R.T.; Ledingham, J.G.G.; Smith, J.C.; Johnston, H.H.: Urinary tract in schoolgirls with covert bacteriuria. Archs Dis. Childh. *50*: 253–258 (1975).

3 Smellie, J.; Edwards, D.; Hunter, N.; Normand, I.C.S.; Prescod, N.: Vesico-ureteric reflux and renal scarring. Kidney int. *8*: suppl. 4, pp. S65–S72 (1975).

4 Shah, K.J.; Robins, D.G.; White, R.H.R.: Renal scarring and vesicoureteric reflux. Archs Dis. Childh. *53*: 210–217 (1978).

5 Bailey, R.R.: The relationship of vesico-ureteric reflux to urinary tract infection and chronic pyelonephritis – reflux nephropathy. Clin. Nephrol. *1*: 132–141 (1973).

6 Rolleston, G.L.; Maling, T.M.J.; Hodson, C.J.: Intrarenal reflux and the scarred kidney. Archs. Dis. Childh. *49*: 531–539 (1974).

7 Ransley, P.G.; Risdon, R.A.; Reflux and renal scarring. Br. J. Radiol. suppl. 14 (1978).

8 Hodson, C.J.; Maling, T.M.J.; McManamon, P.J.; Lewis, M.G.: The pathogenesis of reflux nephropathy (chronic atrophic pyelonephritis). Br. J. Radiol. suppl. 13 (1975).

9 Normand, I.C.S.; Smellie, J.M.: Prolonged maintenance chemotherapy in the management of urinary infection in childhood. Br. med. J. *i*: 1023–1026 (1965).

10 Cardiff-Oxford Bacteriuria Study Group: Sequelae of covert bacteriuria in schoolgirls: a four-year follow-up study. Lancet *i*: 889–894 (1978).

11 Cardiff-Oxford Bacteriuria Study Group: Long-term effect of bacteriuria on the urinary tract in schoolgirls. Radiology *132*: 343–350 (1979).

12 McRae, C.U.; Shannon, F.T.; Utley, W.L.F.: Effect of renal growth of reimplantation of refluxing ureters. Lancet *i*: 1310–1312 (1974).

13 Scott, J.E.S.: The management of ureteric reflux in children. Br. J. Urol. *49*: 109–118 (1977).

14 Edwards, D.; Normand, I.C.S.; Prescod, N.; Smellie, J.M.: Disappearance of vesicoureteric reflux during long-term prophylaxis of urinary tract infection in children. Br. med. J. *ii*: 285–288 (1977).

15 Bailey, R.R.; Roberts, A.P.; Gower, P.E.; Wardener, H.E. de: Prevention of urinary-tract infection with low-dose nitrofurantoin. Lancet *ii*: 1112–1114 (1971).

16 Smellie, J.M.; Katz, G.; Grüneberg, R.N.: Controlled trial of prophylactic treatment in childhood urinary-tract infection. Lancet *ii*: 175–178 (1978).

17 Chantler, C.; Barratt, T.M.: Estimation of glomerular filtration rate from plasma clearance of ^{51}Chromium-edetic acid. Archs. Dis. Childh. *47*: 613–617 (1972).

18 Edelman, C.M.; Barnett, H.L.; Stark, H.; Boichis, H.; Soriano, J.R.: A standardized

test of renal concentrating capacity in children. Am. J. Dis. Childh. *114*: 639–644 (1967).
19 Robins, D.G.; White, R.H.R.; Rogers, K.B.; Osman, M.S.: Urine microscopy as an aid to detection of bacteriuria. Lancet *i*: 476–478 (1975).
20 Eklöf, O.; Ringertz, H.: Kidney size in children: a method of assessment. Acta radiol. (Diag.) *17*: 617–625 (1976).
21 Tanner, J.M.; Whitehouse, R.H.; Takaishi, M.: Standards from birth to maturity for height, weight, height velocity and weight velocity. British Children, 1965. Archs. Dis. Childh. *41*: 454–471 (1966).
22 National Heart, Lung and Blood Institute: Task Force on Blood Pressure Control in Children. Standards for children's blood pressure. Pediatrics, Springfield *59*: 802–803 (1977).
23 McCrory, W.W.: Developmental Nephrology, pp. 79–122 (Harvard University Press, Cambridge 1972).
24 Verrier Jones, K.; Asscher, A.W.; Verrier Jones, E.R.; Mattholie, K.; Leach, K.; Thomson, G.M.: Glomerular filtration rate in schoolgirls with covert bacteriuria. Br. med. J. *285*: 1307–1310 (1982).
25 Savage, D.C.L.; Wilson, M.I.; Fee, W.M.: Renal concentrating ability in 5-year-old girls with covert bacteriuria. Archs Dis. Childh. *47*: 141–143 (1972).
26 Uehling, D.T.: Effect of vesicoureteral reflux on concentrating ability. J. Urol. *106*: 947–950 (1971).
27 Smellie, J.; Normand, C.: Reflux nephropathy in childhood; in Hodson, Kincaid-Smith, Reflux nephropathy, pp. 14–20 (Masson, New York 1979).
28 Scott, J.E.S.: The role of surgery in the management of vesico-ureteric reflux. Kidney int. *8*: suppl. 4, S73–S80 (1975).
29 Britton, K.: Radionuclides in renal imaging. Br. J. Hosp. Med. *20*: 140–146 (1978).
30 O'Grady, F.: Initiation and ascent of urinary tract infection; in Williams, Chisholm, Scientific foundations of urology, vol. I, pp. 177–183 (Heinemann, London 1976).
31 Donckerwolcke, R.A.; Chantler, C.; Brunner, F.P.; Brynger, H.A.O.; Gurland, H.J.; Hathway, R.A.; Jacobs, C.; Selwood, N.H.; Wing, A.J.: Combined report on regular dialysis and transplantation of children in Europe, 1977; in Robinson, Hawkins, Proc. Eur. Dial. Transpl. Ass., vol. XV, pp. 77–114 (Pitman, London 1978).
32 Wallace, D.M.A.; Rothwell, D.L.; Williams, D.I.: The long-term follow-up or surgically treated vesicoureteral reflux. Br. J. Urol. *50*: 479–484 (1978).
33 International Reflux Study Committee: Medical versus surgical treatment of primary vesicoureteral reflux: a prospective international reflux study in children. J. Urol. *125*: 277–283 (1981).
34 Orisaka, S.; Takamura, T.; Inada, F.; Tsuji, I.: Effect of vesicoureteral reflux on renal growth. J. Urol. *119*: 25–30 (1978).
35 Ransley, P.G.; Risdon, R.A.: Reflux nephropathy: effect of anti-microbial therapy on the evolution of the early pyelonephritic scar. Kidney int. *20*: 733–742 (1981).
36 Vargas, A. de; Evans, K.; Ransley, P.; Rosenberg, A.R.; Rothwell, D.; Sherwood, T.; Williams, D.I.; Barratt, T.M.; Carter, C.O.: A family study of vesicoureteric reflux. J. med. Genet. *15*: 85–96 (1978).

Richard H.R. White, The Children's Hospital, Ladywood,
Birmingham BI 6 SET (England)

Contr. Nephrol., vol. 39, pp. 186–189 (Karger, Basel 1984)

Discussion on Chapter 15

Dr. *W. Asscher*: Dr. *White*, I want to ask you about the new scars. You did everything 'blindly'. You had a 'blind' radiologist and 'blind' everything else. I am very familiar with this. But having done it 'blindly', when you talk about 'new scars' did you compare the first with the final radiographs?

It is exceedingly difficult sometimes to diagnose an early scar until the tissue around it grows. Secondly, when you say 'extension of scars', do you mean previous scarring involved more adjacent tissue, or that fresh scars appeared elsewhere?

Dr. *R. White*: 'Extension or progression of scarring', we defined as a measurable further reduction of parenchymal thickness overlying the existing scar.

As regards the 'new scars', we mean fresh areas involved after careful comparison with previous radiographs. Sometimes when we went back to the original films and concluded they were substandard. We had to exclude those patients from the study for this very reason, so we would only accept new scars if we were reasonably satisfied the first films were normal But I don't think you can necessarily totally eliminate an early scar by radiography and it is possible that all 5 of those patients had an original scarring process which was not radiologically apparent.

Dr. *J. Hodson*: You are right! It is not possible to exclude an early scar by radiography, as these inflammatory lesions commence with swelling and end in a contracted state. In between they pass through a phase when the affected tissue is of normal dimensions. Later, when the shrinkage has continued until the affected parenchyma is only 2 mm thick, it may be surrounded by hillocks of hypertrophied tissue. But these remarks only refer to moderate and smaller-sized scars with little papillary retraction. In the late stages of large scars, providing the calyx is fully filled with contrast, there should be a high index of certainty. Tomography, which I don't advise, would settle the point, but a radionucleide parenchymal scan is preferable.

As for 'progression of scarring', as Dr. *Asscher* just said, it can mean further contraction of original scarring, or it can mean new tissue is involved. This distinction is commonly not made clear by writers, even when they recognize the differing significance.

Dr. *R. White*: We accept that this is a weakness of any study of this type and possibly the more reproducible aspect is the renal length. But even then there is no difference emerging between operative and non-operative groups.

Dr. *R. Weiss*: Dr. *White*, in your measurement did you include the midzone parenchymal thickness? As midzone hypertrophy in the presence of bipolar scarring may give a false impression of length reduction.

Dr. *R. White*: No, we haven't done that.

Dr. *R. Weiss*: Secondly, did you divide the recurrences into symptomatic and asymptomatic groups?

Dr. *R. White*: No. We lumped the two together as episodes of urinary tract infection (UTI), with or without symptoms.

Dr. *R. Weiss*: And was there any difference between the symptomatic and the asymptomatic groups in terms of renal growth?

Dr. *R. White*: We haven't divided them up in that way. I can't tell you.

Dr. *J. Hodson*: Do you think they should?

Dr. *R. Weiss*: Presumably, if we all agree on the concept that renal parenchymal infection may interfere with renal growth and that asymptomatic UTI which may or may not involve the renal parenchyma, does not, I think such a distinction would be very useful.

Dr. *R. White*: In our child population, flank pain and constitutional symptoms are really quite rare. The majority have nothing more than dysuria or a reversion to 'wetting', or they may be a little off their food. It is very unusual indeed to see the acute pyelonephritis picture in the young child, and rarely over the age of 10 years.

Dr. *M. Taylor*: I agree. I can only think of 1 of our patients who has had to be hospitalized acutely and required intravenous antibiotics.

Dr. *R. Weiss*: That's distinctly different from the population we are entering into our progressive study, because most of them present with true clinical acute pyelonephritis. The younger children may have nothing more than constitutional symptoms, but I think high fever is one that they all share. I am wondering, therefore, whether or not we are collecting a different group of patients in our study than you are in yours. In other words, when you allocate patients it is usually on the basis of UTI but, if I understood correctly, it is rare for them to have full-blown acute pyelonephritis at onset.

Dr. *R. White*: Children come to us with a variety of symptoms. Some have fever. It is very uncommon to find one with tenderness in the loin. Some have acute upper respiratory infection together with UTI, and it is difficult to determine which is giving rise to the fever. Some have presented with a variety of symptoms which include fever often enough and are found to have UTIs. Some have even presented with head injuries and have been found to have UTI. I think at home there is now a very high suspicion index for UTI in nearly every child coming to the Hospital.

Dr. *N. Goldraich*: They usually have abdominal pain, not loin pain.

Dr. *R. White*: Yes, I agree. Abdominal pain much more commonly than loin pain.

Dr. *R. Weiss*: I think we could emphasize that at least at your hospital everybody is quite attuned to the diagnosis of UTI. But in the USA – I don't know about elsewhere – there are many, many infants with acute fever of unknown origin who are not having urine cultures. Some of the reasons for this are: (1) the unreliability of bag urine specimens obtained as we presently do them; and (2) sometimes it is difficult to convince a parent with an otherwise previously-well infant that, just because this infant has had fever for 24–48 h and is now apyrexial, he or she should have suprapubic bladder aspiration to look for UTI.

Yet this is the route everyone has emphasized we should be following to get at the earliest manifestations of vesicoureteral reflux (VUR), and I think we should all redouble our efforts to convince the general physicians who care for infants that the obtaining of a culture is a matter of urgency, not one to be left day after day.

Dr. *J. Hodson*: The method of home culture described by Dr. *Randolph* in our last Workshop in 1978 [Reflux nephropathy; in Hodson, Kincaid Smith, Chapter 8, Masson, New York] has had further remarkable results which Dr. *Klauber* has kindly consented to summarize in a short addition at the end of the book since this whole question of early diagnosis is so important – as is the requirement for a simple means of home monitoring for UTI (see pp. 378–382).

It also seems to me that facing us all now is the decision, in a study like the International one, which to me is a very precious thing and one on which vast amounts of time and money are being spent on both sides of the Atlantic, as to whether one is going to rely on clinical, or isotopic data and which of the two is the more reliable? To me there is no doubt that the isotope method is more objective.

Dr. *J. Conway*: I'm just confused. I'm new to this sort of thing. I just can't understand these children without pain or symptoms, other than fever, and who yet have rip-roaring pyelonephritis. I'm not sure I am even convinced by your definition of pyelonephritis. I also do not think the radiographic definition of reflux nephropathy (RN) is always reliable, as we have a half dozen children who had renal vein thrombosis secondary to umbilical catheterization and who have hypertension and scarred kidneys, on urography.

Dr. *J. Hodson*: But, Dr. *Conway*, by definition RN in children is scarring due to VUR!

Dr. *J. Conway*: Well, some of them may have VUR because a percentage of all children have VUR. I'm uncertain.

Dr. *J. Hodson*: Very well, then, if you don't accept the clinical diagnostic criteria, can your improve on them? What about the gallium scan?

Dr. *J. Conway*: I think the gallium scan is one way to go, because it is an absolute sign of an inflammatory or infected process. But in the clinical sense there is no question in my mind that the gallium scan or, even better, white blood cell labelling is an absolute indicator of an infectious process.

Dr. *J. Hodson*: White blood cell labelling?

Dr. *J. Conway*: Labelled white blood cells (WBCs). If you take the patients' WBCs and label them with indium oxine and inject them i.v., they settle in the infection site itself, and if it is in the kidney then you can say that this is an infection in the kidney.

Dr. *J. Hodson*: I'd like to bring all these things that have been mentioned back to reality. Here are Dr. *White* and his colleagues in the middle of a highly complex, very well organized, very detailed, survey of children with VUR and UTI and how to treat them, and, with two other similar and larger international efforts now under way, you are suggesting that these new modalities are more reliable as means of diagnosis. I think they *may* be more reliable than clinical signs alone. But to include them at this stage in these surveys, with so many children already involved, means a lot more money and a lot more people who will be required to introduce them. I don't think that any responsible Meeting like this should promote new concepts unless their absence invalidates the study as a whole, which, with the small amount of thinking we have had time to apply to the problem, is yet to be proven. We have to think in terms of hard cash when looking after these children, particularly in Britain. But, nevertheless, you think that if a child is suspect of a scar, has a doubtful urine culture, and is clinically indefinite, he should have a gallium scan?

Dr. *J. Conway*: Absolutely.

Dr. *P. Kincaid-Smith*: Can I just say that it may be different in children, but in the case of pregnant women who have UTI the sign which is most indicative of renal involvement and correlates well with other studies is the leukocyte (WBC) count in the urine. If the average count is, say, 10,000 WBCs/ml for 6 months and then suddenly it starts to climb to 20–30–40–50,000 WBCs/ml, this is usually followed by acute symptomatology of pyelonephritis. I wonder if Dr. *White* is looking at the urine WBC count in his children?

Dr. *R. White*: All our own patients get WBC counts on random clinical specimens in terms of WBCs/ml. We have less tight control over about 45% of the patients which are under the care of outside clinicians, and I cannot vouch for this group. To ensure absolute accuracy that would enormously increase the organization.

Dr. *J. Hodson*: I don't think people who haven't been involved in these complex surveys understand what it is to add in something new. The organizers are so bogged down already with complexities and getting everybody to conform, the last thing they want is some disturbing or revolutionary new idea.

There followed a discussion in which a number of items, such as: urine concentration test; a 1-desamino-8D arginine vasopressin (DDAVP)-induced concentration test; concentration tests combined with ureteral compression to give results for each kidney; the value of urinary leukocyte excretion rates; estimation of radiographic renal area by planimetry, which relates closely to glomerular filtration rate (GFR), and finally radionuclide cystography and parenchymal imaging.

It was accepted that perhaps a properly conducted concentration capacity test was at present the *most sensitive indication of early renal damage* in children of a cooperative age. But, whether combined with DDAVP, or reciprocal single ureteral compression, or carried out without such aids, its results are subject to a high degree of compliance on the part of the child, parents, nursing staff, etc. Furthermore, it was not applicable to the younger age groups but could be used to estimate progress in ongoing studies if its applications could be adequately controlled. Like all these tests it took time to perform properly, and active UTI precluded its use. Dr. *Winberg*, in particular, sounded dubious about its practicality on a large scale involving several different centers.

The concensus was that the imaging modality which appeared to hold out most promise was nuclear medicine, as physiologic, real-time cystography could be combined with cystometry on the one hand, and focal disease identified by dimercaptosuccinic acid (DMSA), glucoheptonate, or gallium scans (in the case of active inflammatory disease) on the other, and function by hippiurate or ^{51}Cr-EDTA. Their practicality was another thing, but at least subjective human factors were largely eliminated.

The question of radiation exposure was raised, and it was pointed out that radionuclide studies were likely to involve less radiation than the usual radiographic techniques.

It was also reemphasized that whereas most studies to date were based on traditional radiographic techniques, no convicing data were available about their reliability. Drs. *Conway* and *Hodson* were both convinced of the unreliability of the micturating cystourethrogram, as the results depended on too many variable factors, both human and technical, for it to provide a reliable basis for grading VUR. The intravenous urogram was also notoriously unreliable with regard to the quality of images obtainable in any but the most carefully controlled situations and this unreliability increased inversely with the age of the patient unless the three basic criteria: (1) visible nephrograms, (2) distinct renal outlines, (3) complete calicine filling (obtainable across the board only by the use of effective ureteral compression), could be achieved regularly. Neither could a recent acute lesion be excluded, nor progressive scarring be measured with any degree of accuracy. These old modalities have served their turn but appear now to be superceded in every respect but one, by isotope techniques. The exception might be the baby in whom adequate imaging with the latter was often partly negated by movement.

It was concluded that a turning point had been reached in the realm of technical definition, which promised to put both diagnosis and follow-up on a new basis of accuracy.

Section V: Pressure, Voiding Dysfunction and Treatment

Contr. Nephrol., vol. 39, pp. 190–210 (Karger, Basel 1984)

16. Bladder-Sphincter Dysfunction, Urinary Infection and Vesico-Ureteral Reflux with Special Reference to Cognitive Bladder Training

Jan D. van Gool[a], *Rene H. Kuitjen*[a], *Raymond A. Donckerwolcke*[a], *Anton P. Messer*[b], *Marianne Vijverberg*[b]

[a]Department of Paediatric Nephrology and [b]Department of Child Psychology, University Children's Hospital, Het Wilhelmina Kinderziekenhuis, Utrecht, The Netherlands

Introduction

Overactivity of both bladder and striated urethral muscles is an established cause for bladder-sphincter dysfunction in children [62]. This overactivity is usually associated with dysfunctional symptoms like urgency, frequency and daytime wetting, and with urinary tract infections (UTI) – with or without vesico-ureteral reflux (VUR) [1, 3, 13, 18, 28, 34, 39, 47]. The symptoms of over-activity-induced dysfunction and associated UTIs have been blamed in the past on either the bladder muscle or the urethral closure mechanism, resulting in two different concepts of diagnosis and treatment. Cystometric findings of uninhibited detrusor contractions (UDCs), in children with recurrent UTIs and symptoms like urgency and daytime wetting, were variously interpreted as 'persistent infantile bladder' [37], 'occult neuropathic bladder' [27, 44, 68], 'isolated neurogenic bladder' [31] or 'subclinical neurogenic bladder' [9]. Treatment accordingly consisted of rehabilitation programmes and anticholinergic drugs. Cystoscopy and voiding cystourethrography (VCU), on the other hand, revealed abnormalities labelled as 'wide bladder neck anomaly' or 'spinning top urethra' [46, 58], 'distal urethral stenosis' [38], 'external sphincter spasticity' [60], 'sphincter hyperkinesia' [45], or 'sphincter dyssynergia' [41], popularizing the concept of urethral dysfunction, and thus of urethral dilatation or urethrotomy as treatment modalities [17, 24, 32].

Table I. Diagnostic labels used in neurologically normal children with bladder-sphincter dysfunction

Bladder outlet	
	Wide bladder neck anomaly [46, 58]
	Distal urethral stenosis [38]
	External sphincter spasticity [60]
	Striated urethral sphincter hyperkinesia [45]
	Vesical sphincter dyssynergia [41]
	Non-neurogenic neurogenic bladder [1]
	Dysfunctional voiding [2, 3]
	Hypertonic internal sphincter [12, 56]
	Internal sphincter dyssynergia [12, 56]
	Hyperactive external sphincter/pelvic floor [12, 13, 56]
	Urethral over-activity [13, 16]
Detrusor	
	Uninhibited paediatric bladder [12, 37, 56]
	Persistent infantile bladder [37]
	Occult neuropathic bladder [27, 44, 68]
	Isolated neurogenic bladder [31]
	Subclinical neurogenic bladder [9]
	Non-neurogenic neurogenic bladder [1]
	Detrusor hyperactivity [13]
	Hypertonic detrusor [12, 56]
	Unstable bladder [5, 62]
	Detrusor over-activity [13, 16]

Urodynamic Investigation Findings

The Two Main Patterns of Dysfunction

Urodynamic studies designed to show the interaction between bladder and sphincter by simultaneous registration of bladder pressure and sphincter EMG activity at first only added still more labels to the two controversial concepts (table I), thus widening the range of therapeutic implications [12, 42, 56]. But recent reviews [2, 5, 20, 35] now support the idea that most labels can be brought down to two patterns of bladder-sphincter over-activity (with or without bladder symptoms). In one pattern, strong UDCs starting early in the filling phase are counteracted by sphincter contractions and hold-manoeuvres, like heel squatting, to prevent premature voiding. In the other pattern, incomplete relaxation of striated urethral and pelvic floor muscles interrupts the voiding act, causing a staccato urinary flow.

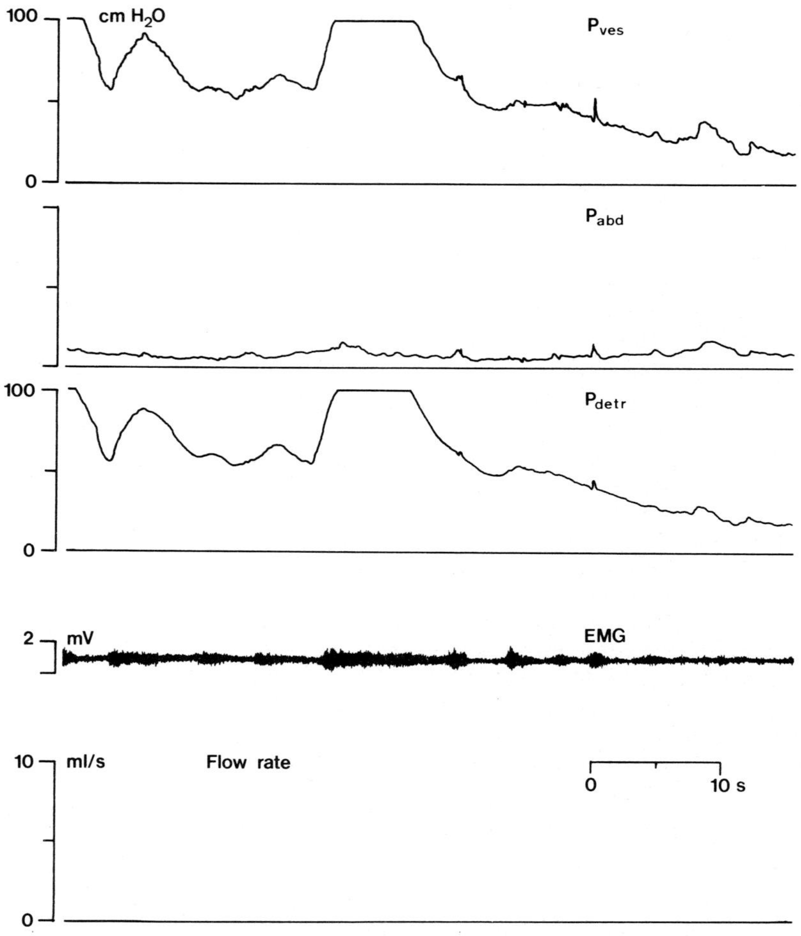

1a

Fig. 1. a 3-week-old male with uncomplicated UTI. Recording of the end of bladder filling phase showing sphincter over-activity 1 week after the UTI had been cured. Simultaneous pictorial recording of cysto-urethrogram (70 mm film) and digital print-out of bladder pressure seen in *b*. Pressure of 213 cm H_2O. Peak pressures are not recorded on tracing as they top the scale used. Marked frequency was present, 'dry' intervals lasting only 30 min or less [40]. VUR was absent. Bladder pressure = recorded intravesical minus abdominal pressures.

Both patterns, with the bladder working against a forcefully closed urethra, generate exceptionally high bladder pressures – during bladder filling, during bladder emptying, or both – which can be transmitted directly to both kidney pelvis and parenchyma in the presence of VUR [3, 15, 23, 34] and uretheral dilatation.

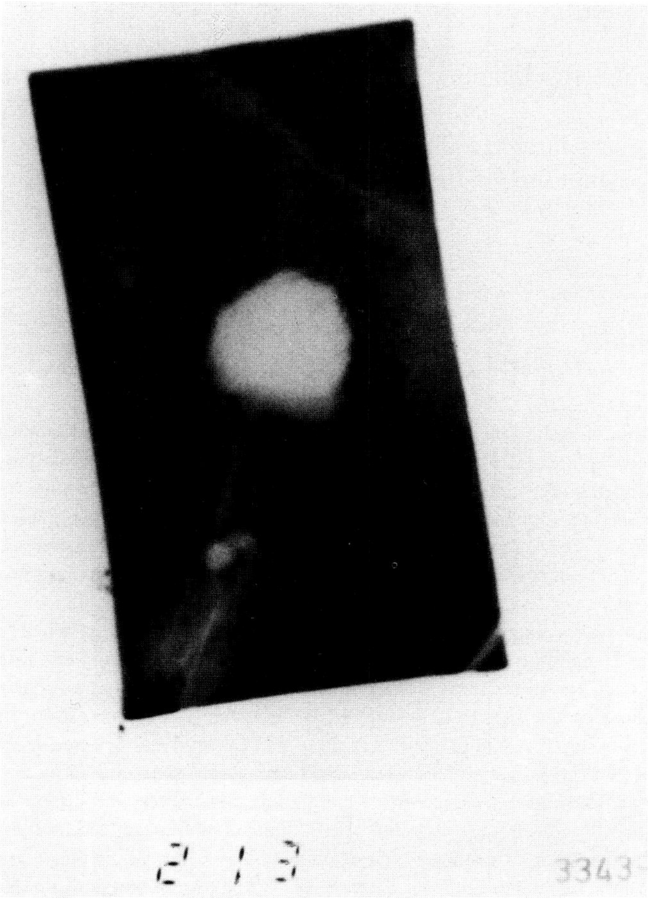

1b

It has been demonstrated that bladder-sphincter over-activity can be induced by UTI. Symptoms like urgency and frequency vary with the degree of over-activity during and after UTI, and in a proportion of children with recurrent UTIs both over-activity and symptoms of dysfunction tend to persist between recurrences [13, 48]. Figure 1a illustrates these findings in an infant with uncomplicated UTI, and surely constitutes a strong argument for incorporation of bladder pressure registration in the radiological workup of every child with symptomatic UTI (fig. 1b).

UTI and high bladder pressure, occurring in association with bladder-sphincter over-activity, play an increasingly well-documented role in the pathogenesis of reflux nephropathy (RN) [3, 15, 34]. As the patterns of bladder-sphincter over-activity are detectable with urodynamic techniques, and as several effective treatment modalities for such dysfunction are available [18, 22, 41, 42, 57, 65], we decided to investigate prospectively a selected group of school-age children, with persistent daytime wetting as the presenting symptom.

Patients and Method

In our children's hospital, the Departments of Paediatric Nephrology and Child Psychology combined their experiences – with intensive training for nocturnal enuresis [43] together with paediatric urodynamics – to meet the urgent demands for treatment of daytime wetting. 37 children (ages ranging from 5 to 14 years) have been followed to date for more than 1 year. The children were referred to our training programme for daytime wetting because of failure of previous treatment, and as such the group was selected by the presenting symptom of persistent daytime wetting.

For every child a documented history of UTI was available; all the children had had full uroradiological investigations (intravenous urography, IVU, and VCU), and these investigations were made available for review. Our part of the comprehensive evaluation consisted of (1) full psychological interviews with both children and parents, (2) elaborate history-taking with emphasis on voiding habits and reactions to urge, and (3) urodynamic studies.

Each urodynamic investigation comprises simultaneous recording of bladder pressure, rectal pressure, electromyographical activity of external anal sphincter, and urine flow rate when voiding occurs. Recordings are repeated several times, both during bladder filling and emptying, without anaesthesia or sedation. At or near the end of the filling phase the child (if of suitable age) is asked to change from a supine to a sitting or standing position to detect detrusor instability; bladder emptying is recorded with the child in the appropriate voiding position. Rectal pressure is substracted electronically from bladder pressure, to differentiate true detrusor acitivity from the effects of abdominal straining. One single infant feeding tube (Ch 04) is used as a catheter both to fill the bladder and to measure its pressure. The pressure gradient created by filling through gravity is measured between two pressure transducers and compensated electronically: this feature enables us to record all events continuously, without having to ask the child to interrupt the important transition phase between filling and voiding [13, 15].

The training programme for diurnal enuresis was based on three principles: (1) the children (re)learned to concentrate on the first sensation of urge by means of a modified enuresis alarm; (2) a cognitive element was provided by registration of urine flow rate and voided volume of each micturition (recording could be done by the children themselves) and (3) the flow rate registration served as a feedback mechanism, indispensable in any training programme. The children are trained in the hospital during a 7-day period, in pairs, to add an element of competition. During follow-up they keep their own records, and they have to phone in the results at regular intervals to the training person, who plays a crucial role in the whole programme, from history-taking to follow-up.

Table II. Enuresis diurna in 14 boys and 3 girls without bladder-sphincter over-activity; mean age at investigation 8.0 years (5–12 years)

Urge: imperative	2/17
Daytime voiding: 'frequency'	unclear
Enuresis nocturna	16/17
UTI	0/17
Radiological abnormalities:	
Wide proximal urethra	0/17
VUR	0/17
Bladder wall trabeculation	0/17
Urodynamic findings	
Urethral over-activity during voiding	0/17
EP_{max} during voiding (range 25–130, n = 20)	49 cm H_20
Detrusor over-activity during filling	4/17
EP_{max} during filling (range 25–140, n = 15)	43 cm H_20
Behavioural problems	
Hyperkinetic, impulsive	9/17
Special schooling programme	8/17
Custodial care	2/17
Encopresis	6/17
Results cognitive training, 1-year follow-up	
100% success	8/17
50% success	5/17
Failure	4/17 (23%)

Results

Based on our comprehensive evaluation of this selected group of children, two categories with daytime wetting emerge, distinctly different in many aspects (tables II, III).

The 'Avoider' Category: An Unsatisfactory Outlook, and Negative Workup:

Those belonging to the category summarized in table II were termed 'avoiders': 14 boys and 3 girls ignored sensations of urge, or even denied them on questioning; and in all of them behavioural problems were a consistent feature, reflected by the high incidence of the need for special schooling. In this category daytime wetting, nighttime wetting and sometimes encopresis were addressed as specific problems, but turned out to be part of a reactive behaviour, possibly originated by maladaption to toilet training.

Table III. Enuresis diurna with urethral over-activity and/or detrusor over-activity in 20 girls; mean age at investigation 8.0 years (4–10 years)

Urge: imperative, 'urgency'	20/20
Daytime voiding: 'frequency'	14/20
Enuresis nocturna	12/20
Recurrent UTIs	20/20
Radiological abnormalities	
Wide proximal urethra	12/20
VUR	9/20
Bladder wall trabeculation	7/20
Urodynamic findings	
Urethral over-activity during voiding	10/20
EP_{max} during voiding (range 30–70, n = 17)	64 cm H_20
Detrusor instability during filling	15/20
EP_{max} during filling (range 20–50, n = 4)	77 cm H_20
Behavioural problems	
Hyperkinetic, impulsive	0/20
Special schooling programme	0/20
Custodial care	0/20
Encopresis	1/20
Results cognitive training, 1-year follow-up	
100% success	18/20
50% success	1/20
Failure	1/20 (5%)

UTI in this category was conspicuously absent, as were abnormalities in the radiological assessment (IVUs and VCUs). 1 boy had had cystoscopy and urethral dilatation.

With urodynamic investigation *no abnormal findings could be recorded*, apart from mild detrusor over-activity during bladder filling in 4 children. During voiding, values for bladder pressure and flow rate were normal, as were flow patterns. The mean percentage difference between measured values for cystometric bladder capacity and calculated normal values for age [21] was −45%.

The failure rate of the training programme, after a 1-year follow-up period, was high (23%), and the effect of intensive training depended heav-

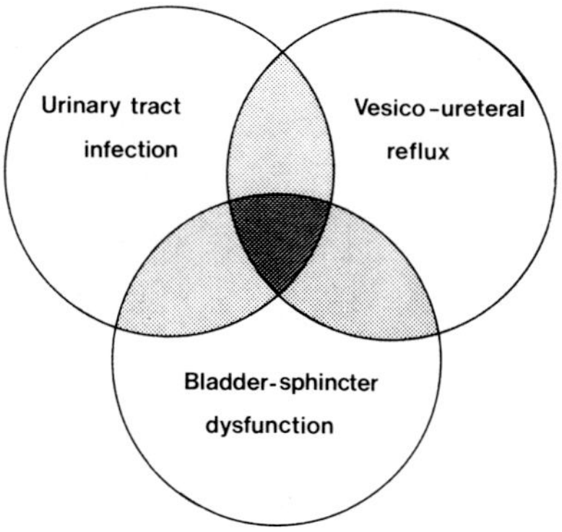

Fig. 2. Venn diagram showing the associations between UTI, VUR and bladder-sphincter dysfunction. The hatched areas are not proportional to real prevalences. The darkest area – high bladder pressures in the presence of VUR and UTI – represents children at risk of developing RN.

ily on the child's personality and his or her ability to cope with emotional stress – the children in this category tended to avoid emotional stress, either by acting out and being over impulsive, or by withdrawing from social contacts and being over-sensitive.

The 'Positive' Category: Positive Cultures, Positive Workups, Positive Attitude, and Positive Results to Therapy

20 children – all of them girls – were placed in the second category, which is summarized in table III. Behavioural problems were absent, both at home and at school. Children and parents alike were highly motivated to get help for their specific problem: persistent daytime wetting interfered continuously with everyday life, and in 4 children this had caused secondary behavioural idiosyncrasies, like elaborate camouflaging or adaptive behaviour to social rejection.

Every child in this category had a documented history of recurrent UTI; 9 girls had had cystoscopy with urethral dilatation or urethrotomy. Of 24 IVUs reviewed only 1 had signs of RN. The most important findings on review of the 22 VCUs were a wide proximal urethra during voiding (60%), an irregular contour of the bladder wall (35%) and VUR grades II–III (45%). Due to differences in technique, exact grading of VUR proved impossible. 4 girls had had surgical correction of VUR.

All the children complained of imperative urge, often described as a painful sensation, felt several times at short intervals just prior to voiding,

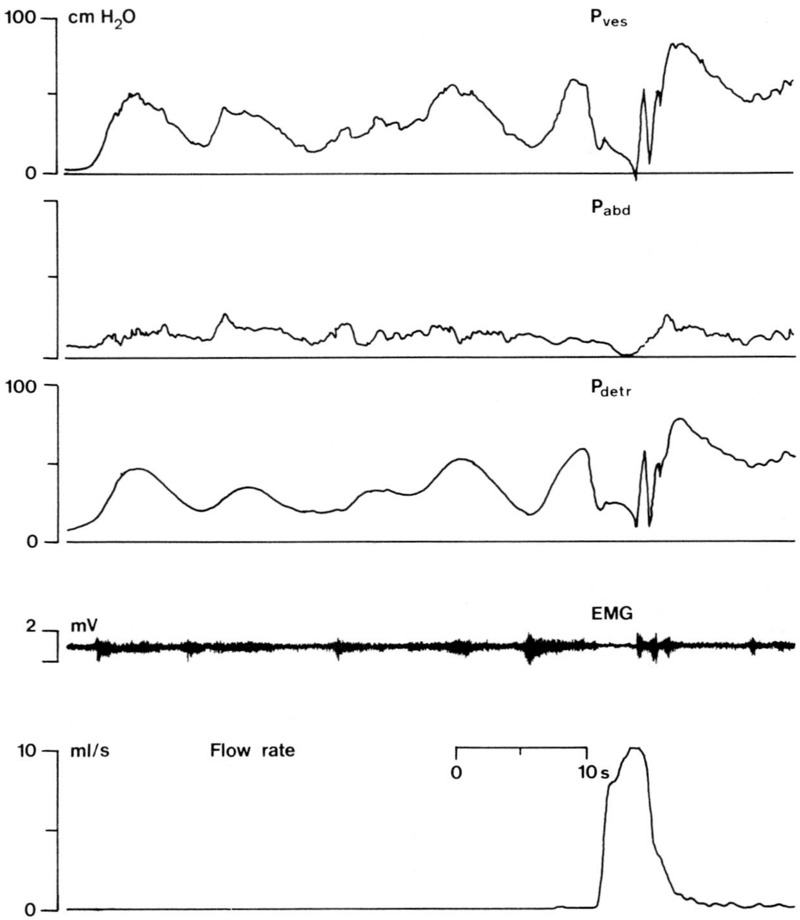

Fig. 3. Urgency: detrusor over-activity, countered with pelvic floor contractions (EMG). 5-year-old girl with recurrent UTI and secondary diurnal enuresis. Detrusor contractions started at bladder volumes of 45 ml and voiding is prevented by forceful contractions of the pelvic floor. High bladder pressures, both before and after actual voiding, are the result. Frequency is reflected in the small cystometric capacity of the bladder, and each time this capacity is reached, the recorded events start again.

and all were unable to reach a suitable place to void without wetting their pants. Wetting was generally worse in the afternoon while, during the morning, most children could cope with the desire to void. None of the children could inhibit the bladder in a normal way: they all tried to hold back by forceful contraction of their pelvic floor muscles, with such concentration that all other activities had to be interrupted. 7 children used to apply extra compression to the bladder outlet by squatting down on one heel (curtsey sign) [11, 29, 63].

A 'Filling' Abnormality

The urodynamic pattern of detrusor overactivity with opposing pelvic floor contractions and correlating with urgency in 15 children, is illustrated in figure 3. Detrusor contractions start early in the filling phase, and each time the child tries to prevent voiding by pelvic floor contraction, very high bladder pressures result. During voiding, bladder pressures and urine flow rate are normal, striated pelvic floor and urethral muscles relax completely, and urine flow is not interrupted. Once complete, the act is immediately followed by another series of strong detrusor contractions which are synchronous with pelvic floor contractions and indicate that voiding *has been stopped prematurely*. In some children a complete voiding act takes two or three small voids one after the other. Mean percentage difference between measured values of bladder capacity and calculated normal values for age [21] was −52%.

An 'Emptying' Abnormality

In 10 of the 20 children multiple interruptions of the urinary stream during voiding were a constant finding in 4 with, and in 6 without, signs of detrusor over-activity. Urine flow was interrupted by short staccato bursts of activity of striated pelvic floor and urethral muscles (fig. 4) which coincided with peaks in bladder pressure. If the short bursts of muscle activity were strong enough, the bladder muscle contracted momentarily against a completely closed urethra, so generating peaks of high pressure during voiding, and forcing the proximal urethra to dilate ('wide bladder neck anomaly', 'spinning top urethra'). Similar events in the filling phase seemed less disturbing, because they served to prevent voiding.

This latter category of bladder-sphincter over-activity and dysfunction responded surprisingly well to cognitive training: the failure rate after 1 year follow-up was 5% (table III). The children learned to concentrate on the sensation of urge, and to use conscious inhibition of detrusor activity instead of the typical hold-manoeuvres; they also learned to relax their pelvic floor muscles during voiding. Recording the urine flow rate proved to be a most effective feedback mechanism in the training process which most children could appreciate, and it provided a data base for progress records.

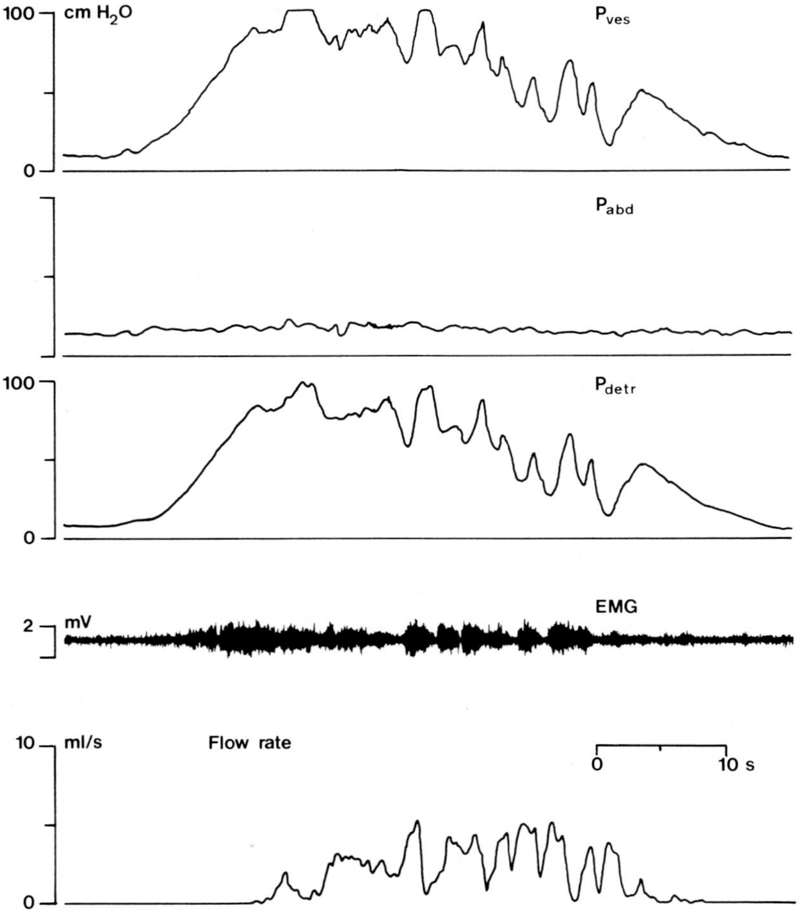

Fig. 4. 'Dyssynergic' voiding: short bursts of over-activity (EMG) of striated urethral and pelvic floor muscles can interrupt urine flow. Steep rises in bladder pressure coincide with interruptions of urine flow during each act of micturition in a 6-year-old girl with long-standing urgency, recurrent UTI, and secondary diurnal enuresis.

In the 2 girls who failed to remain dry, relapse was due to recurrences of UTI. None of the remaining 18 girls have had recurrences of their UTIs so far. After completing the training chemoprophylaxis was discontinued in all of them, often after years of symptomatic UTI and antibiotic treatment regimes.

Discussion

The pattern with bladder-sphincter *over-activity during filling* is probably best described with terms like 'detrusor over-activity' or 'detrusor instability' [5, 26, 62] – the (over)activity of the urethral closure mechanism is secondary to contractions of the unstable detrusor. The terms 'hyper-reflexive bladder' [40] and 'uninhibited bladder' [34, 56] imply a neurological cause for what is registered urodynamically, and should be reserved only to denote true neurogenic bladder dysfunction [25]. Terms like 'hypertonic bladder' [56] denote a property of the bladder wall: a hypertonic bladder may be overactive, underactive, or have normal activity.

Most authors agree on the very high prevalence of detrusor instability in toddlers and young children, and incomplete voluntary control over the voiding reflex is thought to be the basis for this age-dependent finding [5, 35]. As soon as central control of the voiding reflex has been developed a child learns how to postpone voiding without counteracting detrusor contractions with the voluntary activity of striated muscles [4, 69]. Rigorous toilet training – a culture-dependent element [64] – can interfere with this learning process and may lead to the persistence of detrusor instability with the symptoms mentioned above. Although detrusor instability is associated with abnormally high bladder pressures, the presence of UDCs on their own do not seem to have grave pathophysiological consequences. However, when UTI complicates the learning process, bladder-sphincter over-activity is reinduced and reinforced. Exteroceptive stimuli from the inflamed bladder wall then cause extreme detrusor instability, while the child will try to prevent voiding with forceful pelvic floor contractions for fear of both dysuria, and of getting wet again. In a proportion of children with recurrent UTIs, detrusor instability and dysfunctional symptoms persist between actual UTIs [13, 15], aided by the development of detrusor hypertrophy [18].

Although this pattern was thought to produce results similar to obstructive uropathy by generating high bladder pressures many times a day over periods of months or years, recent studies fail to corroborate this. No statistically significant positive correlation was found between detrusor instability and (bilateral) upper tract deformities [16]. Nor could a significant negative correlation be demonstrated between detrusor instability and resolution of VUR [61]. This indicates that in the pathophysiology of VUR and RN other factors than simply bladder pressure are involved in order to transmit it to the renal pelvis and on into the renal papillae and collecting tubules.

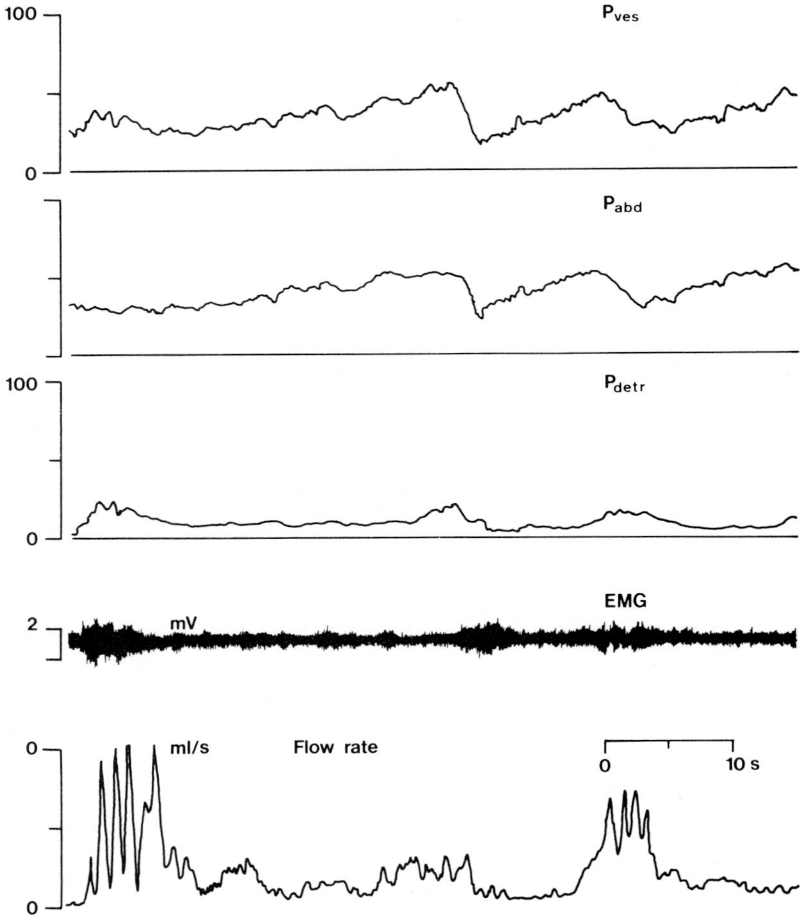

Fig. 5. Straining may mimick 'dyssynergic' voiding: without abdominal pressure recording these pressure/flow tracings would have been mistaken for bladder-sphincter dysfunction during voiding. The recording was made during urodynamic investigation of a 6-year-old girl with diurnal and nocturnal enuresis, who tried to comply with every parental demand to void.

The pattern of bladder-sphincter over-activity *during voiding* is urodynamically indistinguishable from detrusor-sphincter dyssynergia in true neurogenic bladder dysfunction. This explains the widespread use of terms like 'dyssynergic voiding' or 'striated sphincter spasticity', and 'non-neurogenic neurogenic bladder'. This pattern, and its resemblance to true neurogenic dyssynergia, were first described in 1967 by *Scott* et al. [54], and it is now widely felt that the word 'dyssynergia' should be reserved for hyper-reflexive striated urethral muscles during micturition in patients with organic neurogenic bladder dysfunction [8, 26, 55]. For such dysfunction during voiding, in children who are normal neurologically, we prefer the term 'urethral over-activity' [15, 16] as the striated muscles of urethra and pelvic floor contract periodically during micturition, instead of showing complete relaxation (fig. 5). This urethral over-activity may or may not occur with detrusor instability. Although it is tempting to regard both patterns as parts of a continuum [2, 15, 20], analogous with neurogenic bladder dysfunction, at least one recent study failed to demonstrate a statistically significant correlation between the two patterns in a group of children similar to ours [16].

Clinically there are many similarities, however, as both detrusor instability and urethral over-activity in children can correlate with urgency, frequency and daytime wetting, and with UTI. In our material we did not find the association with emotional disturbances and psychosocial problems, originally described in children with so-called 'non-neurogenic neurogenic bladders' [1]. Behavioural problems in our category with bladder-sphincter dysfunction (table III) were clearly secondary, and were adaptive reactions to minor degrees of social rejection, while in the children categorized as 'avoiders' (table II) no abnormalities in bladder-sphincter function were detected, apart from occasional effects of straining in the child who tries to comply with demands to void (fig. 5), and mild detrusor over-activity.

The peaks of high bladder pressures generated by sudden isometric episodes in detrusor activity during voiding in children with urethral over-activity create a waterhammer effect in the refluxing upper tract, and in all available studies this pattern of bladder-sphincter over-activity has a statistically significant correlation with RN, both in children [2, 5, 16, 20, 35] and in adults [10, 30, 33, 36, 51, 52, 67].

Prevalence

Differences in the recorded prevalence of urethral over-activity in children are in part the result of selection of the patient material in the various studies and in part of differences in urodynamic techniques [14, 66]. Exteroceptive stimuli applied to the very sensitive zone of urethral mucosa, directly overlying the urethral sphincter area, will always elicit reflex activity in pelvic floor muscles. Such stimulation is likely to occur when occluding-type catheters are placed transurethrally to measure pressure in bladder or urethra. Normal proprioceptive stimuli, such as flow turbulence, will also trigger contractions of urethral and pelvic floor muscles when the sensitivity of the urethral mucosa is increased by UTI [13, 60]. In our study, urethral over-activity could always be confirmed by numerous non-invasive flow-rate recordings made during the training programme.

Relationship to Experimental Work in Animals

A number of assumptions have been made by stating that bladder pressure is transmitted to the renal pelvis and papillae in the presence of VUR. First of all, experimental work on pyelotubular backflow suggests that there is a threshold value for the pressure with which urine is forced back into the collecting tubules in intrarenal reflux (IRR) [50]. This threshold is usually determined with static pressures rising stepwise, and little is known about the effect on threshold values and IRR of steep and fast pressure rises – as found in urethral over-activity, and to a lesser extent in detrusor instability. Secondly, changes in papillary morphology during infancy and childhood have to be taken into account [49, 59], as well as the influence of bladder wall stress and bladder pressure on ureterovesical resistance to flow [7]. And thirdly, as a conduit for retrograde flow and pressure transmission a strongly muscular ureter must obviously differ in physical properties from a thin-walled dilated ureter.

Results of Treatment

The excellent results of cognitive training in the 20 children with bladder-sphincter dysfunction indicate that both detrusor instability and urethral over-activity result to a certain extent from incorrect learning processes which are acutely aggravated by UTI. Both the cognitive element and the feedback of the training programme serve to reorientate children with disturbed voiding habits. The fact that nocturnal wetting, occurring in 12 of the 20 children with bladder-sphincter dysfunction, resolved spontaneously after training for daytime wetting, may illustrate this.

At the start of the training programme for diurnal enuresis, a disproportionate number of children turned out to be 'avoiders', and this may give a false impression of the prevalence of children with daytime wetting due to behavioural problems versus bladder-sphincter dysfunction (tables II, III). In the available epidemiological studies, children with behavioural problems and wetting are relatively rare. The predominance of girls in the category with bladder-sphincter dysfunction is the same in our material as in larger, less selective, populations [6, 53].

Table IV. Checklist for detection of bladder-sphincter over-activity in school-age children with daytime wetting

		yes 1	unclear 2	no 3
Daytime wetting				
Damp pants only	1.1	•		
Pants soaking wet	1.2			•
Normal early morning voiding	1.3	•		
Wetting, in afternoons especially	1.4	•		
Wetting throughout the day	1.5			•
How many times per day	1.6	0–1	1–2	>2
Nighttime wetting				
Damp bedsheet only	2.1	•		
Bedsheets soaking wet	2.2			•
Wetting early in the night	2.3			•
Wetting throughout the night	2.4	•		
Waking up at night to void	2.5	•		
Hard to wake up to make void	2.6			•
Micturition				
Daytime voiding frequency	3.1	1–4	4–7	>7 •
Voiding sloppy, stopped too soon	3.2		•	
Straining during voiding	3.3		•	
Interrupted or staccato urine flow	3.4	•		
Two or more voidings per time	3.5	•		
Pain associated with voiding	3.6	•		
Urge and reactions on urge				
Urge is imperative and immediate	4.1	•		
Hold manoeuvre successful	4.2			•
Two or more times urge prior to voiding	4.3	•		
Squatting or squeezing on urge	4.4	•		
Urge felt but ignored	4.5			•
Urge suppressed	4.6			•
Pain felt prior to voiding	4.7	•		
Behavioural problems				
Excessively sensitive, withdrawn	5.1			•
Excessively impulsive, hyperkinetic	5.2			•
Special school, remedial teaching	5.3			•
Custodial care	5.4			•
Encopresis	5.5		•	
Techniques for camouflage	5.6	•		
Adaptation problems (family, school)	5.7	•		
Secondary social isolation	5.8	•		

Pattern Detection by History Taking

Based on our comprehensive evaluation of 37 children with daytime wetting a checklist has been developed based on a simple, accurate, history-taking, which will provide a simple method for detecting the patterns of bladder-sphincter over-activity, and will help to avoid unnecessary more complex studies in children with enuresis (table IV). Only a proportion of children with bladder-sphincter over-activity will have dysfunctional symptoms like urgency and wetting, depending on the amount of motivation they can muster to remain dry during the day.

A checklist to detect urethral over-activity or detrusor instability can be very helpful as a means of assessment of bladder function in the diagnosis and management of VUR [19]. In children with bladder-sphincter dysfunction surgical correction of VUR meets with a high incidence of complications, whereas its detection may help to find the correct indications for antireflux surgery. Cognitive bladder training may prove an important tool in the conservational management of children with VUR. High bladder pressures of this aetiology will then no longer contribute to the pathogenesis of RN, once the underlying dysfunction is corrected.

Conclusions

Continuous recording of urodynamic parameters over 12- or 24-hour periods in infants and toddlers with uncomplicated UTI is required fully to elucidate its role in the aetiology of bladder-sphincter dysfunction which, in the presence of VUR at this age, carries the highest risk for future development of RN.

Despite the fact that the transmission of bladder pressure in the presence of VUR to the upper urinary tract and into the kidney is not a straightforward affair, much more can be learned about this whole process from simultaneously conducted bladder pressure readings and radiographic documentation.

Detection of bladder-sphincter over-activity rather than dysfunction seems essential in children with VUR, because of the contribution of high bladder pressures to the pathogenesis of kidney damage, and because of the possible beneficial role of cognitive bladder training in the management of VUR.

References

1 Allen, T.D.: The non-neurogenic bladder. J. Urol. *117*: 232–238 (1977).

2 Allen, T.D.; Bright, T.C.: Urodynamic patterns in children with dysfunctional voiding problems. J. Urol. *119*: 247–249 (1978).

3 Allen, T.D.: Vesicoureteral reflux as a manifestation of dysfunctional voiding; in Hodson, Kincaid-Smith, Reflux nephropathy (Masson, New York 1979).

4 Apley, J.; McKeith, R.: The child and his symptoms (Blackwell, Oxford 1962).

5 Bauer, S.B.; Retik, A.B.; Colodny, A.H.; Hallett, M.; Khoshbin, S.; Dyro, F.M.: The unstable bladder of childhood. Urol. Clins N. Am. *7*: 321–336 (1980).

6 Berg, I.; Fielding, D.; Meadow, R.: Psychiatric disturbance, urgency, and bacteriuria in children with day and night wetting. Archs Dis. Childh. *52*: 651–657 (1977).

7 Coolsaet, B.L.R.A.; Vanrooij, G.E.P.M. van; Blok, C.: Detrusor pressure versus bladder wall stress in relation to ureterovesical resistance. Neurourol. Urodyn. *1*: 105–112 (1982).

8 Diokno, A.C.; Koff, S.A.; Hender, L.F.: Periurethral striated muscle activity in neurogenic bladder dysfunction. J. Urol. *112*: 743–749 (1974).

9 Dorfman, L.E.; Bailey, J.; Smith, J.P.: Subclinical neurogenic bladder in children. J. Urol. *101*: 48–54 (1969).

10 Farrar, D.J.; Osborne, J.L.; Stephenson, T.P.; Whiteside, C.G.; Weir, J.; Berry, J.; Milroy, E.J.G.; Turner Warwick, R.: A urodynamic view of bladder outflow obstruction in the female: factors influencing the results of treatment. Br. J. Urol. *47*: 815–822 (1976).

11 Fielding, D.; Berg, I.; Bell, S.: An observational study of postures and limb movements of children who wet by day and at night. Devl Med. Child Neur. *20*: 453–461 (1978).

12 Firlit, C.F.; Smey, P.; King, L.R.: Micturition urodynamic flow studies in children. J. Urol. *119*: 250–253 (1978).

13 Gool, J.D. van; Tanagho, E.A.: External sphincter activity and recurrent urinary tract infection in girls. Urology *10*: 348–353 (1977).

14 Gool, J.D. van; Schmidt, R.A.; Tanagho, E.A.: Development of reflex activity of detrusor and striated sphincter muscles in experimental paraplegia. Urol. int. *33*: 293–303 (1978).

15 Gool, J.D. van: Bladder infection and pressure; in Hodson, Kincaid-Smith, Reflux nephropathy (Masson, New York 1979).

16 Griffiths, D.J.; Scholtmeijer, R.J.: 'Detrusor-sphincter dyssynergia' in neurologically normal children. Neurourol. Urodyn. *2* (in press, 1983).

17 Hendry, W.F.; Stanton, S.L.; Williams, D.I.: Recurrent urinary infections in girls: effects of urethral dilatation. Br. J. Urol. *45*: 72–83 (1973).

18 Hinman, F., Jr.; Baumann, F.W.: Vesical and ureteral damage from voiding dysfunction in boys without neurologic or obstructive disease. J. Urol. *109*: 727–732 (1973).

19 Hinman, F., Jr.; Baumann, F.W.: Complications of vesicoureteral operations from incoordination of micturition. J. Urol. *116*: 638–643 (1976).

20 Hinman, F., Jr.: Syndromes of vesical incoordination. Urol. Clins N. Am. *7*: 311–320 (1980).

21 Hjalmas, K.: Micturition in infants and children with normal lower urinary tract. A urodynamic study. Scand. J. Urol. Nephrol. *11*: suppl. 37, pp. 1–106 (1977).

22 Hjalmas, K.; Hellstrom, A.L.: Habilitation of dysfunctional bladder in children. Proc. Int. Continence Soc. (1981).

23 Hutch, J.A.; Miller, E.R.; Hinman, F., Jr.: Vesicoureteral reflux. Am. J. Med. *34*: 338–349 (1963).
24 Immergut, M.A.; Gilbert, E.C.: Internal urethrotomy in recurring urinary tract infection in girls. J. Urol. *109*: 126–127 (1973).
25 International Continence Society: First, second and third reports on the standardization of terminology of lower urinary tract function. J. Urol. *121*: 551–554 (1979).
26 International Continence Society: Fourth report on the standardization of terminology of lower urinary tract function – terminology related to neuromuscular dysfunction of the lower urinary tract. Br. J. Urol. *53*: 333–335 (1981).
27 Johnston, J.H.; Farkas, A.: Congenital neuropathic bladder: practicalities and possibilities of conservational management. Urology *5*: 719–727 (1975).
28 Johnston, J.H.; Koff, S.A.; Glassberg, K.I.: The pseudo-obstructed bladder in enuretic children. Br. J. Urol. *50*: 505–510 (1978).
29 Jonge, G.A. de: The urge syndrome; in Kolvin, McKeith, Meadow, Bladder control and enuresis (Heinemann, London 1973).
30 Jorgensen, T.M.; Djurhuus, J.C.; Schroder, H.D.: Idiopathic detrusor-sphincter dyssynergia in neurologically normal patients with voiding abnormalities. Eur. Urol. *8*: 107–110 (1982).
31 Kahmi, B.; Horowitz, M.I.; Kovetz, A.: Isolated neurogenic dysfunction of the bladder in children with urinary tract infection. J. Urol. *106*: 151–153 (1971).
32 Kaplan, G; Sammons, T.A.; King, L.: A blind comparison of dilatation, urethrotomy, and medication alone in the treatment of urinary tract infections in girls. J. Urol. *109*: 917–919 (1973).
33 Kaplan, W.E.; Firlit, C.R.; Schoenberg, H.W.: The female urethra syndrome: external sphincter spasm as etiology. J. Urol. *124*: 48–49 (1980).
34 Koff, S.A.; Lapides, J.; Piazza, D.H: Association of urinary tract infection and reflux with uninhibited bladder contractions and voluntary sphincter obstruction. J. Urol. *122*: 373–376 (1979).
35 Koff, S.A.: Bladder-sphincter dysfunction in childhood. Urology *19*: 457–461 (1982).
36 Lapides, J.; Costello, R.T., Jr.: Uninhibited neurogenic bladder: a common cause for recurrent urinary tract infection in normal women. J. Urol. *101*: 539–544 (1969).
37 Lapides, J.; Diokno, A.C.: Persistence of the infant bladder as a cause for urinary infection in girls. J. Urol. *103*: 243–248 (1970).
38 Lyon, R.P.; Smith, D.R.: Distal urethral stenosis. J. Urol. *89*: 414–421 (1963).
39 Lyon, R.P.; Marshall, S.: Urinary tract infections and difficult urination in girls: long-term follow-up. J. Urol. *105*: 314–317
40 Mahony, D.T.; Laferte, R.O.; Blais, D.J.: Studies of enuresis. IX. Evidence of a mild form of compensated detrusor hyperreflexia in enuretic children. J. Urol. *126*: 520–523 (1981).
41 Maizels, M.; King, L.R.; Firlit, C.F.: Urodynamic feedback: a new approach to treat vesical sphincter dyssynergia. J. Urol. *122*: 205–209 (1979).
42 Mann, C.M.; Ellis, D.G.: Voiding abnormalities in children: methods of evaluation and results of treatment. J. pediat. Surg. *16*: 785–789 (1981).
43 Messer, A.P.: Zeer moeilijk eten en moeilijk beinvloedbaar bedplassen; thesis, Leiden (Swets & Zeitlinger, Lisse 1980).
44 Mix, L.W.: Occult neuropathic bladder. Urology *10*: 1–9 (1977).

45 Mulholland, S.G.; Yalla, S.V.; Raezu, D.M.; Duckett, J.W., Jr.: Primary external urethral sphincter hyperkinesia in a boy. Urology *4*: 577–580 (1974).

46 Murphy, J.J.; Schoenberg, H.W.; Tristan, T.A.: Diagnosis and management of lower urinary tract dysfunction in children. J. Urol. *89*: 192–197 (1963).

47 Nesbitt, R.E.: Urethrovesical malfunctions and urinary incontinence in female children and adolescents. Pediat. Clins N. Am. *19*: 705–716 (1972).

48 Randolph, M.F.; Mooris, K.E.: The first urinary tract infection in the female infant. J. Pediat. *65*: 57–66 (1964).

49 Ransley, P.G.; Risdon, R.A.: Renal papillary morphology in infants and young children. Urol. Res. *3*: 111–113 (1975).

50 Hodson, C.J.; Maling, T.M.J.; McManamon, P.J.; Lewis, M.G.: The pathogenesis of reflux nephropathy. Br. J. Radiol. suppl. 13 (1975).

51 RAZ, S.; Smith, R.B.: External sphincter spasticity syndrome in female patients. J. Urol. *115*: 443–446 (1976).

52 Rees, D.L.P.; Whitfield, H.N.; Islam, A.K.M.S.; Doyle, P.T.; Mayo, M.E.; Wickham, J.E.A.: Urodynamic findings in adult females with frequency and dysuria. Br. J. Urol. *47*: 853–860 (1975).

53 Schmitt, B.D.: Daytime wetting (diurnal enuresis). Pediat. Clins N. Am. *29*: 9–20 (1982).

54 Scott, F.B.; Quesada, E.M.; Cardus, D.: The use of combined uroflowmetry, cystometry and electromyography in evaluation of neurogenic bladder dysfunction; in Boyarsky, The neurogenic bladder (Williams & Wilkins, Baltimore 1967).

55 Siroky, M.B.; Krane, R.J.: Neurologic aspects of detrusor-sphincter dyssynergia, with references to the guarding reflex. J. Urol. *127*: 953–957 (1982).

56 Smey, P.; Firlit, C.F.; King, L.R.: Voiding pattern abnormalities in normal children: results of pharmacological manipulation. J. Urol. *120*: 574–577 (1978).

57 Stanton, S.L.; Cardosa, L.: The use of bio-feedback in the treatment of detrusor instability. Proc. Int. Continence Soc. (1978).

58 Stanton, L.; Williams, D.I.: The wide bladder neck in children. Br. J. Urol. *45*: 60–64 (1973).

59 Tamminen, T.E.; Kaprio, E.A.: The relation of the shape of the renal papillae and collecting duct openings to intrarenal reflux. Br. J. Urol. *49*: 345–354 (1977).

60 Tanagho, E.A.; Miller, E.R.; Lyon, R.P.; Fisher, R.: Spastic striated external sphincter and urinary tract infection in girls. Br. J. Urol. *43*: 69–82 (1971).

61 Taylor, G.M.: Unstable bladder activity and the rate of resolution of vesico-ureteric reflux (this volume).

62 Turner-Warwick, R.T.: Clinical problems associated with urodynamic abnormalities; in Lutzeyer, Melchoir, Urodynamics – upper and lower urinary tract (Springer, Berlin 1973).

63 Vincent, S.A.: Postural control of urinary incontinence: the curtsey sign. Lancet *ii*: 631–632 (1966).

64 Vries, M.W. de; Vries, M.R. de: Cultural relativity of toilet training readiness: perspective from East Africa. Pediatrics, Springfield *60*: 170–177 (1977).

65 Wear, J.B.; Wear, R.B.; Cleeland, C.: Biofeedback in urology using urodynamics: preliminary observations. J. Urol. *121*: 464–468 (1979).

66 Wein, A.; Barrett, D.M.: Etiologic possibilities for increased pelvic floor electromyography activity during cystometry. J. Urol. *127*: 949–952 (1982).

67 Whiteside, C.G.; Arnold, E.P.: Persistent primary enuresis: a urodynamic assessment. Br. med. J. *i*: 364–367 (1975).
68 Williams, D.I.; Hirst, G.; Doyle, D.: The occult neuropathic bladder. J. pediat. Surg. *9*: 35–41 (1975).
69 Yeates, W.K.: Bladder function in normal micturition; in Kolvin, McKeith, Meadow, Bladder control and enuresis (Heinemann, London 1973).

Jan D. van Gool, Department of Paediatric Nephrology, University Children's Hospital, Het Wilhelmina Kinderziekenhuis, Nieuwe Gracht 137, NL-3512 LK Utrecht (The Netherlands)

Contr. Nephrol., vol. 39, pp. 211–220 (Karger, Basel 1984)

17. The Uninhibited Bladder in Children: Effect of Treatment on Vesicoureteral Reflux Resolution

Stephen A. Koff, Daniel Murtagh

Section Pediatric Urology, Ohio State University, College of Medicine, Columbus, Ohio; University of Michigan Medical Center, Ann Arbor, Mich., USA

Introduction

In 1979 [1] we reported on the association of urinary tract infection (UTI) and vesicoureteral reflux (VUR) with uninhibited bladder contractions (UDC) in neurologically normal children, and hypothesised that UTI and VUR were manifestations of urinary tract obstruction which occurred during UDCs. Unfortunately, the data were insufficient to establish a causal relationship between UDCs and VUR, or to estimate the effect that treatment of the former would have on the progression or resolution of VUR. The following study evolved in an attempt further to examine this relationship and to determine whether the treatment of a purely urodynamic disorder could influence dysfunction of the ureterovesical junction causing VUR.

The pattern of bladder and sphincter dysfunction which accounts for obstruction during uninhibited contraction has been termed 'dyssynergia'. This means simply that the usual synergy between bladder contraction and sphincter relaxation is disrupted and instead there is simultaneous and pathologic constriction of the urinary sphincter muscles during bladder contraction. The obstruction which results is as severe and significant as an anatomic obstruction, and high intravesical pressures often exceeding a 150-cm H_2O have been documented [2]. It must be recognized that this type of dyssynergia is intimately related to 'toilet training' and to the development of urinary control in infancy. For the infant to develop the adult pattern of urinary control, at least three separate but related events must take place for the complete maturation of bladder form and function. First, the capacity of the bladder must increase in order for it to function as a satisfactory reservoir. Second, voluntary control over the striated muscle sphincter must occur to allow for decisive starting and stopping of micturition. Third, direct voluntary control over the spinal cord micturition reflex arc must occur for the child voluntarily to initiate or inhibit voiding at any degree of bladder filling.

By the age of 2–4 years most children have completed toilet training and have developed the adult pattern of urinary control. However, for unknown reasons some children fail to gain complete voluntary control over their micturition reflex arc. It is not clear whether this represents a failure of nerve maturation or a developmental regression, but it is not due to any form of neuropathy. As a result, whenever the bladder fills to a specific threshold volume it contracts just as it did throughout infancy. These contractions have been termed UDCs. In this report we will deal only with them and with the specific type of dyssynergia which they cause. These contractions are so common in infancy and childhood that they often are not considered an abnormality at all because they in fact represent the normal mechanism for infant voiding. Clearly if UDCs are viewed only as a pattern of bladder hyperactivity their pathologic features will be overlooked. The significance of UDCs *depends entirely on the child's voluntary response to them*. Once the child has passed through the age of toilet training and has learned the significance of continence, the only alternative to urinary leakage during a UDC is tight voluntary constriction of the urinary sphincter muscles. However, because the UDC is unsuppressable it results in simultaneous bladder and sphincter contraction or, in other words, dyssynergia. It must be emphasized that this type of obstruction occurs only during the bladder storage phase when the child is not voiding, because *this is the only time when true UDCs occur*. During voluntary voiding there will be no obstruction and urine may in fact proceed at increased flow rates because the normal reflex coordination between the bladder and sphincter is functioning properly. In addition, the fact that UDCs are normal and physiologic before the age of toilet training means that they may not be incriminated as a pathologic process accounting for urinary tract dysfunction in this age group.

Clinical Material

Having defined this specific urodynamic abnormality, we attempted to investigate its role in VUR and UTI in 1976 by beginning a prospective controlled study to compare the rates of VUR and UTI resolution in different subgroups of children. The patient population was composed of 62 children, 60 girls and 2 boys, who underwent a complete evaluation for recurrent UTI and in whom VUR was demonstrated radiographically at least 2 weeks after their UTI was eradicated. Their ages ranged between 2 and 14 years and *all were toilet trained prior to the development of UTIs*. The initial evaluation consisted of a history and physical examination, urinalysis and culture, voiding cystourethrogram (VCU), intravenous urogram (IVU) and cystoscopy. In addition all children underwent complete urodynamic studies, which included combined cystometry and periurethral striated muscle electromyography during bladder filling and, more recently, during bladder emptying according to previously described techniques [3, 4]. The follow-up evaluation consisted of clinical and urinary examinations performed at 3-monthly intervals. An IVU was done every other year and a VCU annually until VUR disappeared on two consecutive studies. Low dose antibiotic prophylaxis was prescribed for all children as long as their VUR persisted. The drugs used were furadantin or cotrimoxazole at 25–50% of their weight-adjusted recommended daily dose. Children were placed on a bowel program and treated for constipation, and were encouraged to void every 3 h while awake and to reduce their fluid intake in order to avoid bladder overdistension. Patients with UDCs were treated additionally with anticholinergic drugs, usually oxybutynin, given 3 times daily with the dose based on body weight and adjusted according to symptomatic response and side effects.

The indications for surgical intervention in these children were determined in 1976 and continued throughout the study. They include UTI while on therapy, discontinuation of antibiotics, non-compliance with treatment or follow-up protocol, and the development of puberty.

Results

The patient population was divided into 3 groups based on urodynamic findings. All children had normal renal function and no child displayed obstructive uropathy, overt neurologic disease, *or dyssynergia during voiding*. Group 1 was composed of children with UDCs who were maintained satisfactorily on anticholinergic drugs. There were 26 patients with 43 refluxing ureters. Group 2 consisted of children with UDCs who failed to take their anticholinergic drugs, either because of side effects or medication frequency. There were 8 patients with 12 ureters in this group. Group 3 was an age-matched control group having normal cystometric findings and consisted of 28 children with 47 refluxing ureters. In each group the children were all toilet-trained prior to presentation and of a comparable age: the mean age for children with uninhibited contractions was 5.4 years and the mean age for control group children was 5.8 years.

Cystoscopy failed to demonstrate obstruction in any patient. Examination of the ureteral orifices in each group of children demonstrated minor degrees of ureteral ectopia and configuration abnormality associated with the lower grades of VUR, while with higher grades of VUR there tended

Table I. Recurrent UTIs while on antibiotics

	group					
	1		2		3	
		%		%		%
Asymptomatic	3/26	12	3/8	38	9/28	32
Febrile	1/26	4	2/8	25	11/28	39
Total	4/26	16	5/8	63	20/28	71

$p < 0.001$.

to be more significant and severe abnormalities of ureteral positioning and configuration. This trend was independent of the presence of UDCs.

The prevalence of RN at presentation was similar to both groups of children. In those with UDCs it was present in 30%, while its prevalence in children with normal cystometrograms was 38%. At the conclusion of the study 2 kidneys in the UDC group and 3 control kidneys had developed new scars. Symptoms differed significantly among the groups. 74% of children with UDCs had daytime urinary incontinence, compared with 21% of children with normal cystometrograms. Nocturnal incontinence was found in 79% of children with UDCs and in only 21% of normals. The period of follow-up ranged between 1.5 and 7 years, with a mean value of 3.9 years for children in whom VUR still continued. In 7 cases VUR was absent in one cystogram only to be present the following year on a subsequent study.

29 children (46%) developed a UTI while on prophylactic antibiosis. Table I illustrates the frequency of UTIs broken down into asymptomatic, and febrile UTIs. The overall UTI rate in group 1 was 16%, 63% in group 2, and 71% in group 3. These were was highly significant (<0.001). Asymptomatic and febrile UTIs occurred in roughly the same proportions among each of the groups.

The rates of VUR resolution are illustrated in table II. In patients with treated UDCs, VUR resolved in 44% and improved to grade I in another 16%. This contrasts with a 33% resolution rate in group 2 and a 17% resolution rate in group 3, in both of which no improvements to grade I were observed. Comparison of the resolution rate of VUR in children with

Table II. VUR resolution – treatment groups

Group	Resolved (%)	Improved to grade I (%)	Continues (%)	Surgery (%)
1 43 ureters	19 (44)*	7 (16)	3 (7)	14 (33)
2 12 ureters	4 (33)	0	0	8 (67)
3 47 ureters	8 (17)	0	12 (26)	27 (57)

*$p < 0.05$.

treated UDCs to normal controls was significant ($p < 0.05$). Table III describes the relationship between grade of VUR and resolution in each of the treatment groups. Although the numbers are small and not statistically significant, a trend exists which suggests that in children with treated UDCs, improvement and *resolution of VUR is relatively independent of the severity of the VUR*. This contrasts with the other groups where higher grades of VUR were less likely to show spontaneous resolution.

In order to estimate the reduction in bladder capacity caused by the UDCs, the bladder volume at which they occurred was measured and compared to an estimate of bladder capacity using the formula: bladder capacity in ounces equals the age of the child in years plus 2 [5]. The results indicated that *the average bladder capacity in children with uninhibited bladders was 54% of the mean age capacity*.

Discussion

Voluntary constriction of the urinary sphincter in an attempt to keep from wetting is the mechanism by which UDCs cause bladder sphincter dyssynergia and urinary obstruction and produce repetitively high intravesical pressure [1, 2, 6]. The results of this study indicate that treatment of UDCs will reduce the rate of recurrent UTIs in these children and enhance their VUR resolution. This suggests that UDCs persisting after the age of toilet training amount to a pathologic mechanism which is responsible in

Table III. Reflux resolution – grade of reflux

	At diagnosis	Resolved	Improved to grade I	Continues	Surgery
Group 1					
Grade I	9	5	0	1	3
II	10	3	4	1	2
III	11	7	1	0	3
IV	10	2	2	1	5
V	3	2	0	0	1
Totals	43	19	7	3	14
Group 2					
Grade I	3	0	0	0	3
II	4	1	0	0	3
III	3	2	0	0	1
IV	2	1	0	0	1
V	0	0	0	0	0
Totals	12	4	0	0	8
Group 3					
Grade I	3	1	0	0	2
II	11	3	0	3	5
III	17	4	0	6	7
IV	9	0	0	3	6
V	7	0	0	0	7
Totals	47	8	0	12	27

some degree for UTI and for perpetuating and possibly initiating VUR. This situation is identical to that which occurs in children with spina bifida or other neuropathy where dyssynergia causes profound changes in bladder anatomy and results in trabeculation, diverticula and VUR. The only differences are that in children with UDCs, the sphincter contriction is purely voluntary whereas in neurologic disease it occurs reflexly, and that the dyssynergia which occurs with UDCs is transient and temporary, as most children will outgrow their tendency for UDCs in several months, or years, after diagnosis. Until they resolve, however, the kidney is just as vulnerable to VUR, high pressures, and UTI as in cases of spina bifida and must therefore be protected.

The uninhibited bladder is actually a common childhood condition which has been estimated to occur in up to 60% of children with recurrent UTIs [6, 7]. In attempting to identify these children, it is obvious that symptoms of bladder hyperactivity predominate and the majority may have daytime and nighttime incontinence. However, *up to 30% of children do not have incontinence*, because their sphincters are strong enough to overcome the UDCs, but unfortunately at the expense of raised intravesical pressure [1, 2]. Also unfortunately, at least 20% of children with normal bladders have daytime and nighttime wetting and this further reduces the specificity of these symptoms. One sign which has been particularly useful in diagnosis is Vincent's 'curtsey', a maneuver where the child squats down and actually compresses the perineum and urethra with a heel to prevent urinary incontinence. Our experience suggests that this maneuver is almost pathognomonic for UDCs [8].

Examination of the occurrence of UTI on therapy (table I) indicates that children with supposedly normal bladder function have a much higher incidence of recurrent UTI than do children with abnormal bladder function. At first glance this seems paradoxical, but what actually is demonstrated is that children in whom a mechanism for UTI can be identified and successfully treated have a lower rate of reinfection than do children in whom no such mechanism can be identified. Since children with UDCs characteristically void to completion, without a residue, the mechanism for UTI appears to be elevated intravesical pressure and relative bladder overdistension due do frequent obstructed UDCs and a reduced functional bladder capacity. Although the explanation for such a high rate of recurrent UTI in the controls is not exactly clear, it is obvious that anticholinergic/antispasmodic drugs, such as oxybutynin, afford children with UDCs protection against recurrent UTIs. Anticholinergic drugs work by shifting the cystometric curve to the right, so raising the threshold for uninhibited contractions, and thereby enlarging the functional capacity of the bladder [9]. Because these agents do not totally eliminate UDCs, however, other measures, such as reduction in fluid intake and frequent bladder emptyings, are necessary in order to keep the bladder urine volume below the threshold for UDCs. Unfortunately this aspect of treatment goes against the grain of many patients, and physicians who treat UTIs and have observed how important excessive fluid intake is in a successful treatment program. However, while increased fluids are very useful in treating acute

UTIs, *they are specifically disadvantageous in children with UDCs* because of rapid bladder overfilling, and an attempt to force fluids on these children can quickly undermine an otherwise successful treatment program.

In addition to producing UTI, the repetitive obstruction and raised intravesical pressures produce a spectrum of intravesical anatomic distoritions which include trabeculation, diverticula, and saccules which can interfere with vesicoureteral function and, combined with elevated pressures, contribute to VUR. *The occurrence of VUR in up to 50% of children with uninhibited bladders has been noted* [1, 2]. The results of this study strongly support a causal relationship between UDCs and VUR by demonstrating that the resolution rate of the latter is enhanced in children with treated uninhibited bladders compared to their untreated mates and to peers with normal bladder function.

The factors that have been considered most important in determining the resolution of VUR in children with so-called 'primary' VUR have been anatomic factors relating to the maturation of the ureterovesical junction [10–13]. These include the obliquity of the ureter as it passes through the bladder, the length of the intramural ureter, and its valvular competence. With these, the severity of the VUR, the presence of ureteral dilatation, and the appearance of the ureteral orifice have been useful predictors of ureterovesical junction maturation and indicators to the disappearance or persistence of VUR. As a result of maturation, spontaneous VUR resolution has been shown to occur in a significant proportion of children [12–14], and *Edwards* et al. [13] have documented the actual rate at which VUR disappears to be in the range of 20–30% of affected ureters in each 2-year period.

Our experience with children having UDCs with VUR requires that we reassess the traditional view that anatomic factors are the only cause for VUR in children with so-called primary VUR and laterally placed orifices. We believe instead that these children are not a homogenous population, and that the perpetuation and resolution of their VUR may be strongly influenced by urodynamic factors, such as dyssynergia with high intravesical pressures. Although the overall VUR resolution rate in our entire group was approximately 18% per 2-year period, a value comparable to that described by *Edwards* et al. [13], the variation within the group was great and ranged from 35% per 2-year period for children with treated UDCs to 7% per 2-year period for children with normal cystometrograms. This indicates that maturation of the ureterovesical junction does occur in children, and that VUR resolves at a predictable rate, but that maturation is not entirely an anatomic process. Instead, it is significantly affected by neurophysiologic maturation with elimination of disordered patterns of urinary control. Consequently, VUR resolution can be enhanced by treatment of specifically identified urodynamic abnormalities.

As a result of these findings, we suggest that the currently used criteria for VUR, which are based upon the degree of pelvicalyceal and ureteral dilation and on the appearance and location of the ureteral orifices are not sufficiently physiologic fully to assess the potential for VUR resolution in many children. In order to complete the physiologic evaluation, some assessment of bladder function and pressure must be made and should be included in any meaningful classification or prognostic formula. We suggest further that so-called 'primary' VUR can no longer be considered the expression of a single pathologic process, i.e. lateral ureteral ectopia. Instead it should be subdivided, or subclassified, in recognition of the fact that the prevalence and variability of bladder dysfunction in neurologically normal children causes different subgroups of refluxers to behave differently and to have altogether different prognoses.

In the past, urodynamic studies have had a rather insignificant role in the prognostication and management of neurologically normal children with VUR and, in fact, the currently ongoing International Reflux Study in children does not include a urodynamic assessment of bladder function [11, 12]. We believe strongly that because urodynamics are readily available and sufficiently well standardized, it is time to change this attitude and to include urodynamic studies in the evaluation of neurologically normal children with recurrent UTIs and VUR, particularly before surgical treatment is initiated. It has not been long since the management of UTI and VUR in children with spina bifida – myelomeningocele was improved significantly by obtaining careful urodynamic information and by treating the underlying bladder dysfunction. The result has been improved rates of spontaneous resolution of VUR and an improved ability surgically to treat VUR successfully [15, 16]. The same situation applies to children who do not require wheelchairs. If dyssynergia can be identified as a mechanism for high intravesical pressure and can be incriminated in the pathogenesis of UTI and VUR, its specific therapy is required before surgically correcting the latter. No less would or should be done for cases of anatomic obstruction, or in instances of overt neuropathy with obstructive sequelae. The results of this study suggest strongly that the uninhibited bladder is a significant prognostic factor in children with VUR which, successfully treated, can alter the disease course in a significant number of patients and may make surgical correction unnecessary. As a result we now consider that the evaluation of the child with VUR and UTI is not complete until there has been a thorough evaluation of lower urinary tract function.

References

1 Koff, S.A.; Lapides, J.; Piazza, D.H.: Association of urinary tract infection and reflus with uninhibited bladder contractions and voluntary sphincteric constriction. J. Urol. *122*: 393 (1979).

2 Koff, S.A.; Lapides, J.; Piazza, D.H.: Reflux nephropathy; 1st ed. (Masson, New York 1979).

3 Koff, S.A.; Kass, E.J.: Abdominal wall electromyography: a new non-invasive method for improving pediatric urodynamic accuracy. J. Urol. *127*: 736 (1982).

4 Diokno, A.C.; Koff, S.A.; Bender, L.F.: Periurethral striated muscle activity in neurogenic bladder dysfunction. J. Urol. *114*: 743 (1974).

5 Koff, S.A.: Estimating bladder capacity in children. Urology (in press).

6 Lapides, J.; Diokno, A.C.: Persistence of the infant bladder as a cause for urinary infection in girls. Trans. Am. Ass. gen.-urin. Surg. *61*: 51 (1969).

7 Bauer, S.B.; Retik, A.B.; Colodny, A.H.; Hallett, M.; Khoshbim, S.; Dyro, F.M.: The unstable bladder of childhood. Urol. Clins. N. Am. *7*: 321 (1980).

8 Vincent, S.A.: Postural control of urinary incontinence. The curtsey sign. Lancet *ii*: 631 (1966).

9 Dionko, A.C.; Lapides, J.: Oxybutynin: a new drug with analgesic and anticholinergic properties. J. Urol. *108*: 307 (1972).

10 Lyon, R.P.; Marshall, S.; Tanagho, E.A.: The ureteral orifice: its configuration and competency. J. Urol. *102*: 504 (1969).

11 International Reflux Study Committee: Medical versus surgical treatment of primary vesicoureteral reflux. Pediatrics, Springfield *67*: 392 (1981).

12 International Reflux Study Committee: Medical versus surgical treatment of primary vesicoureteral reflux: a prospective international reflux study in children. J. Urol. *125*: 277 (1981).

13 Edwards, D.; Normand, I.C.S.; Prescod, N.; Smellie, J.M.: Disappearance of vesicoureteric reflux during long-term prophylaxis of urinary tract infection in children. Br. med. J. *ii*: 285 (1977).

14 Aladjem, M.; Boichis, H.; Hertz, M.; Herzfeld, S.; Raviv, U.: The conservative management of vesicoureteric reflux: a review of 121 children. Pediatrics, Springfield *65*: 78 (1980).

15 Kass, E.J.; Koff, S.A.; Diokno, A.C.: Fate of vesicoureteral reflux in children with neuropathic bladders managed by intermittent self catheterization. J. Urol. *125*: 63 (1981).

16 Sullivan, T.; Purcell, M.M.; Gregory, J.G.: The management of vesicoureteral reflux in the pediatric neurogenic bladder. J. Urol. *125*: 65 (1981).

Stephen A. Koff, MD, Associate Professor Surgery, Head Section Pediatric Urology, Ohio State University, College of Medicine, Columbus, OH (USA)

Contr. Nephrol., vol. 39, pp. 221–237 (Karger, Basel 1984)

18. Vesico-Ureteral Reflux in Children with Spina bifida and Detrusor-Sphincter Dyssynergia

Jan D. van Gool

Department of Paediatric Nephrology, University Children's Hospital, Het Wilhelmina Kinderziekenhuis, Utrecht, The Netherlands

Introduction

Of growing concern to all who care for children with meningomyelocele (MMC) are two still largely unsolved urological problems: incontinence, compromising quality of life, and upper urinary tract damage, influencing life expectancy [1, 16, 17]. The incidence of upper urinary tract damage increases with age in children with MMC [16, 19, 25], and indicates the need for early assessment and classification of the primary disorder – neurogenic bladder dysfunction.

To define the nature and extent of motor-neuronic abnormalities of bladder innervation, information is needed about the detrusor muscle (visceromotor) and the main component of urethral resistance, the striated urethral muscles (somatomotor) – both during filling of the bladder and during voiding. Urodynamic techniques are accepted tools for obtaining this information, usually given in terms of reflex activity of detrusor and striated urethral muscles. Although urodynamic investigations are not yet routine procedures in children with MMC [3, 8, 10, 18, 20, 22, 23], they are at least complementary to the much widely used uroradiological investigations and so provide a valuable new dimension to our knowledge of the pathophysiology of neurogenic bladder dysfunction: the relation between functional obstruction of the bladder outlet, and upper urinary tract damage [21]. This relationship is illustrated in figure 1, showing intrarenal reflux in a 2-year-old MMC patient, with bladder pressures in excess of 150 cm H_2O and a cystometric bladder capacity of less than 50 ml.

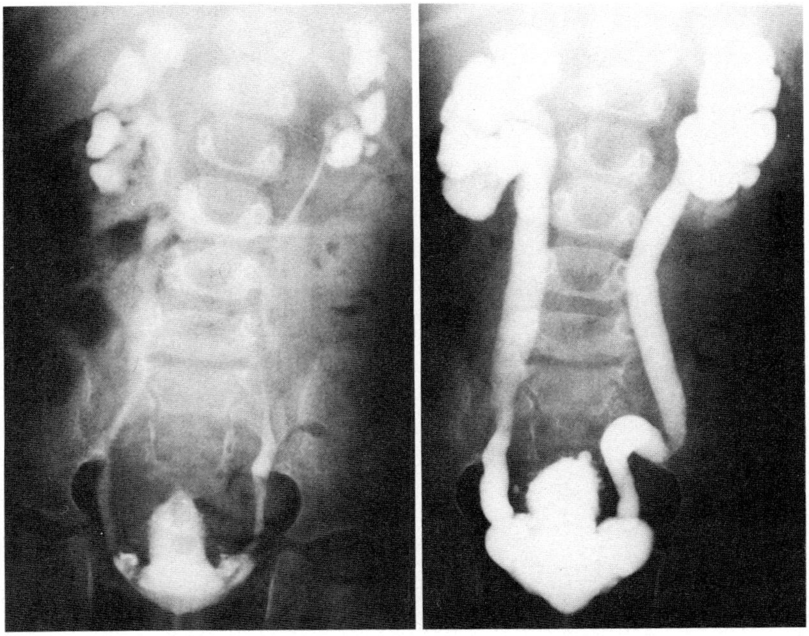

a b

Fig. 1. VUR in a 2-year-old girl with myelomeningocele, hyper-reflexic activity of detrusor muscle, and functional infravesical obstruction. *a* At the beginning of retrograde bladder filling, bilateral VUR develops. *b* The bladder is filled with 40 ml, detrusor activity starts, and the VUR changes dramatically in appearance. Intrarenal reflux is now visible in both upper and lower poles of the left kidney. On subsequent urodynamic investigation maximal bladder pressure during voiding was in excess of 150 cm H_2O. Follow-up on these findings is not available yet.

Patients and Methods

In an attempt to base urological care on the pathophysiology of neurogenic bladder dysfunction, we started out to do full urodynamic studies on children with MMC in 1973 [10]. From 1975 on these studies were performed on all infants with MMC under the age of 1 year. From 1973 through 1980, 140 urodynamic investigations have been carried out on 91 unselected children with MMC (fig. 2). The mean age at the time of the first investigation was 3.2 years (range 2 weeks to 16 years), the mean interval between first and repeat investigations was 3.2 ± 2.4 years. Together with uroradiological and neurological examinations, urodynamic investigations now form the basis of a comprehensive management programme for all our patients with neurogenic bladder dysfunction.

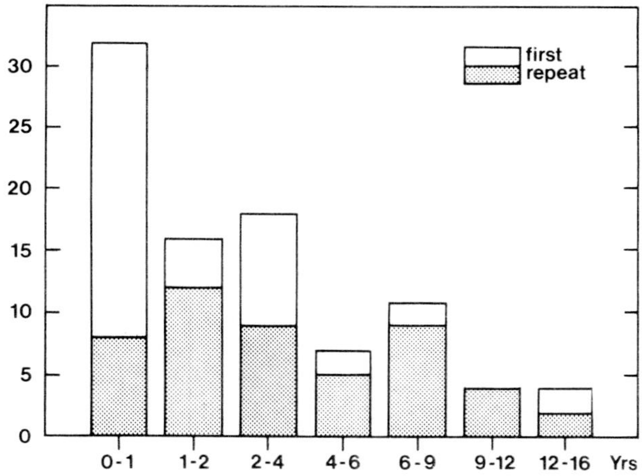

Fig. 2. Age distribution for 140 urodynamic investigations in 91 children with MMC. Mean age at first investigation was 3.2 years, ages ranging from 0.04 to 16.1 years. Mean interval between first and last investigation was 3.2 years (range 0.16–9.38 years). Clinical follow-up varied between 1.5 and 10 years.

Each urodynamic investigation consists of simultaneous registration of bladder pressure, rectal pressure, electromyographic activity of external anal sphincter, and urine flow-rate whenever possible. Several recordings are made, both during bladder filling and bladder emptying. Abdominal pressure artefacts, superimposed on the bladder pressure tracting, are cancelled by electronic subtraction of rectal pressure from bladder pressure, and obstruction of the bladder-outflow tract is minimized by using one single Ch 04 infant feeding tube, both to fill the bladder transurethrally and to measure bladder pressures. The pressure difference caused by filling through gravity is measured between two pressure transducers and compensated electronically.

The urodynamic setup has been described in detail in 1976 [10], and has not been changed since the studies started in 1973. Urodynamic techniques and terminology in this study comply with standards set by the International Continence Society [14].

All uroradiological examinations – intravenous urography (IVU) and voiding cysto-urethrography (VCU) – were done in the Paediatric X-Ray Department of the Wilhelmina Children's Hospital.

Prevalence of vesico-ureteral reflux (VUR), VUR grades, and urological management will be given in tabulated form: VUR confined to the ureter only is designated grade I; VUR reaching ureter, pelvis and calices is designated grade II; while grade III covers VUR with moderate to gross dilatation of ureter, pelvis and calices [15]. The development of upper tract dilatation and reflux nephropathy (RN) will be illustrated with tracings of all available IVUs of the children with VUR [13]. The tracings are dated in decimal years, and placed on a horizontal layout, together with markings for VUR and treatment modality.

Table I. 4 main patterns of neurogenic bladder dysfunction in 91 children with MMC

Bladder dysfunction pattern	n (%)	P_{max} cm H_2O	VUR n (%)
No recognizable pattern	4 (4.4)	–	–
1 Normal bladder function	6 (6.6)	41.6 ± 14.0	–
2 Detrusor: hyper-reflexia Pelvic floor: areflexia	5 (5.5)	39.0 ± 21.0	–
3 Detrusor: areflexia Pelvic floor: areflexia	35 (38.5)	37.0 ± 11.1	4
4 Detrusor: hyper-reflexia Pelvic floor: hyper-reflexia	31 (34.0)	72.0 ± 27.0	8
5 Detrusor: areflexia Pelvic floor: hyper-reflexia	10 (11.0)	63.0 ± 23.0	3
	91 (100)		15 (16)

Results

Based on 4 combinations of reflex activity of detrusor and pelvic floor muscles [5, 8, 9, 14, 24], 4 patterns of neurogenic bladder dysfunction emerged: their relative frequencies are shown in table I. These patterns could be demonstrated at a very early age, and all repeat investigations proved them to be consistent. Also, the urodynamic studies yielded values for maximal bladder pressure during bladder emptying (P_{max}), given as mean values in table I. For comparison, normal values will be quoted for one of the few available urodynamic studies in normal children [12].

VUR was the most common abnormality detected by uroradiological investigation. Its overall prevalence on initial VCUs was 16%; these were usually performed at about the same time as the urodynamic investigations. In table I, the number of children with VUR is given for each pattern of bladder dysfunction. None was found either in the 6 children with normal bladder function (table I, pattern 1), or in the 5 with the combination of

Table II. VUR prevalence (9%) and management in 35 MMC children with areflexia of both detrusor and pelvic floor muscles. Numbers indicate renal units, number of patients in parentheses

VUR catgories	Initial VCU	Follow-up VCU	Dilatation on initial IVU	Dilatation on follow-up IVU	Reflux nephropathy	Urological management (n)
No VUR	65	62	–	1[a]	–	intermittent catheterization (5)
Grade I	1	–	–	–	–	
Grade II	4	–	–	–	–	diversion (1)
Grade III	–	1[a]	–	1[a]	1[a]	intermittent catheterization (1)

detrusor hyper-reflexia and pelvic floor areflexia (table I, pattern 2), and these categories will not be described any further. Attention will thus be focussed on VUR in children with hyper-reflexia of pelvic floor muscles (detrusor-sphincter dyssynergia, causing functional bladder outflow obstruction, table I, patterns 4 and 5), as opposed to children with areflexia of pelvic floor muscles (inert striated urethral sphincter; low urethral resistance, table I, pattern 3).

Areflexia of both detrusor and pelvic floor muscles was found in 34 children (table I, pattern 3). Bladder emptying was usually performed by manual expression, but in selected cases intermittent catheterization was used. Values for P_{max} during bladder emptying ranged from 22 to 60 cm H_2O. At VCU, a wideopen bladder neck and urethra were a constant finding during manual expression of the bladder, and bladder wall contours were smooth, without signs of hypertrophy. Functional infravesical obstruction in this group was ruled out by the normal values for P_{max} and by the normal configuration of the bladder outflow tract during manual expression.

3 children had VUR on initial examination (9%), in a total of 5 renal units. VUR grades, management, and results at follow-up are summarized in table II. In 1 patient with bilateral VUR grade II, urinary diversion had been carried out in 1973, because of incontinence and UTI. In another patient bilateral VUR grade II resolved spontaneously. In the remaining one, unilateral VUR grade III with bilateral upper tract dilatation was recently detected at follow-up after a prolonged period of untreated UTI. With the

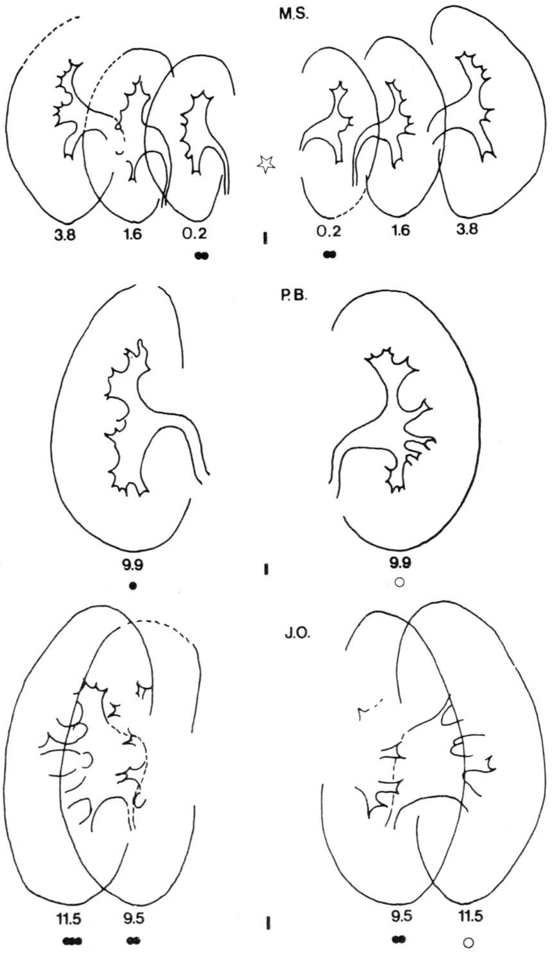

Fig. 3. Kidney growth and contours in 3 children with VUR and areflexia of both detrusor and pelvic floor muscles (table II). Kidneys are traced from IVUs, and placed on a horizontal line. Ages are in decimal years. VCUs are marked by dots: ○ = absence of VUR; ● = presence of VUR; the number of dots indicate the grade of reflux (I–III). ☆ = urinary diversion.

possible exception of this patient (table II), kidney growth remained normal in this group, and RN did not develop during follow-up. Details are given in figure 3.

Hyper-reflexia of both detrusor and pelvic floor muscles was found in 31 children (table I, pattern 4). Pelvic floor hyper-reflexia – causing detrusor-sphincter dyssynergia during detrusor contractions – was substantiated in all these children by the finding of isolated reflex activity in sacral spinal cord segments on neurological examination. In some, electromyographic activity of pelvic floor muscles was continuously present, without any relation to detrusor contractions or changes in abdominal pressure. In most children this activity occurred either in short bursts during voiding, or increased and decreased synchronously with every detrusor contraction, both during filling and voiding (fig. 4a).

On VCU, ballooning of the proximal urethra during reflex micturition was a prominent feature, with a narrow zone at the level of the pelvic floor indicating functional infravescial obstruction. Bladder wall contours in this group were irregular, with multiple diverticula illustrating the degree of detrusor hypertrophy (fig. 4b). Correspondingly, the values for P_{max} during voiding were nearly twice as high as normal: 72.0 ± 27.0 cm H_2O (range: 37–150 cm H_2O), versus 37.0 ± 4.1 cm H_2O [12].

Table III summarizes VUR prevalence, VUR grades and management in the 31 children in this group. 8 showed VUR (28%) on initial evaluation, in a total of 9 renal units. In figure 5, the development of upper tract dilatation and RN is given in detail. Tracings of all available IVUs of the 8 children with VUR are dated in years, and placed on a horizontal layout, on which VUR and treatment are also marked [13, 15]. Signs of RN developed in 5 of the 9 refluxing units, 2 of which showed impaired kidney growth at follow-up. 7 of the 9 refluxing units had dilated pelves and calices initially, compared with 5 at follow-up – 4 with and 1 without RN.

Management during the follow-up period consisted of antimicrobial prophylaxis and treatment of UTI, and of surgical procedures in cases with bladder outflow resistance; a temporary increase in incontinence directly following these procedures was accepted. In boys, the procedure was urethrotomy by endoresection (sphincterotomy), in girls, with mild dyssenergia, urethral dilatation was also used. Selected cases were put on a regimen of clean intermittend catheterization (table III). Whenever the effects of urethrotomy or urethral dilatation diminished, the procedures were repeated or – preferably – clean intermittent catheterization was started.

Hyper-reflexia of pelvic floor muscles, combined with areflexia of the detrusor muscle was found in 10 children (table I, pattern 5). Hyper-reflexic, or dyssynergic, pelvic floor activity could be corroborated by other signs of isolated reflex activity in sacral spinal cord segments. Bladder emptying occurred mainly by straining, or with manual expression. During these manoeuvres electromyographic activity of the pelvic floor muscles

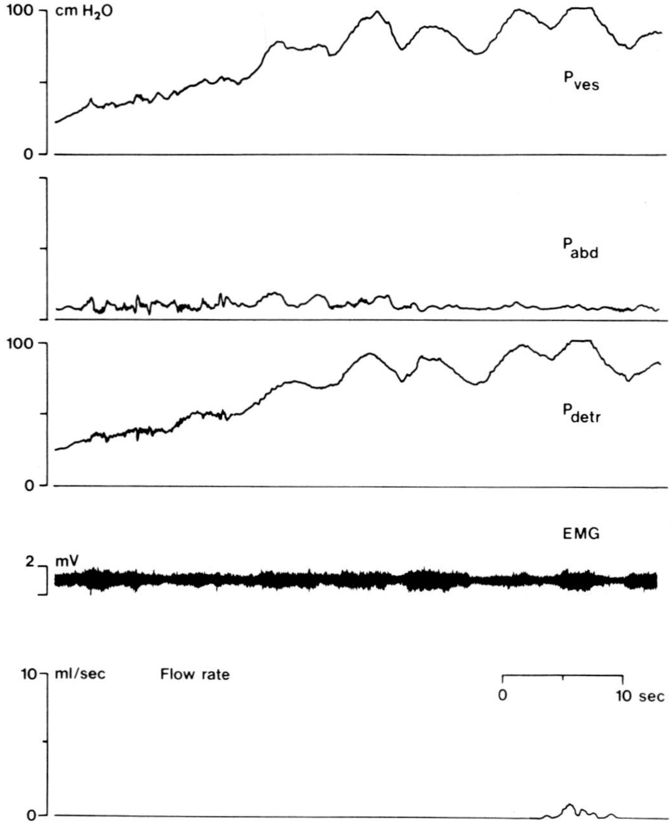

4a

Fig. 4. a Detrusor-sphincter dyssynergia with detrusor hyper-reflexia in a 6-year-old girl with MMC. P_{ves} = Bladder pressure; P_{abd} = rectal pressure; P_{detr} = bladder pressure minus rectal pressure. Dyssynergic pelvic floor activity (EMG) increases and decreases with every detrusor contraction, during bladder filling and voiding, without any sensation of urge. Voiding occurs as a series of urine leakages at extremely high bladder pressures, with dribbling incontinence as a result. During follow-up (the first investigation was done at 2 months) dyssynergia did not change, but maximal bladder pressures during voiding gradually became higher. VUR and UTI could not be demonstrated. Although bladder capacity was only 120 ml at the last investigation, incontinence was cured with clean intermittent catheterization. *b* VCU of a child with detrusor-sphincter dyssynergia and detrusor hyper-reflexia. Note diverticula of the bladder wall (detrusor hypertrophy), wide proximal urethra and narrow segment at the level of the pelvic floor.

Table III. VUR prevalence (28%) and management in 31 MMC children with hyper-reflexia of both detrusor and pelvic floor muscles. Numbers indicate renal units, number of patients in parentheses

VUR categories	Initial VCU	Follow-up VCU	Dilatation on initial IVU	Dilatation on follow-up IVU	Reflux nephropathy	Urological management (n)
No VUR	53	59	–	1	–	urethrotomy (3) intermittent catheterization (6)
Grade I	–	2	–	–		
Grade II	2	–	–	–	1	urethrotomy (6) intermittent catheterization (5)
Grade III	7	1	7	4	4	diversion (1)

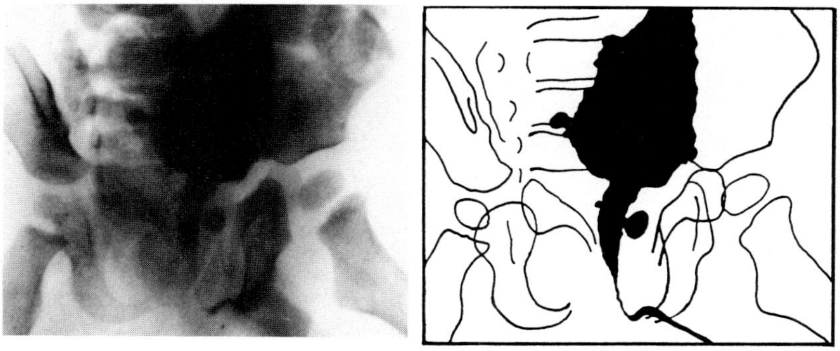

4b

was either continuously present, without apparent relation to pressure changes in abdomen and bladder, or it waxed and waned with the changes in these pressures (fig. 6a).

On VCU, ballooning of the proximal urethra could be provoked by straining or expression, while during filling of the bladder the bladder neck was completely closed. Bladder wall contours were smooth, and no signs of bladder wall hypertrophy could be detected (fig. 6b). The values of P_{max} during bladder emtpying in this group were higher than normal: 62.0 ± 23.0 cm H_2O (range 45–120 cm H_2O) versus 37.0 ± 11.1 cm H_2O [12].

Table IV states prevalence, grades and management in the 10 children in this group: 3 had VUR on initial evaluation – a total of 4 renal units. A

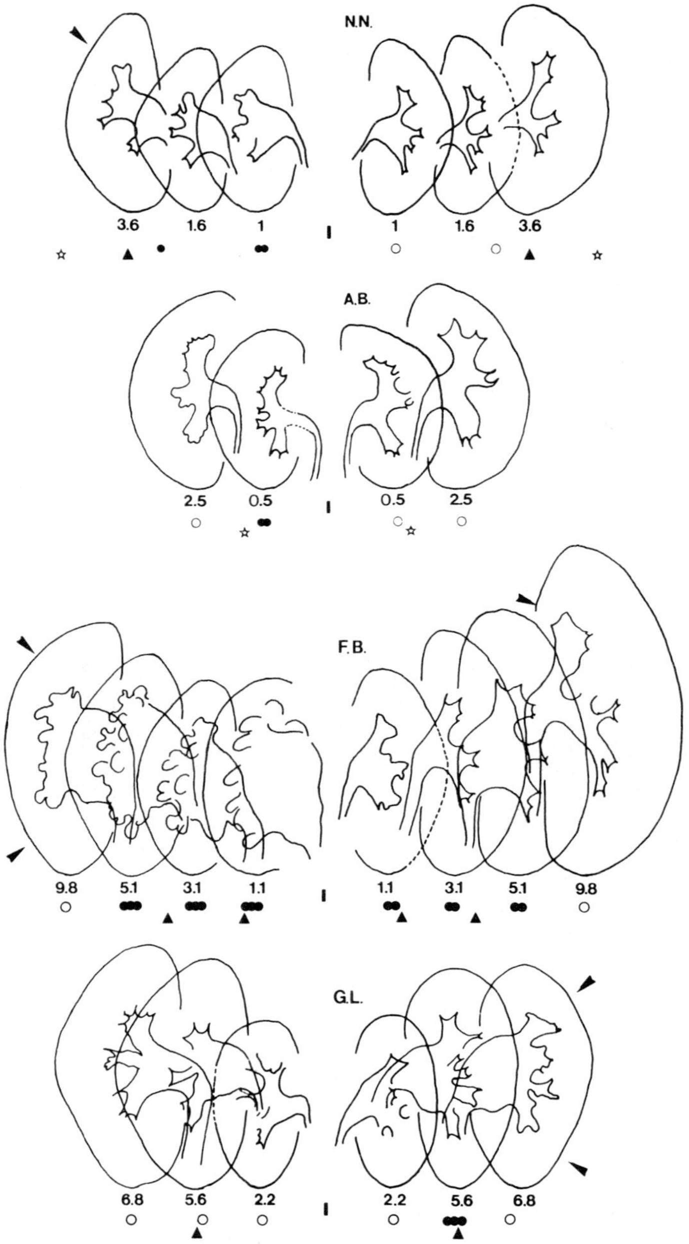

Fig. 5. Kidney growth and contours in 8 children with VUR and detrusor-sphincter dyssynergia combined with detrusor hyper-reflexia (table III). Kidney outlines are traced from IVUs and positioned symmetrically on a horizontal line, with respective ages in decimal years [13]. Symbols as in figure 3. Parenchymal scars are indicated by arrows. Follow-up of the 2 chil-

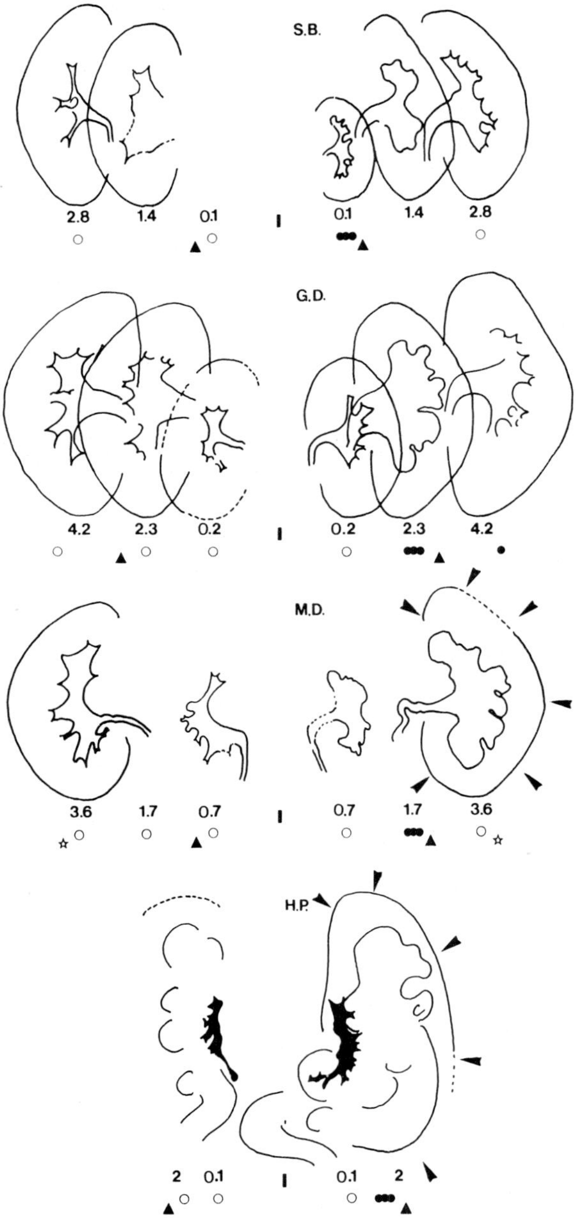

dren with diffuse thinness of parenchyma and generalized caliectasis (F.B. and G.L.) did not take place in our hospital: timing of initial evaluation and treatment was different, and high pressure VUR persisted for a longer period of time than in the other 6 children. In H.P. (horseshoe kidney), bilateral caliectasis has been followed with ultrasonography and is diminishing.

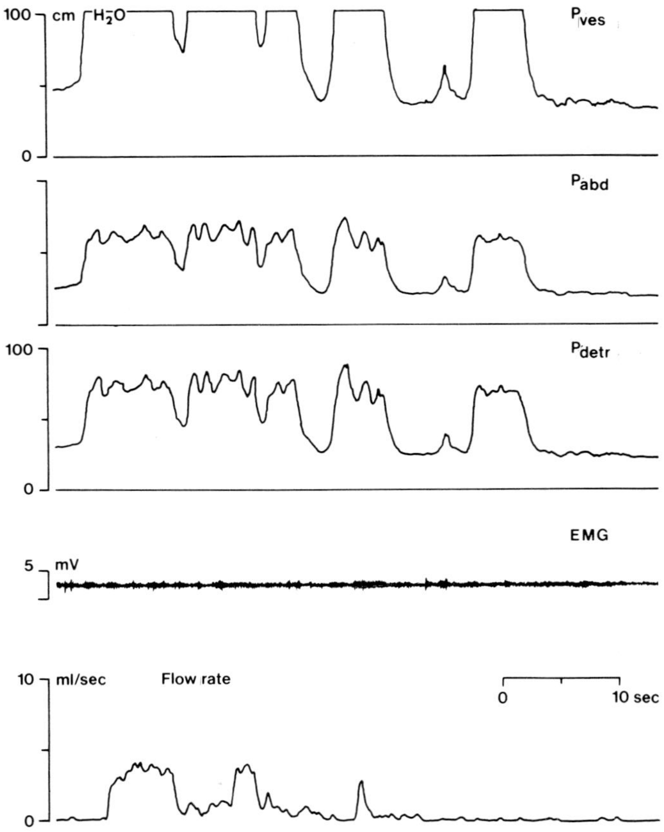

6a

Fig. 6. a Dyssynergia pelvic floor activity with detrusor areflexia in a 14-year-old boy with MMC. During manual expression of the bladder at 145 ml volume (arrows), bladder pressure is much higher than abdominal pressure. Very high bladder pressures generate poor urine flow, due to dyssynergic pelvic floor activity (EMG). Overflow incontinence started at volumes of 150 ml; stress incontinence was prevented by reflex activity of pelvic floor muscles during coughing and straining. With clean intermittent self-catheterization, complaints about overflow-incontinence disappeared completely. *b* VCU in a child with detrusor-sphincter dyssynergia and detrusor areflexia. Signs of detrusor hypertrophy are absent: bladder wall contour is smooth. With straining, bladder neck and proximal urethra open up; the urethra at the level of the pelvic floor remains narrow.

Table IV. VUR prevalence (30%) and management in 10 MMC children with detrusor areflexia and hyperreflexia of pelvic floor muscles. Numbers indicate renal units, number of patients between brackets (n)

VUR categories	Initial VCU	Follow-up VCU	Dilatation on initial IVU	Dilatation on follow-up IVU	Reflux nephropathy	Urological management	(n)
No VUR	16	19	4	–	–	diversion urethrotomy	(2) (1)
Grade I	–	–	–	–	–		
Grade II	1	–	–	–	–	diversion urethrotomy	(1) (2)
Grade III	3	1	2	2	2		

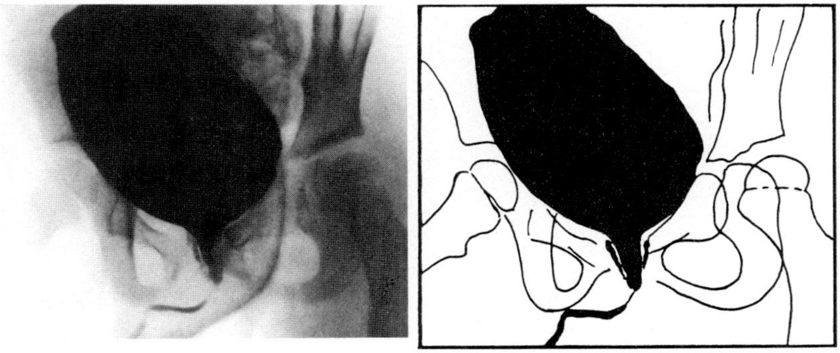

6b

detailed account of upper tract dilatation associated with RN is given in figure 7, where IVU tracings of the 3 children with VUR are placed on a horizontal time-scale, together with symbols for VUR and treatment [13, 15]. RN developed in 2 renal units, without impairment in kidney growth. 6 renal units showed upper tract dilatation, 2 with and 4 without VUR. At follow-up, dilatation had disappeared in the 4 non-refluxing units, as a result of urinary diversion. The urinary diversions mentioned in table IV have all been carried out prior to 1975, and reflect the urological attitude at that time.

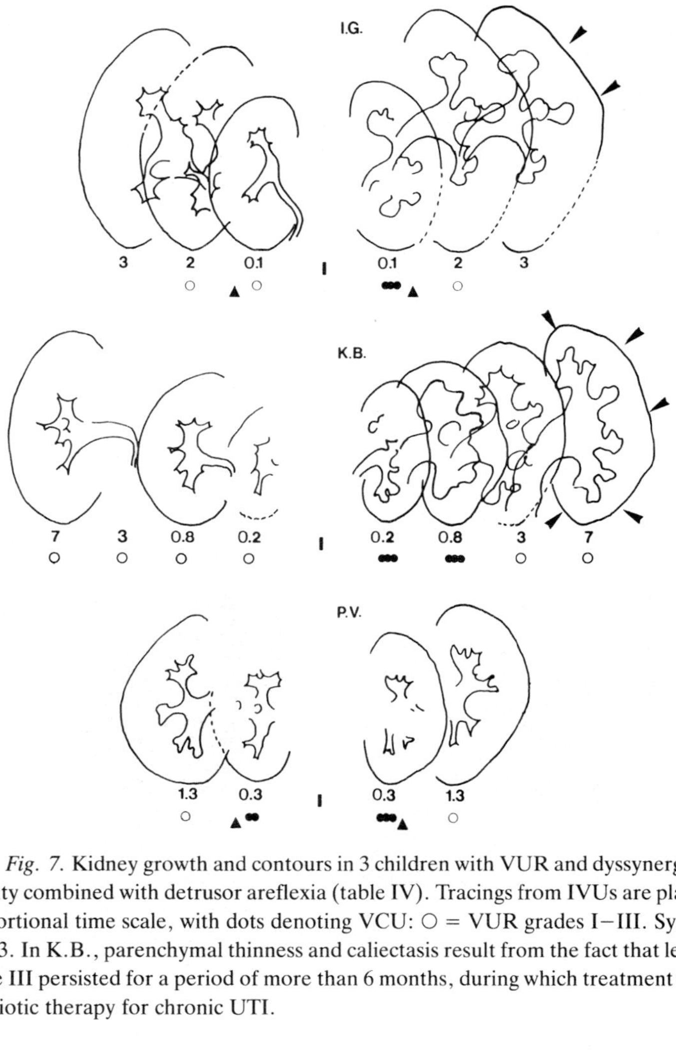

Fig. 7. Kidney growth and contours in 3 children with VUR and dyssynergic pelvic floor activity combined with detrusor areflexia (table IV). Tracings from IVUs are placed on a non-proportional time scale, with dots denoting VCU: ○ = VUR grades I–III. Symbols as in figure 3. In K.B., parenchymal thinness and caliectasis result from the fact that left-sided VUR grade III persisted for a period of more than 6 months, during which treatment was limited to antibiotic therapy for chronic UTI.

Discussion

The most important diagnostic modality gained from urodynamics proved to be pattern recognition: 4 patterns of neurogenic bladder dysfunction could be demonstrated at a very early age, and all repeat investigations proved the pattern to be consistent. The 4 patterns are based upon the complex neurological lesion occurring in MMC. In 1 dysplastic segment of the spinal cord some areas may have intact but isolated motor neuron function, while others have no efferent output at all. Consequently, detrusor (visceromotor) and pelvic floor (somatomotor) muscles can exhibit areflexia or hyper-reflexia, independent of each other. Areflexia of pelvic floor muscles usually leads to incontinence, while hyper-reflexia denotes obstruction – both can occur in combination with hyper-reflexia or areflexia of detrusor muscle [5, 7–10, 14, 24].

In both patterns with detrusor-sphincter dyssynergia due to hyper-reflexic pelvic floor activity, values for 9_{max} were significantly higher than normal, in contrast with the patterns showing areflexia of pelvic floor muscles. These high pressures, generated by hyper-reflexic detrusor activity or by manual expression of an areflexic bladder, indicate the clinical importance of detrusor-sphincter dyssynergia. As a functional infravesical obstruction dyssynergia is wholly comparable with anatomical obstructions in its effects on bladder wall and upper urinary tract.

In a hyper-reflexive bladder, dyssynergia will cause detrusor hypertrophy, giving rise to still higher pressures, until detrusor decompensation and retention ensue. In an areflexic bladder with functional obstruction due to dyssynergia, overflow incontinence and retention will be obvious features right from the start. This is reflected by the fact that upper tract dilatation – in the absence of VUR – occurs mainly in the group where dyssynergia is combined with detrusor areflexia.

The most important clinical effect of obstructive uropathy is brought about by high bladder pressures in the presence of VUR: the prevalence of VUR and RN is significantly higher in the two groups with dyssynergia than in the children with pelvic floor areflexia. Our management, aimed at relief of functional infravesical obstruction, resulted in a substantial resolution rate of VUR and a lower overall prevalence of VUR than is found in the literature. More important, VUR prevalence in our series does not show the reported increase with age. The same management might also benefit the results of antireflux surgery in MMC [4].

Current opinions on the importance of the sympathetic innervation of urethral smooth muscle differ, most being based on animal experiments. However, bladder outflow resistance in the patient mentioned in figure 1 could be lowered significantly by the administration of α-adrenergic blocking agents, indicating urethral smooth muscle as an important component of outflow resistance in this case.

The 3 children with detrusor-sphincter dyssynergia and VUR who developed extensive RN and generalized caliectasis (fig. 5b, 7) have in common the long period of time over which high pressure VUR persisted, and a history of chronic UTI. This stresses the importance of early detection of detrusor-sphincter dyssynergia, and the preventive value of lowering urethral resistance in the presence of high-pressure VUR as soon as possible.

Early urodynamic assessment in children with MMC, complementary to uroradiological investigations, should make it possible to detect and monitor the risks for RN, before upper tract damage becomes irreversible [8, 19, 21].

References

1 Althouse, R.; Wald, N.: Survival and handicap of infants with spina bifida. Archs Dis. Childh. *55*: 845–850 (1980).

2 Anderson, J.T.; Bradley, W.E.: The syndrome of detrusor-sphincter dyssynergia. J. Urol. *116*: 493–495 (1976).

3 Bauer, S.B.; Labib, K.B.; Dieppa, R.A.; Retik, A.B.: Urodynamic evaluation of boy with myelodysplasia and incontinence. Urology *10*: 354–362 (1977).

4 Bauer, S.B.; Colodny, A.H.; Retik, A.B.: The management of vesicoureteral reflux in children with myelodysplasia. J. Urol. *128*: 102–105 (1982).

5 Bors, E.; Comarr, A.E.: Neurological urology: physiology of micturation, its neurological disorders and sequelae (Karger, Basel 1971).

6 Diokno, A.C.: Evaluation of the neurogenically obstructed patient; in Krane, Siroky, Clinical neurology, pp. 111–121 (Little & Brown, Boston 1979).

7 Emery, J.L.; London, R.G.: Clinical implications of cord lesions in neurospinal dysraphism. Devl. Med. Child Neur. *13*: suppl. 25, pp. 1–14 (1972).

8 Festge, O.-A.; Tischer, W.; Rosenbaum, K.-D.; Gross, W.: Zur urodynamischen Diagnostik neurogener Blasenentleerungsstörungen bei Kindern. Zentbl. Chir. *102*: 711–723 (1977).

9 Gibbon, N.O.K.: Nomenclature of neurogenic bladder. Urology *8*: 423–431 (1976).

10 Gool, J. van; Ridder, A.L.A. de; Kuijten, R.H.; Donckerwolcke, R.A.M.G.; Tiddens, H.A.: Measurement of intravesical and rectal pressures simultaneously with electromyography and anal sphincter in children with myelomeningocele. Devl. Med. Child Neur. *18*: 287–301 (1976).

11 Gosling, J.A.; Dixon, J.S.: A comparative study of the human external sphincter, periurethral and levator ani muscles. Br. J. Urol. *53*: 35–41 (1981).

12 Hjalmås, K.: Micturition in infants and children with normal lower urinary tract. A urodynamic study. Scand. J. Urol. Nephrol. *11*: suppl. 37, pp. 1–106 (1977).

13 Hodson, C.J.: Reflux nephropathy: scoring the damage; in Hodson, Kincaid-Smith, Reflux nephropathy chapter (Masson, New York 1979).

14 International Continence Society: Fourth report on the standardization of terminology of lower urinary tract function – terminology related to neuromuscular dysfunction of the lower urinary tract. Br. J. Urol. *53*: 333–355 (1981).

15 International Reflux Study Committee: Medical versus surgical treatment of primary vesicoureteral reflux: a prospective international reflux study in children. J. Urol. *125*: 277–282 (1981).
16 Laurence, K.M.: Effect of early surgery for spina bifida on survival and quality of life. Lancet *i*: 301-305 (1974).
17 Lorber, J.: Spina bifida cystica. Results of treatment of 270 consecutive cases with criteria for selection for the future. Archs. Dis. Child. *47*: 854–873 (1972).
18 Mayo, M.E.; Chapman, W.H.; Shurtleff, D.B.: Bladder function in children with meningomyelocele: comparison of cine-fluoroscopy and urodynamics. J. Urol., pp. 303–314 (1979).
19 McGuire, E.J.; Woodside, J.R.: Prognostic value of urodynamic testing in myelodysplastic patients. J. Urol. *126*: 205–209 (1981).
20 Meunier, P.; Mollard, P.: Manometric and electromyographic assessment of urethral resistances in children. Br. J. Urol. *49*: 303–314 (1977).
21 Mollard, P.; Meunier, P.: Urodynamics of neurogenic bladder in children. A comparative study with clinical and radiological conclusions. Br. J. Urol. *54*: 239–248 (1982).
22 Pekarovic, E.; Robinson, A.; Zachary, R.B.; Lister, J.: Indications for manual expression of the neurogenic bladder in children. Br. J. Urol. *42*: 191–196 (1970).
23 Thomas, G.G.; Zachary, R.B.; Lister, J.: Serial follow-up studies of bladder pressure in spina bifida infants. J. pediat. Surg. *9*: 471–476 (1974).
24 Wein, A.: Classification of neurogenic voiding dysfunction. J. Urol. *125*: 605–609 (1981).
25 Wilcock, A.R.; Emery, J.L.: Deformities of the renal tract in children with meningomyelocele and hydrocephalus, compared with those of children showing no such deformities. Br. J. Urol. *42*: 152–157 (1970).

Jan D. van Gool, Department of Paediatric Nephrology, University Children's Hospital, Het Wilhelmina Kinderziekenhuis, Nieuwe Gracht 137, NL-3512 LK Utrecht (The Netherlands)

Contr. Nephrol., vol. 39, pp. 238–246 (Karger, Basel 1984)

19. Unstable Bladder Activity and the Rate of Resolution of Vesico-Ureteric Reflux[1]

C.M. Taylor

Department of Nephrology, The Birmingham Children's Hospital, Birmingham, England

Introduction

Unstable bladder activity (UDC) has been previously demonstrated in children with vesico-ureteric reflux (VUR) and urinary tract infection (UTI) [1–4]. In our study [3] of 37 girls with severe, primary VUR we showed that the commonest urodynamic abnormality was UDC. This was found in 75% of cases and correlated well with urge incontinence, urgency of micturition and nocturnal enuresis. The correlation between dynamics and symptoms, which paralleled urodynamic observation in adult females [5], supported the view that the finding of UDC in a child of school age, able to cooperate fully during dynamic study, was in fact a significant abnormality. The detrusor contractions of UDC may occur at relatively low bladder volume, small detrusor radius and against an outflow tract voluntarily closed in an attempt to retain continence. This results in an isometric contraction often capable of generating intravesical pressures in excess of those found during voiding [1, 3]. It is therefore relevant to question whether this particular bladder abnormality can lead to delay in the spontaneous resolution of VUR that normally occurs with time. This report concerns the urodynamic findings in 33 girls and 14 boys undergoing non-operative management of severe VUR over a 2-year observation period.

[1] This work was supported by The Medical Research Council (UK), Grant No. G. 977/406.

Patients and Methods

The patients had been referred to the Birmingham Children's Hospital and were participants in a prospective trial of operative versus non-operative management of VUR [6]. All had been shown to have VUR of either grade II or III [7]. Uroradiological and urodynamic investigations were performed when the child was free from UTI. In every patient physical examination excluded neurological abnormality, and the radiological appearance of the urethra showed no evidence of obstruction.

The Urodynamic Study

This was performed without sedation, after preparatory explanation to the child by the nurse assistant, and was well tolerated. First the patient voided naturally at voluntary capacity into a Disa mictiometer [8] and the flow-rate was displayed on a multi-channel SE Laboratories. (EMI) ultraviolet recorder. Voided urine volume and maximal urinary flow rate were recorded and repeated until consistent results were obtained. The child was then catheterized with a 3.5 French gauge recording, and a 5 French gauge filling catheter. The volume of any residual urine was noted and a rectal catheter inserted. Rectal and vesical pressures were measured with SE Laboratories (EMI) dometype pressure transducers via fluid-filled manometer lines. The rectal pressure was electronically subtracted from the recorded vesical pressure to give the true substracted detrusor pressure; all three pressures being simultaneously displayed on the multi-channel recorder. Cystometrograms were obtained while the bladder was filled at 10 ml/min with the child supine and then at 40 ml/min in the erect posture. Finally, pressure/flow voiding studies were performed after removal of the filling catheter.

Definition of Urodynamic Parameters

The terminology used in the text conforms to the standardization produced by the International Continence Society [9]. A diagnosis of unstable bladder refers to any substracted vesical pressure rise above 15 cm H_2O occurring during bladder filling which the patient cannot inhibit. Voiding pressure is the substracted vesical pressure observed at maximal urinary flow rate during voiding. Urethral resistance was calculated from the formula:

$$\text{Resistance} = \frac{\text{voiding pressure}}{\text{maximal urine flow rate}} \quad [10].$$

In all the girls urethral resistance calculations were derived from the simultaneously recorded voiding pressure and maximal urinary flow. Boys, voiding past a urethral catheter, not infrequently achieved flow rates below those seen during their free voiding studies. In these cases urethral resistance was calculated from voiding pressure and the highest urinary flow rate observed, whether in free voiding or during the pressure-flow study.

All patients were treated with continuous low-dose chemoprophylaxis during the 2-year observation period, and the urine was monitored for UTI at 3-monthly intervals, or more often if suggestive symptoms occurred. After 2 years IVUs and VCUs were repeated.

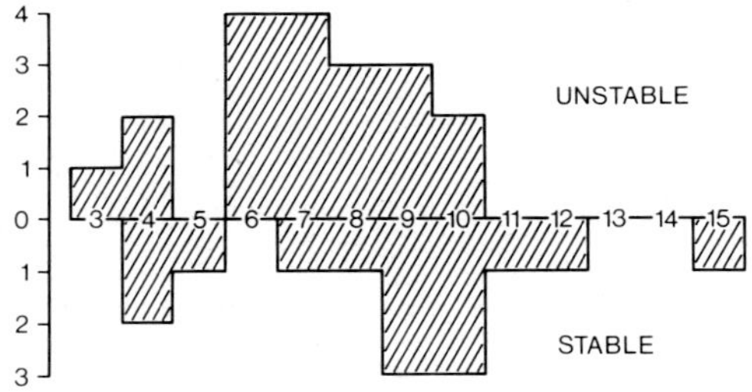

Fig. 1. Girls: bladder stability related to age in years at time of urodynamic investigation.

Table I. Girls: bladder stability and initial VUR grade

	Stable	Unstable
Number of patients	14	19
Number of ureters	27	38
VUR grade III	14	15
II	7	11
I	0	2
0	6	10

Results

Girls

We have previously shown that girls with radiologically defined primary VUR typically have normal outflow tract resistance [3]. Urethral resistance was measured in all but 3 cases and gave values in the normal range of < 0.58 cm H_2O/ml/s or (0.5 mm Hg/ml/s) accepted by *Zatz* [10] and confirmed by ourselves. The mean urethral resistance was 0.27 cm. H_2O/ml/s, standard deviation (SD) ± 0.1, range 0.12–0.53.

14 girls had stable and 19 unstable bladders (fig. 1). The former were older, their mean age being 9.1 years: for those with unstable bladders the mean age was 7.3 years, $t = 1.7147$, $p = 0.05$. 15 of the 19 girls with instability suffered from urge incontinence, 2 developing this during the observation period. No girl with a stable bladder had urge incontinence. The bladder capacity of those with stable bladders was significantly greater than

Table II. Girls: bladder stability and change in VUR grade over 2 years

Bladder stability	VUR grade (ureters)					
	initial		after 2 years			
			III	II	I	0
Stable	III	14	10	1	2	1
	II	7	2	–	3	2
	I	0	–	–	–	–
	0	6	1	–	1	4
Unstable	III	15	8	2	4	1
	II	11	1	2	2	6
	I	2	1	–	1	–
	0	10	–	–	3	7

of those with unstable ones: mean capacity ± standard error, stable 429 ± 47, unstable 246 ± 18 ml, t = 3.6323, p = 0.001.

The grades of VUR in both groups are shown in table I. 1 child with a stable bladder had a solitary kidney, explaining the odd number of ureters in the groups. The change of VUR over 2 years is demonstrated in table II. For comparable grades of VUR at entry *there was no significant difference in the rate of resolution of VUR between stable and unstable groups*. The rate of resolution observed was broadly similar to that observed in the Birmingham Reflux Study [6] and in other reports [11].

Boys

14 boys were studied. The mean age at urodynamic investigation was 7.7 years, range 5.1–13.1 years. All but 3 had unstable bladders generating intravesical pressures betwen 20 and 60 cm H_2O during bladder filling. The grades of VUR at entry to the observation period and after 2 years are shown in table III. The overall rate of resolution of VUR in these children was poor in this relatively short time interval, and no significant difference in outcome between stable and unstable bladders could be shown.

With regard to excretory urodynamics, the boys were not a homogenous group and differed in this respect from the girls. 2 boys generated high intravesical pressures during voiding and a third failed to void to completion (table IV). Outflow tract resistance was calculated in these boys under-

Table III. Boys: bladder stability and change in VUR grade over 2 years

Bladder stability	VUR grade (ureters)					
	initial		after 2 years			
			III	II	I	0
Stable	III	4	4	–	–	–
	II	2	–	2	–	–
Unstable	III	10	6	3	–	1
	II	4	2	1	–	1
	0	8	0	1	1	6

Table IV. Boys with abnormal excretory urodynamics

Patient No.	1	2	3
Age, years	6.5	11.8	13.1
Maximal urine flow rate, ml/s	12	23	12
Residual urine, ml	170	30	410
Bladder capacity, ml	415	420	630
Stable/unstable	unstable	unstable	stable
Voiding pressure, cm H_2O	200	96	36
VUR grade at entry	III III	II II	III III
VUR grade at 2 years	III III	III III	III III

going non-operative management and in a further 9 treated operatively. Discounting the urethral resistance value from patient 1 (1.29 cm H_2O/ml/s), the mean value ± 2 SD obtained from the boys was 0.41 ± 0.19 cm H_2O/ml/s. The mean voiding pressure ± 2 SD was 54.5 ± 31 cm H_2O. 3 boys with the lowest free-voiding maximal urinary flow rate, which was 12 ml/s in each case, include patients 1 and 3 (table IV) and a 13-year-old boy with chronic renal insufficiency, whose calculated urethral resistance exceeded the mean by more than 2 SD. Cases 1 and 3 also voided with interrupted flow.

Patient 1 was studied on two occasions, 1 year apart, with consistent results. Radiological appearance of the bladder demonstrated a fundal ring which gave the bladder an hour-glass appearance during systole (fig. 2).

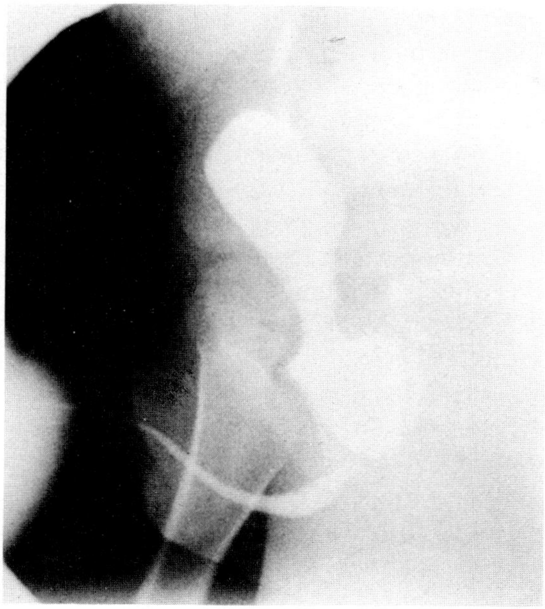

Fig. 2. Male patient 1; micturating cysto-urethrogram.

Bladder pressure was recorded from the trigonal region of the bladder. This boy had some urgency of micturition, urge incontinence and nocturnal enuresis. Further follow-up at 5 years showed that his VUR had improved to grade II on the left and grade I on the right. He demonstrated no renal scarring.

Patient 2 had nocturnal enuresis but no other micturition disturbance. He also had no focal renal scarring. In the out-patient clinic, patient 3 was repeatedly found to have a palpable bladder after voiding. In the pressure-flow voiding study, detrusor systole faded before complete evacuation, leaving a large residuum. This boy had no scarring on the right, but the left kidney showed uniform parenchymal loss with calyceal dilatation.

Discussion

Many children with VUR receive continuous antibiotic prophylaxis until it resolves and the most appropriate use of chemoprophylaxis in the prevention of reflux nephropathy continues to be evaluated. The rate of resolution of VUR is higher in those children with less severe grades of VUR, but appears not to be influenced by sex, age or intercurrent UTI [11]. It seems important to try to identify more precisely those children in whom VUR is likely to persist, so that the treatment choices may be made more rationally. This had been a stimulus towards examining the outcome in defined urodynamic subgroups.

Although girls with UTI have been shown to have abnormal *voiding* dynamics [4], we have very rarely seen this in our series of girls referred because of gross VUR. The voluntary sphincter obstruction accompanying an uninhibited detrusor contraction, which is seen both clinically [10] and at urodynamic study [1, 2, 4, 14], is an appropriate response on the part of the patient to maintain continence. In girls referred primarily because of VUR, it is uncommon to find that the pelvic floor tone and activity are so abnormal that volitional voiding is interrupted, or outflow tract resistance inappropriately increased [3, 10]. In this context the term bladder/sphincter dyssynergia gives rise to confusion, as it can refer to either the socially appropriate voluntary sphincter contraction accompanying uninhibited detrusor systole during urine storage, or to inappropriate sphincter contraction during micturition, giving rise to the pathological consequence of outflow tract obstruction; bladder hypertrophy, decompensation, residual urine and upper tract changes. UDC is the commonest urodynamic abnormality of both girls and boys with VUR. However, it appears from this study that the finding of instability itself at a single investigation has little, if any, effect upon the rate of resolution of VUR in girls. The smaller number of boys in this study, the short observation period, and the complication of excretory abnormalities demand further studies before reaching a conclusion for males.

In clinical practice there is no indication for urodynamic studies in the investigation of girls with VUR. The history may suggest UDC and symptomatic treatment may be indicated, urodynamic investigation being reserved for those patients whose response to treatment is unsatisfactory. In boys, it is clear from this study that cysto-urethrography cannot be relied upon to demonstrate functional abnormalities and the term ‘primary’ VUR may need to be revised to accomodate urodynamic classification. Although a palpable bladder was a relevant physical sign in patient 3, the high voiding pressure of patients 1 and 2 had not been anticipated clinically. Voiding studies are an inexpensive and easily performed out-patient screening test for abnormal excretory function and may be usefully applied to boys.

The dynamic abnormalities of the 3 boys detailed resemble other reported cases [14–17]. We are not aware of an association betwen the fundal ring abnormality seen in patient 1 and functional obstruction. Patient 2 appears to be an example of the 'supervoiders' described by *Gleason* et al. [18], and patient 3 bears some resemblance to a 12-year-old boy described by *Allen* [17]. The effect of these and similar excretory bladder function disturbances on the resolution of VUR deserves further study.

References

1 Koff, S.A.; Lapides, J.; Piazza, D.H.: Association of urinary tract infection and reflux with uninhibited bladder contractions and voluntary sphincter obstruction. J. Urol. *122*: 373–376 (1979).

2 Tanagho, E.A.; Miller, E.R.; Lyon, R.P.; Fisher, R.: Spastic striated external sphincter and urinary tract infection in girls. Br. J. Urol. *43*: 69–82 (1971).

3 Taylor, C.M.; Corkery, J.J.; White, R.H.R.: Micturition symptoms and unstable bladder activity in girls with primary vesicoureteric reflux. Br. J. Urol. *54*: 494–498 (1982).

4 Gool, J. van; Tanagho, E.A.: External sphincter activity and recurrent urinary tract infection in girls. Urology *10*: 348–353 (1977).

5 Farrar, D.J.; Whiteside, C.G.; Osborne, J.L.; Turner-Warwick, R.T.: A urodynamic analysis of micturition symptoms in females. Surgery Gynec. Obstet. *141*: 875–881 (1975).

6 The Birmingham Reflux Study Group: A prospective trial of operative versus non-operative treatment of severe vesico-ureteric reflux: two years' observation in 96 children (Chapter 15, this volume).

7 Rolleston, G.L.; Shannon, F.T.; Utley, W.L.F.: Relationship of vesicoureteric reflux to renal damage. Br. med. J.: 460–463 (1970).

8 Rowan, D.; McKenzie, A.L.; McNee, S.C.; Glen, E.S.: A technical and clinical evaluation of the Disa uroflowmeter. Br. J. Urol. *49*: 285–291 (1977).

9 International Continence Society: Second report on the standardization of terminology of lower urinary tract infection. Br. J. Urol. *49*: 207–210 (1977).

10 Zatz, L.M.: Combined physiologic and radiological studies of bladder function in female children with recurrent urinary tract infection. Invest. Urol. *3*: 278–308 (1965).

11 Edwards, D.; Normand, I.C.S.; Prescod, N.; Smellie, J.M.: Disappearance of vesicoureteric reflux during long-term prophylaxis of urinary tract infection in children. Br. med. J. *ii*: 285–288 (1977).

12 Dejonge, G.A.: The urge syndrome in bladder control and enuresis: clinics in developmental medicine, vol. 48/49. chap. 8, pp. 66–69 (Heinemann, London 1973).

13 Bradley, W.E.; Anderson, J.T.: Techniques for analysis of micturition reflux disturbance in childhood. Pediatrics, Springfield *59*: 546–556 (1977).

14 Williams, D.I.; Hirst, G.; Doyle, D.: The occult neuropathic bladder. J. pediat. Surg. *9*: 35–41 (1974).

15 Hinman, F.: Urinary tract damage in children who wet. Pediatrics, Springfield *54*: 142–150 (1974).

16 Hinman, F.; Baumann, F.W.: Vesical and ureteral damage from voiding dysfunction in boys without neurological or obstructive disease. J. Urol. *109*: 727–732 (1973).
17 Allen, T.D.: The non-neurogenic bladder. J. Urol. *117*: 232–238 (1977).
18 Gleason, D.M.; Bottaccini, M.R.; Reilly, R.J.; Byrne, J.C.: The residual stream energy is a diagnostic index of male urinary outflow obstruction. Investve Urol. *10*: 72–77 (1972).

C.M. Taylor, Department of Nephrology, The Birmingham Children's Hospital, Ladywood Middleway, GB-Birmingham B16 8ET (England)

Contr. Nephrol., vol. 39, pp. 247–251 (Karger, Basel 1984)

Discussion on Chapters 16–19

Dr. *P. Ransley*: I think the importance of this morning's session has been that for the first time we see urodynamics applied to the vesicoureteral reflux (VUR) problem other than for a single physiological act, and we have been shown that the various VUR groups behave differently and have different prognoses.

If I can summarise, what the speakers appear to have said is that there is a group of primary refluxers; another group with the unstable, uninhibited type of bladder, the so-called dyssynergic group; there are boys with non-specifically abnormal lower tracts – as described by Dr. *Taylor* – with some features which don't allow them to be classified with straighforward primary refluxers; and then there are those with true neuropathic bladders, known spinal lesions, which are further subdivisible into distinct subgroups. The essence is that in the first two groups, the 2-year VUR remission rate was certainly less than 20% overall while in the unstable uninhibited group it was certainly more than 30%, with Dr. *Koff*'s cases added in, more than 40%.

The only snag is that in Dr. *Koff*'s group are children who are perhaps most at risk of renal damage because they have the worst bladders. But in fact they had less in the way of recurrent urinary tract infection (UTI) on follow-up. By comparison the apparently safest group, who have supposedly normal bladders, were those who had the highest incidence of breakthrough UTI on the follow-up period. So there seemed to be a slight contradiction in these results.

I think the 3 cases Dr. *Taylor* showed us have to be regarded as urologically abnormal, both as regard the cystographic appearances and the bladder capacities. They seem to fit into a grey zone between normality and something like a pseudo-prune belly syndrome: perhaps some mild form of dysplasia.

The new clinical grouping concept, and Dr. *Conway*'s ability to prognose from his isotope cystograms, the reflux-bladder-volume correlating with the eventual disappearance of VUR, may hopefully lead to a time when two studies, carried out say a year, 18 months or 2 years apart, will enable us to predict what will happen in the future, and so reduce the number of studies required.

Dr. *J. van Gool*: One further point about UTI: we noted that in the group of girls that were screened after UTI had been eradicated the bladder pressures returned to normal. We also noted that most of the mothers also stopped administering prophylactic treatment, reasoning that as the symptoms had gone no more medication was required. And up to now we have not seen any recurrence of UTI in that group.

Dr. *P. Ransley*: In other words, as this bladder abnormality was cured, they stopped getting UTIs.

Dr. *J. van Gool*: Maybe. It's difficult to prove. It could be the other way around, the bladder abnormality being both initiated and prolonged by UTI.

Dr. *P. Ransley*: Yes. But I think it's a true concept that, when the bladder problem is treated, further UTIs cease.

Dr. *P. Avis*: It seems to me there is some contradiction between the role of bladder pressure and VUR. I think that Dr. *Conway* indicated that bladder pressure didn't have a great deal to do with whether VUR occurred or not, while some of the other speakers seemed to indicate that without high bladder pressure VUR wouldn't occur.

Dr. *P. Ransley*: I think it was a question of what they were actually monitoring. One study was concerned with bladder volume and not pressure, and the other was concerned with pressure and not volume.

Dr. *J. Conway*: At the present time we're recording both pressure and volume. In searching the literature there seems to be no question that probably as much as 70–90% of all VUR occurs at low pressure and low bladder volume. These are also our findings. Not only that, but the symptoms that the patients experience, whether of urgency to void, or feeling of fullness, have nothing to do with VUR. This is our conclusion.

Dr. *J. van Gool*: One of the factors explaining this problem might be that, as Dr. *Conway* pointed out, there was no correlation between uninhibited bladder activity and VUR. But he did not measure simultaneous rectal pressure. What might have been read as uninhibited bladder contractions might have been straining or something like that. One has to be very careful in making conclusions just from the bladder pressure alone.

Dr. *S. Koff*: The other point that has to be defined is the effect of the single pressure spike compared to the chronic effect of increased bladder pressure. Although VUR may not occur at a single pressure spike, the repetitive effect of high pressure spikes, as in the neuropathic bladder, can begin to alter the bladder status, so that at different volumes different effects can result, one of them being VUR.

Dr. *J. Hodson*: So now we have two parameters relating to ureteric status. We already have a grading of VUR based on the ureteric and calycine findings, and now there is this newer concept based on pressure. To me it essential to find out whether the former relates directly to the latter. We have to determine this basic fact, because there is no doubt that RN has some association with the grade of the VUR. There are thousands of studies showing it is the higher grades of VUR, as measured by ureteric diameter, which are associated with RN. Can we indeed say that wide ureters are associated with low pressure?

Dr. *P. Ransley*: Dr. *Hodson*, as a radiologist of many years' standing, you must accept the existence of the non-obstructive, non-refluxing megaureter in pediatric patients. I don't think you'd ever succeed in showing that these wide ureters originally resulted from increased pressure.

Dr. *J. Hodson*: This may be so, but it is an area about which virtually nothing is known, and I do not think it is a common entity in the population as a whole. These cases tend to gravitate to specialist centers.

Dr. *P. Ransley*: Infection may be a factor in their causation.

Dr. *J. Hodson*: Yes. But I'm still trying to get down to the fact that there are ongoing international studies in which one of the main measurements of VUR is based on the old idea of ureteric dilatation. Shouldn't it be pressure or, at least, both?

Dr. *P. Ransley*: I think, ideally, it's got to be both. What we heard this morning is, to my way of thinking, a much more physiological approach to the whole concept of VUR. Dr. *Conway* said earlier that, in any refluxing child, he could produce a result which varied between grades 0 and 5 depending on when he decided to take his picture. And although this was probably intended as a rhetorical remark, it underscores the question we are presently discussing.

I think that this morning we have learned that the lower urinary tract function should perhaps become the basis of our assessment of prognosis of VUR for the future.

Dr. *J. Hodson*: Dr. *van Gool*, you frequently used the expression 'pelvic floor contraction'. Do you mean, by this, the external urethral sphincter, or a combination of the external sphincter and other muscles?

Dr. *J. van Gool*: Well, there is still a lot of discussion going on as to whether there *is* such a thing as an 'external sphincter'. That is why I prefer to use the other terms. There is certainly some striated muscle in the urethra and there seems to be a true anal sphincter.

Dr. *R. White*: In this context there is something which has often struck me during the clinical examination of girls with UTI, namely that the ascending colon is always palpable. They either have dyschezia or constipation. I'm quite sure that they never empty their bowels completely. This may be related to an inability to relax the pelvic floor muscles.

Dr. *P. Ransley*: Certainly; treating their bowel problem greatly eases the management of their UTI.

Dr. *P. Kincaid-Smith*: Can anybody give us an idea of the relative importance and frequency of the unstable, uninhibited bladder in relation to VUR. Dr. *Conway* said that most of the VUR is at low pressure, and the other two speakers really dealt mainly with high pressure groups. Has anyone got figures as to the relative incidences of the two groups in the childhood population?

Dr. *M. Taylor*: Well, one can only say that all those patients who are shown to have VUR are a select group, and nobody knows what is the incidence of VUR of any sort in the population as a whole. But in those who have presented with severe symptomatic UTI or a micturition disturbance of some kind, the unstable bladder is a very frequent finding. I would just define what I mean more clearly. I refer to bladder contractions during filling while the urethra remains closed. I am not talking about voiding now, but the filling phase.

Dr. *P. Kincaid-Smith*: What I was trying to get at is that one group of papers suggested the unstable bladder was very common and occurred with low pressures, and the other that it was very rare.

Dr. *P. Ransley*: The two statements are not necessarily mutually exclusive. A bladder which refluxed at low pressure could also give rise to uninhibited contractions.

Dr. *P. Kincaid-Smith*: I judged that from the frequency of those contractions, one would see them during cystometric studies.

Dr. *P. Ransley*: But if contractions are not necessarily giving rise to VUR, which was part of this morning's message, then the pressure spike on a tracing won't necessarily correspond with a surge of isotope up the ureter.

Dr. *R. White*: One thing that we haven't taken into account is that if the bladder is frequently generating pressures at 2 and 3 times the normal voiding pressure presumably, even if VUR isn't occurring at the moment of one of these spikes, the urine coming down the ureter still has to overcome this high pressure to get into the bladder. This obstruction must have some effect on the kidney itself, or am I wrong?

Dr. *P. Ransley*: It has been shown there can be transmission of bladder pressure through a refluxing orifice, but this does not necessarily reach the kidney unless the whole system is full. And in the experimental model, one can see differences between the behavior of two ureteric orifices subjected to the same abnormal bladder pressure. So I think the effect depends on how long the pressure spike persists. If only for a short time there may be transmission to one kidney and not to the other. With a longer, more sustained contraction both kidneys may be affected.

Dr. *J. Hodson*: It is my belief and observation that once a ureter has been dilated, not just distended but dilated, whether as the result of obstruction, or sterile reflux, or pregnancy, and whether in man or animal, it permanently remains extraordinarily distensible by a pressure increase in that ureter. Clinically, if one employs ureteric compression routinely at intravenous urography (IVU) three particular groups can be identified because of this unusual degree of ureteric dilatation: one is the youngster who has moderate or severe VUR, another is the multiparous woman, a third is the patient who, in the past, has had severe ureteric obstruction over a period of months.

And although I'm not sure that one can say that these observations have anything to do at all with what has been postulated today, I think the grading of VUR against ureteric dilatation has to be looked at with very, very great care.

Dr. *J. Conway*: At the start we did a baseline comparison between our isotope cystography and our laboratory cystometry in the same group of patients and we found no differences between the two. That was one of the reasons that we decided that the simultaneous measurement of rectal pressure is not significant.

Secondly in a general population being screened for voiding dysfunction, the uninhibited bladder patient – which is determined only during filling – occurs in probably less than 15% of patients. I am excluding cases of meningomyelocele, as in this disease the incidence is much higher. As well, many of our patients with uninhibited bladder contractions have never had VUR.

As regards the dilated ureter and increased pressure, equating the two, in a sense, is of concern. From the experience of a large number of diuretic isotope renograms our overall experience is that the dilated ureter, generally speaking, is not obstructed. In fact, the ones I worry about are those which are not dilated. These are the ones that I think may transmit pressures more so than the ones that are dilated; this opposes the concept that the wider the ureter, the greater risk ot the kidney.

Dr. *M. Taylor*: Going back to the question of classification. Do patients with primary VUR have normal bladders? If so, we certainly have to change the present classification based on radiologic criteria.

Dr. *P. Ransley*: I agree with you entirely. Maybe one can divide cases on the basis of inferred urodynamic abnormalities from their history alone. What we need to know is the outcome of these groups in terms of renal damage. None of the speakers have told us the proportion of renal dysplasia and/or scarring present in any of these groups at the time of presentation and what they are like 5 years later. And because we didn't have that information at the start of our own study we may have to start again from scratch.

Dr. *J. Conway*: Two grave concerns: one is the fact that several of the presentation were using different bladder capacity standards. I don't understand that. Does each laboratory have its own bladder standard capacities? We searched the literature before reporting our data and found that there are a few classifications that we could standardize and these fit the formula that we described.

The second thing is the use of radiologic cystography as a basis for grading VUR. As several speakers have pointed out, this technique has an inbuilt degree of error that in simple truth renders it meaningless. So I think that the sooner that we get onto a more physiologic way of measuring VUR the better.

Dr. *J. van Gool*: I would like to support the statement that it is perfectly possible to detect bladder instability from the clinical history and we therefore do not need invasive techniques for screening purposes.

Dr. *S. Koff*: I hope, too, the pendulum now doesn't swing so that every child with VUR and UTI gets a full urodynamic study. That would be a disaster. Clearly we have to decide, in each group, which patients are at risk and which require this investigation.

Dr. *P. Ransley*: You mean correlating clinical and simply obtained criteria, such as urine flow rate and voiding pattern, with underlying urodynamic data. And maybe this will show that a good history of the flow rate is a way of sorting these children out.

Dr. *S. Koff*: Or a trial with anticholinergic drugs.

Dr. *J. Conway*: And bladder capacity, our urologists currently feel that that is becoming one of the most important clinical parameters in differentiating patient groups.

Dr. *W. Asscher*: Another whole area on which information is badly needed is the incidence of uninfected VUR on which, at the present, there is virtually none.

Section VI: Bacterial Infection

Contr. Nephrol., vol. 39, pp. 252–272 (Karger, Basel 1984)

20. Initiation of Clinical Pyelonephritis – The Role of P-Fimbriae-Mediated Bacterial Adhesion

Stefan B. Svenson[a,b], *Gunilla Källenius*[a,c], *Timo K. Korhonen*[d], *Roland Möllby*[a,b], *James A. Roberts*[e], *Kjell Tullus*[f], *Jan Winberg*[c]

[a]Department of Bacteriology, National Bacteriological Laboratory, Stockholm, Sweden; [b]Department of Bacteriology, Karolinska Institute, Stockholm, Sweden; [c] Department of Pediatrics, Karolinska Institute, Karolinska Hospital, Stockholm, Sweden; [d]Deparment of General Microbiology, University of Helsinki, Helsinki, Finland; [e]Department of Urology, Delta Primate Research Center, Covington and Tulane University, New Orleans, Lo., USA; [f]Department of Paediatrics, Danderyd Hospital, Stockholm, Sweden

Introduction

The way bacteria reach the renal tissue in patients with acute clinical pyelonephritis long remained an enigma. Vesico-ureteral reflux (VUR) provided a rationale for the ascent of bacteria from the bladder to the pelvis and intrarenal reflux (IRR) for the spread into the renal parenchyma. Gross VUR with IRR into conglomerate papillae has been identified as a main risk factor for progressive renal damage [16, 39, 40, 49]. However, only a minority of infants and children who have an acute attack of clinical pyelonephritis have VUR demonstrable by voiding cysto-urethrography (VCU) and in still fewer IRR is found [62]. Even scarring is found without associated demonstrable VUR.

Furthermore, in some children with VUR, the urinary tract infection (UTI) still seems to be limited to the bladder. Obviously, a mechanistic concept of pathogenesis of pyelonephritis and renal scarring – expressed in the term 'reflux nephropathy' (RN) – needs an amendment and a completion.

In this paper we attempt to analyse the role of bacterial adhesion in the pathogenesis of acute pyelonephritis and renal scarring. Bacterial adhesion to epithelial surfaces is an important step in the establishment of many infections involving mucosal surfaces [2, 12, 19, 50]. In UTIs certain *E. coli*

Table I. Examples of factors associated with virulence of uropathogenic *E. coli*

Factor
Possession of certain 0 serotypes
Amount of K antigens
Possession of certain K antigens*
Resistance to serum bacterial activity
Haemolytic activity
Opsonizing requirement
Adherence to human uroepithelium
Capacity to cause *D*-mannose-resistant haemagglutination

* e.g., K1, K5, K12, K13.

strains which cause pyelonephritis have specific fimbriae (proteinaceous extensions from the bacterial surface) which recognize carbohydrate receptors on the urinary tract epithelium. This receptor-active carbohydrate has been both identified and synthesized. This has made it possible to study on a molecular level the course of events when these UTIs are established. Monkeys possess on their uroepithelial cells the same carbohydrate receptor for pyelonephritogenic *E. coli* as humans. Experimental UTIs in monkeys may therefore shed light on the human infection and its consequences. It is concluded that establishment of UTI is the consequence of a complicated interaction between host and parasite.

Bacterial Virulence Properties in Non-Obstructive Pyelonephritis

Bacterial Virulence Markers. The bacterial aetiology of non-obstructive UTI varies with sex and age [60, 61]. Among girls below 10 years and boys below 1 year of age *E. coli* predominates. Many characteristics of *E. coli* have been proposed as special virulence factors in UTI; some of these are listed in table I.

Presence, amount and type of K antigens, particular O serotypes and resistance to the bactericidal action of normal human serum are some of the factors that have been implicated. Although there is a statistical correlation between the possession of each of the above-mentioned factors and uropathogenicity, the mechanisms through which they aid the bacterium to cause disease is in most instances unknown. For example, the higher prevalence of certain 0-types may be true statistically but the biological significance of carriage of a certain antigenic type of lipopolysaccharide (LPS) is still unclear. It is conceivable that certain 0-types might be genetically linked to other, as yet unidentified, factors which are of direct pathogenic importance (e.g. capsules, toxins, or adhesins). This has been shown to be the case in certain *E. coli* strains causing diarrhoea and pyelonephritis [38, 52].

As regards the capsular K antigens, it is more likely that certain of these extracellular polysaccharides contribute to pathogenicity. Thus, capsular antigens of low immunogenicity (e.g. K1) are often found on pyelonephritogenic *E. coli* [20] and are likely to endow the bacteria with a higher virulence by impairing the hosts' ability to evoke relevant protective immune responses.

Adhesion as a Bacterial Virulence Factor. The adhesive ability of bacteria – those belonging to the normal indigenous flora as well as many pathogens – is essential for the colonization of mucosal surfaces. The differential adhesiveness displayed by different bacteria not only explains the selective tissue colonization and invasion in a given host, but also gives a rationale for understanding the tropism for a particular host species which most bacterial pathogens show [2, 12, 19, 50].

In *E. coli* strains isolated from patients with UTI the most important feature appears to be related to their specific ability to adhere to human uroepithelium. This has been reported to correlate with the clinical severity of the UTI the bacteria had caused [53, 54]. Such an adhesive property is likely to endow the bacteria with an increased resistance to mechanical removal by secretions and the flow of urine. This will facilitate their ascent from the periurethral area and the vagina to the bladder and from there to the upper urinary tract.

Fig. 1. Electron micrograph of a negatively stained preparation of a P-fimbriated *E. coli* (strain JR1). *a* Untreated control (× 75,000). *b* Incubated with antibodies against P-fimbriae (× 60,000). *c* Incubated with higher concentrations of P-fimbriae antibodies (× 75,000).

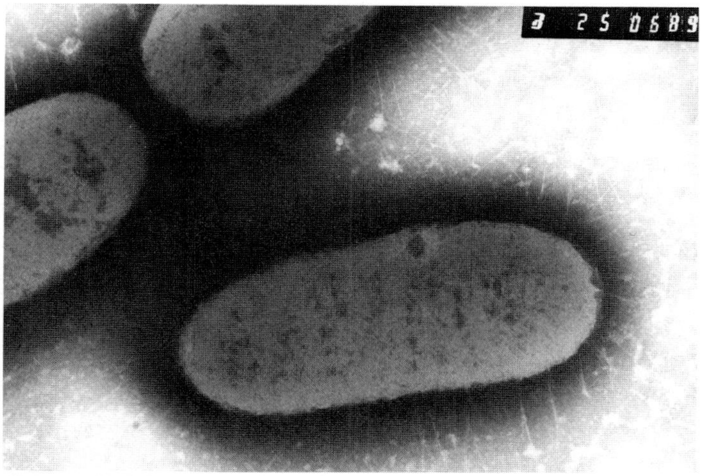

a

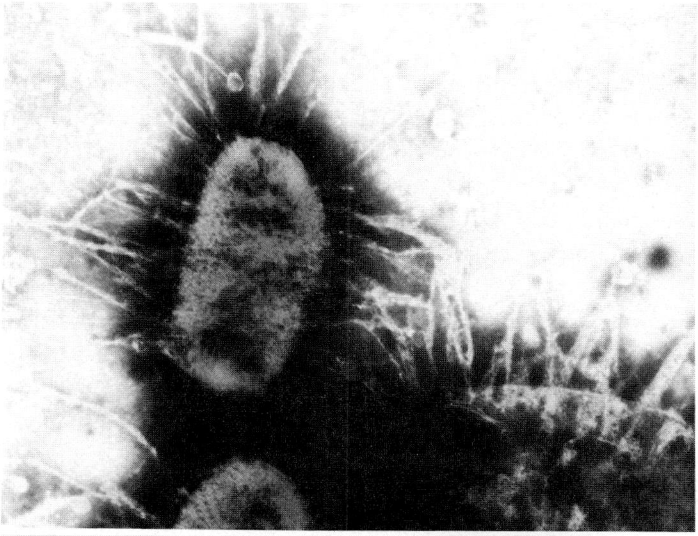

b

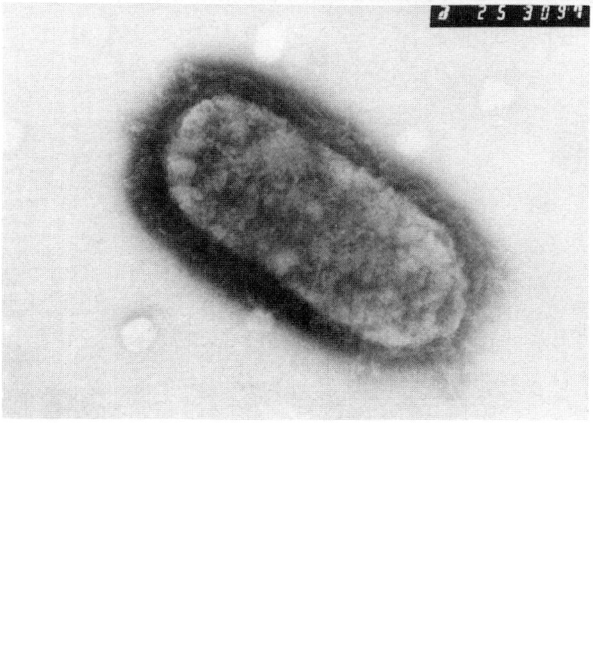

c

Table II. Phenotypes of the human P blood group system

Phenotype	P blood group antigens	Approximate Frequency
P_1	P, P_1, p^k	75%
P_2	P, p^k	25%
P_1^k	P_1, p^k	very rare
P_2^k	p^k	very rare
p	–	very rare

The specific adhesive capacity of bacteria has frequently been associated with the presence on the bacterial cell surface of proteinaceous appendages named fimbriae or pili [3, 5]. Morphologically, fimbriae are rigid filaments 3–7 nm in diameter and up to 2–3 μm long. The fimbriae occur in large numbers on each bacterial cell where they are arranged in a peritrichous fashion (fig. 1a).

Type 1 Fimbriae. The most common class of fimbriae occurring on *E. coli* and other facultative gram-negative bacteria is the so-called *type 1 fimbriae* [7] which recognize and bind specifically to *α-D*-mannopyranosyl group-containing receptors. Such adhesion is accordingly inhibited by addition of *D*-mannose, i.e. mannose-sensitive (MS) adhesion [6]. The clinical relevance of this type of fimbriae is, however, open to question. They are not known to be associated with upper UTI. Furthermore, since more than 85% of all *E. coli* have the genetic potential to express type 1 fimbriae, their pathogenetic importance must be difficult to judge [8].

P Fimbriae. Another type of fimbriae which, as shown below, frequently occurs in pyelonephritogenic *E. coli* is P fimbriae [28]. These are distinct from type 1 fimbriae in that they display *D*-mannose-resistant (MR) adhesion to human kidney and uroepithelial cells [26]. Bacteria possessing these fimbriae also bind to human erythrocytes, inducing a mannose-resistant haemagglutination [23].

From studies of the agglutinability of human erythrocytes of various P blood group phenotypes, it became evident that the receptors which

Table III. Haemagglutination of human erythrocytes of various P phenotypes by P-fimbriated pyelonephritogenic *E. coli* [from ref. 27]

Type of erythrocytes	Haemagglutination titre	Haemagglutination titre with added α-*D*-Gal*p*-(1–4)-β-*D*-Gal*p*-1-0-Me
P_1	4–256[a] (16)	none
P_2	4–256 (16)	none
P_1^k	4–256 (16)	none
P_2^k	4–256 (16)	none
p	none	none

[a] The figures indicate the range of the highest dilution yielding a visible haemagglutination. Figures in parentheses show the median titres.

pyelonephritogenic *E. coli* recognized were related to the antigens of the human P blood group system (table II, III) [24].

P Blood Group Antigens. The P blood group antigens correspond to a series of glycosphingolipids (table IVa). The specificity of the bacterial binding to the carbohydrate moiety of the P^k-antigen glycosphingolipid (trihexosylceramide) was evidenced by haemagglutination inhibition experiments utilizing the isolated and purified oligosaccharide from this glycosphingolipid [24, 25]. Independently *Leffler and Svanborg-Edén* [33] reported that P blood group antigen-related glycosphingolipids were functional as receptors for one pyelonephritogenic *E. coli* strain.

All P blood group antigen-specific glycosphingolipids contain the α-*D*-Gal*p*-(1–4)–β-*D*-Gal*p* carbohydrate structure (table IVa) which we have identified as the minimal receptor for P fimbriae [25, 29, 32]. This structure is present also in the Forssman antigen (table IVb).

By studies of the absolute molecular conformation of the carbohydrate chain of these glycosphingolipids it was found that the most hydrophobic domain of the α-*D*-Gal*p*-(1–4)-β-*D*-Gal*p* configuration was equally well exposed in the intrachain position (globoside and Forssman antigen) as in the terminal position (trihexosylcleramide and the P_1 glycosphingolipid) [57].

Table IV. p^k, P, P^1 and Forssman blood group antigens and corresponding glycosphingolipids isolated from human erythrocyte membranes

	Antigen	Structure of glycosphingolipid
A	p^k	[α-*D*-Gal*p*-(1−4)-β-*D*-Gal*p*-](1−4)-β-*D*-Glc*p*-Cer (trihexosyl ceramide)
	P	β-*D*-GalNac*p*-(1−3)[-α-*D*-Gal*p*-(1−4)−β-*D*-Gal*p*-](1−4)-β-*D*-Glc*p*-Cer (globoside)
	P_1	[α-*D*-Gal*p*-(1−4)-β-*D*-Gal*p*-](1−4)-β-*D*-GlcNac*p*-(1−3)-β-*D*-Gal*p*-(1−4)-*D*-Glc*p*-Cer
B		α-*D*-GalNAc-(1−3)-β-*D*-GalNAc(1−3)-[α-*D*-Gal*p*-(1−4)-β-*D*-Gal*p*-](1−4)-Glc-Cer
		(Forssman antigen)

Minimal receptor structures are boxed.

The final proofs of the fact that the α-*D*-Gal*p*-(1−4)-β-*D*-Gal*p* carbohydrate sequence comprises the molecular conformation needed for recognition and binding of the fimbriae of the pyelonephritogenic *E. coli* strains was achieved by two different experimental approaches, both of which rest on the chemical synthesis of this disaccharide. Firstly, the synthesized soluble β-methylglycoside of this disaccharide was shown to totally inhibit haemagglutination of human P_1, P_2, p^k and p^k_2 erythrocytes (table III), as well as to prevent adhesion of pyelonephritogenic *E. coli* to human uroepithelial cells [27]. Secondly, studies of individuals of the rare p̄ blood group phenotype have been helpful. These individuals lack the glycosyl transferases involved in the synthesis of all P blood group antigens [35] (tables II, IVa). Therefore, they lack receptors for these fimbriae on their erythrocytes and uroepithelial cells. Accordingly, they are deficient in binding P fimbriae. By coating such p̄ phenotype erythrocytes and uroepithelial cells with a synthesized glycolipid containing the key α-*D*-Gal*p*-(1−4)-β-*D*-Gal*p* carbohydrate entity we were able to endow these cells with high ability to bind P-fimbriated *E. coli* [29].

Fimbriae from several P-fimbriated pyelonephritogenic *E. coli* strains have been purified and shown to exhibit the same binding specificities as whole bacteria, i.e. they recognize P blood group antigens containing the α-*D*-Gal*p*-(1−4)-β-*D*-Gal*p* carbohydrate structure [32].

Host Factors in Pyelonephritis

VUR and IRR. Several factors have been considered important in pathogenesis of acute pyelonephritis and renal scarring. The close association between the more severe grades of VUR, with or without IRR and renal scarring, is well established through the pioneering work of *Hodson and Edwards* [15] and has been repeatedly confirmed [for references see 62]. Compound papillae were identified as a prerequisite for IRR [15, 39, 40]. *Hodson and Kincaid-Smith* [17] and *Hodson* et al. [16] found that in the pig (which has a multipapillary kidney similar to man) surgically induced urethral obstruction could cause gross VUR and IRR, with consequent tubular damage and interstitial fibrosis. The morphology of these lesions was similar to that seen in man with 'reflux nephropathy' [17]. These renal lesions were reported to occur also under sterile experimental conditions [16, 41].

However, the clinical significance of sterile VUR in the natural history of renal scarring and end-stage renal failure remains unclear. For example, *Smellie and Normand* [51] have shown that if VUR is present, and continuous antibacterial therapy is maintained so that the patient is kept free of UTI, the VUR itself has not yet caused progressive renal disease in their series. These findings are supported by other authors [13]. They, together with the fact that demonstrable VUR may not occur in children with acute non-obstructive pyelonephritis, whether this leads to later scarring or not [63], suggest that other important predisposing factors involving the host-parasite relationship are likely to exist.

Cell Receptors for Bacteria. The first clues of one such other predisposing host factor came from the findings of *Fowler and Stamey* [10] who studied the adherence of gram-negative bacteria to vaginal epithelial cells in women. They found that cells from UTI-susceptible women bound bacteria more abundantly than vaginal cells from healthy women. *Källenius and Winberg* [22], who studied the attachment of pyelonephritogenic strains of *E. coli* – later shown to be P-fimbriated – to periurethral cells from infants and children, showed that infection-prone girls bound these bacteria more abundantly than matched healthy controls. This, taken together with the fact that more than 90% of cases of acute non-obstructive *E. coli*-induced pyelonephritis in children were caused by P-fimbriated strains [28], suggested that the localization, density and/or accessibility of P fimbriae-specific receptors on target cells in the urinary tract and the kidney could be one such predisposing host factor.

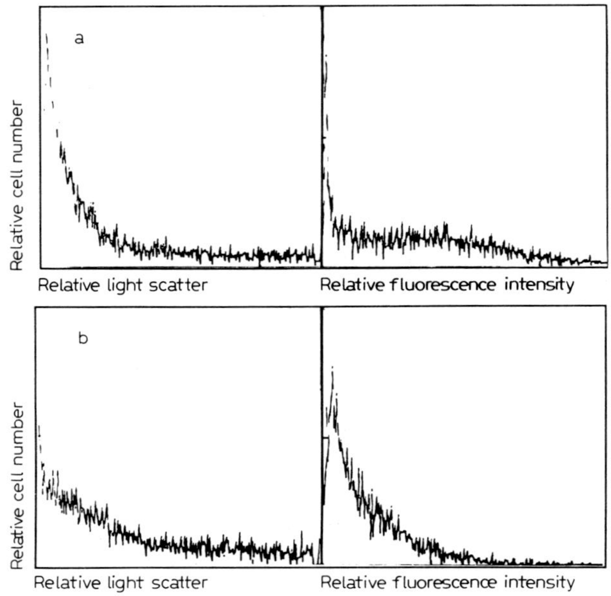

Fig. 2. Light scatter and fluorescence spectra of uroepithelial cells from a UTI-prone woman (*a*) and a healthy woman (*b*). Cells are stained with FITC-labelled *E. coli* JR1 and subjected to FACS analysis [from ref. 58].

Assessment of P Fimbriae Receptors [5]. We have recently developed rapid and sensitive methods for assessment of P-fimbriae receptor localization and density on mammalian cells [58]. The methods have taken advantage of the newly developed fluorescence-activated cell-sorting (FACS) technology, by which huge numbers of cells can be sorted simultaneously for size and relative fluorescence [14]. The method used for determination of P fimbriae receptor densities on cells is based on the ability of the patient's cells to bind fluorescein-labelled P-fimbriated bacteria. The cells are then subjected to FACS analysis. Figure 2 shows two typical fluorescence spectra of voided uroepithelial cells from an infection-prone young female (fig. 2a) and a healthy control (fig. 2b). In each instance 50,000 cells were monitored for binding of P-fimbriated *E. coli*. While most of the uroepithelial cells from the healthy control subject bound very few P-fimbriated bacteria (i.e. showed a large number of cells at low fluorescence levels) most of the cells from the infection-prone female bound the P-fimbriated bac-

Table V. Isolation of P-fimbriated *E. coli* from urine of patients with UTI and/from faeces of healthy controls [modified from ref. 28]

	n	Percent
Febrile symptomatic (clinical pyelonephritis)	35	94
Afebrile, symptomatic (cystitis)	26	19
Afebrile, asymptomatic	36	14
Faeces (controls)	82	7

Table VI. Occurrence of P-fimbriated *E. coli* in periurethral area and in faeces of pyelonephritic patients and healthy controls [modified from ref. 28]

Category	Periurethral occurrence	Faecal occurrence		Dominating faecal strain	
		n	%	n	%
Patients (n = 10)	10	10	100	9	90
Healthy controls (n = 52)	ND	5	10	1	2

ND = Not done.

teria firmly (i.e. most cells exhibited high fluorescence). We suggest that individuals possessing high densities of P fimbriae-specific receptors are at higher risk of contracting UTIs.

Clinical Relevance of P-Fimbriated E. coli Host-Parasite Relationship

P Fimbriation and Level of UTI: Faecal Colonization. While the association between P-fimbriated *E. coli* and acute non-obstructive pyelonephritis in children was found to be over 90%, the corresponding figure for cystitis and asymptomatic UTI was approximately 20 and 15%, respectively. Less than 10% of healthy subjects had P-fimbriated *E. coli* strains in faeces (table V) [28]. In patients with acute pyelonephritis the infecting P-fimbriated *E. coli* dominated the faecal flora in 90% of cases (table VI). In addition they were, in every instance, the predominant strain in the periurethral area. These findings support the concept that these UTIs are caused by bacteria which originate in the faecal reservoir and which ascend to the urinary tract via colonization of the urethral orifice.

Epidemiological Studies. The Role of Faecal Colonization. A crucial question is whether intestinal colonization with P-fimbriated *E. coli* predisposes to pyelonephritis. This is presently being examined in a prospective and a retrospective study. Retrospectively we have found an increased incidence of acute pyelonephritis in a group of children between 0 and 2 years of age who, during the neonatal period, had passed through a particular ward. In 1981–1982 more than 60% of the children with acute pyelonephritis (22 out of 36) in the referral area of this hospital had spent time in this neonatal ward. This incidence of pyelonephritis was 4–5 times higher than expected, since among all children in this referral area only 10–15% had passed through this ward.

Upon screening for P-fimbriated *E. coli* in the faeces of both ward personnel and neonates warded during 1982, more than 50% of the former and up to 85% of the latter were heavily colonized with P-fimbriated *E. coli*. The outbreak of pyelonephritis was traced back to the turn of 1979–1980 and appears to have been caused by a single P-fimbriated *E. coli* clone of 0:6,K5 serotype. This strain may have been maintained in the intestinal reservoir of staff and neonates in this ward for at least 3 years. The findings suggest that a child faecally colonized with potentially pyelonephritogenic P-fimbriated *E. coli* may be at a higher risk for future pyelonephritis. Early detection of a nosocomial spread of P-fimbriated bacteria may thus help to prevent pyelonephritis.

P Fimbriae Receptor-Specific Particle Agglutination Test. For rapid identification of P-fimbriated bacteria we have developed a P fimbriae receptor-specific particle agglutination test (PPA test), which accurately identifies these bacteria by simple slide agglutination [56]. With this test we have been able to detect P-fimbriated *E. coli* directly in centrifuged fresh urine specimens from patients with acute pyelonephritis. This shows that these fimbriae are present on bacteria also in vivo. The test may also be used to trace nosocomial spread of P-fimbriated *E. coli*.

Experimental Pyelonephritis in the Monkey

These clinical data are strongly suggestive that P fimbriae-mediated adhesiveness constitutes a virulence factor for pyelonephritogenic *E. coli* strains. Nonetheless, experimental pyelonephritis in a suitable animal model would provide more information about the pathogenesis of acute pyelonephritis. In most animal models so far tested it has been difficult to produce pyelonephritis with *E. coli*, either by haematogenous or ascending routes, without prior manipulation of the urinary tract [21]. One explanation may be that the *E. coli* strains used have not been able to adhere to the uroepithelial and renal cells of the experimental animal in question due to lack of relevant fimbriae, and/or the cells of the animal model may have lacked the relevant receptor structure(s).

Monkeys – although they possess monopapillary kidneys – are naturally prone to acute pyelonephritis. The incidence of non-obstructive chronic pyelonephritis in monkeys at autopsy was 0.65% [42], which should be compared to the 0.23% incidence found in man [9]. Furthermore, monkeys show an age-related maturation of the competence of the vesico-ureteral junction [45], which seems to parallel that reported for infants and children [31, 46]. Thus, if the monkey has the relevant receptor on its uroepithelial cells, it would fulfill one important criterion for being a suitable experimental animal for the study of the pathogenesis of human pyelonephritis.

Identification of P Fimbriae Receptors in the Monkey. Glycosphingolipids corresponding to the antigens of the human P blood group system are present in the kidney tissue of *Macaca mulatta*, *M. fascicularis*, Green monkeys, chimpanzees and baboons. We have also serologically proved that P blood group antigens are present in *M. fascicularis* erythrocytes. Moreover, P-fimbriated *E. coli* isolated from the urine of patients with pyelonephritis were found to adhere equally well to *M. fascicularis* uroepithelial cells as to those of man. This bacterial adherence was also totally inhibited by the soluble P fimbriae-specific receptor analogue (α-*D*-Gal*p*-(1–4)-β-*D*-Gal*p*-1-OMe). We thus concluded that these monkeys possess P fimbriae-specific carbohydrate receptor(s) [48].

Experimental UTIs in Monkeys with P-, and Type 1, Fimbriated E. coli

(1) Ureteral Inoculation. When monkeys (*Macaca* species) were inoculated into the ureter at normal pressure, *E. coli*, later on shown to be P-fimbriated, induced primarily ureteritis and subsequently, both acute and chronic pyelonephritis. A different *E. coli* strain, later shown to be type 1 fimbriated, inoculated in a similar fashion, did not cause pyelonephritis or did so only rarely [43].

(2) Bladder Inoculation. In another set of experiments, the bladders of 7 monkeys without VUR were inoculated with approximately 10^6 P-fimbriated *E. coli* suspended in 0.5–1 ml saline. 5 of the 7 monkeys so inoculated developed either uni- or bilateral acute and chronic pyelonephritis, whereas no monkey inoculated with type 1-fimbriated *E. coli* developed pyelonephritis.

(3) Vaginal Colonization. The thesis of an ascending route of infection was supported in another set of experiments. 3 adult monkeys were colonized with P-fimbriated *E. coli* in the vagina. Up to date 2 of these monkeys have developed cystitis of which 1 now has progressed to acute pyelitis [unpublished data].

Hence, these unpublished observations relating to ascending UTI in monkeys support the importance of the interplay between bacterial P fimbriae and P fimbriae-relevant receptor structures in the urinary tract. The pathogenesis of UTI in monkeys thus parallels that which occurs in man.

In vivo Infection Blockade Experiments in the Monkey. In further studies conducted in vivo in the monkey model, we tried to block the P fimbriae-mediated bacterial attachment by administration of a synthetic soluble receptor analogue.

Firstly, P-fimbriated *E. coli* bacteria were introduced by retrograde catheterization into the kidney pelvis of *M. fascicularis* monkeys, at high pressures. Such procedures will invariably cause acute pyelonephritis within 48 h. But after administration of P-fimbriated *E. coli* mixed with the synthetic soluble receptor analogue (α-*D*-Gal*p*-(1–4)-β-*D*-Gal*p*-1-OMe), there was no rise in the peripheral white blood cell counts for 48 h after challenge. By contrast, in control monkeys similar inoculation yielded a drastic increase in white cell counts within 2 h after the challenge (fig. 3) [30].

Secondly, P-fimbriated *E. coli* bacteria were introduced into the ureter of baboons at low pressure; after which their excretion time was measured

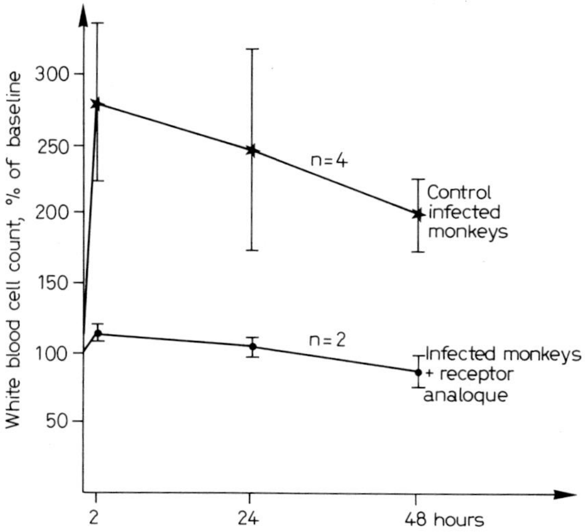

Fig. 3. Peripheral white blood cell count in monkeys infected with a P-fimbriated *E. coli* 04. 4 monkeys were inoculated with 5×10^8 *E. coli* in 0.25 ml physiological saline into the renal pelvis at a perfusion pressure of ~15 mm Hg. 2 monkeys were inoculated in a similar way at pressures of >35 mm Hg, but together with 5 mg of the soluble synthetic receptor analogue α-*D*-Gal*p*(1–4)-β-*D*-Gal*p*-1-0Me [from ref. 30].

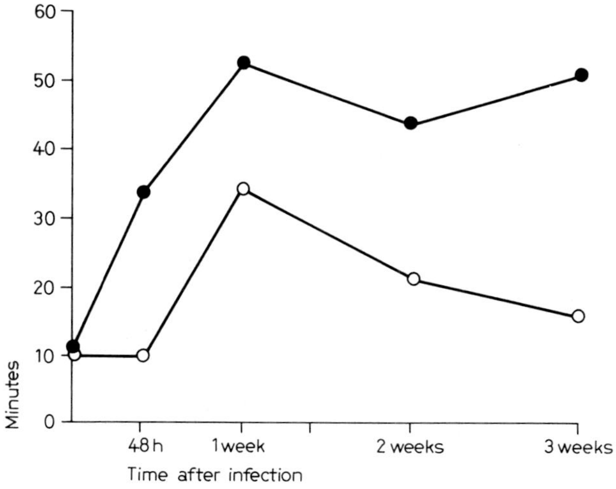

Fig. 4. Excretion time of radionuclide in baboons inoculated with a P-fimbriated *E. coli* 04 (3 monkeys) and with the same strain mixed with a receptor analogue (2 monkeys). ● = Mean for 3 baboons inoculated with P-fimbriated *E. coli* ○ = Mean for 2 baboons inoculated with P-fimbriated *E. coli* plus receptor analogue [from ref. 48].

over a 3-week period. In 3 baboons so infected, without addition of the receptor analogue, the ureteral excretion time, as shown by ^{131}I-hippuran scintiphoto studies [44], more than tripled within 48 h after infection. This is considered to reflect ureteral malfunction. In 2 baboons which were inoculated with a mixture of bacteria and the above-mentioned receptor analogue, no changes in excretion time were noted for 48 h (fig. 4). Hence, the ureteral functional abnormality was apparently prevented by the receptor blockade. Also, of more importance, while the control animals lost 10% of their renal function, as assessed by the measurement of the effective renal plasma flow, there was no change in renal function in the two monkeys subjected to receptor blockade experiments [unpublished].

All baboons were sacrificed 1 month after inoculation. The 3 which were inoculated with bacteria alone showed ureteritis and chronic pyelonephritis, with involvement of 30% of their kidneys. By contrast, there were no signs of ureteritis in the 2 which were similarly inoculated, but with addition of the soluble synthetic P fimbriae-specific receptor analogue. And only 5% of their kidneys showed any inflammatory changes. These in vivo studies also appear to support the relevance of P-fimbriae-mediated adhesion in the pathogenesis of human UTI.

Svanborg-Edén et al. [55] recently reported that globotetrarose, isolated from globoside (for structure see table IVa), interfered with bacterial adhesion and blocked experimental infection in the mouse.

Vaccination Experiments in the Monkey. In order to evaluate the relative importance of the immune response directed towards P fimbriae, we immunized monkeys with highly purified P fimbriae [32]. High titres of antifimbrial antibodies were elicited. In animals whose blood showed anti P-fimbriae antibody titres of 16,000 or more by enzyme-linked immunosorbent assays (ELISA), neither acute nor chronic pyelonephritis occurred although they were inoculated with P-fimbriated bacteria at pressures high enough to induce IRR [unpublished]. We assume that this was because bacterial adhesion did not occur in these animals due to blockage of fimbriae by antifimbrial antibodies. Indeed, when P-fimbriated *E. coli* were exposed in vitro to antifimbrial antibodies, the fimbriae became aggregated (fig. 1b, c). Such treatment interferes with the ability of the bacteria to adhere to erythrocytes and uroepithelial cells. Similar results were obtained in vivo in the vaccinated monkeys. Electron microscopic studies showed that the fimbriae of the few bacteria that were recovered from the urine of these animals were heavily coated with antibodies.

Interplay of Host and Bacterial Factors in Pathogenesis of Non-Obstructive Human Pyelonephritis – A Hypothesis

Based on the above-mentioned and other studies, we propose the following hypothesis for the interplay of host and bacterial factors in renal infection caused by P-fimbriated *E. coli*. Colonization of the intestinal tract and the periurethral area with P-fimbriated *E. coli* precedes ascending infection. Both the colonization and the ascending infection are dependent on the presence of specific receptors on the surface of the urinary tract epithelial cells. Ureteral infection occurs by means of retrograde ascent by VUR and/or by the hypothetical, peripheral juxta-epithelial area of turbulent flow in the ureter.

Bacteria bound to epithelial receptors of the ureter may replicate locally and advance further in retrograde direction through turbulence of flow. Structural damage of the ureter [11] and/or endotoxin inhibition of normal autonomic neurotransmission [4, 34, 36, 37, 59] causes ureteral hold-up of excretion and increased perfusion pressure in the ureter and renal pelvis [18, 43] with possible consequent change of papillary shape [1, 47]. Pyelorenal backflow may occur at low pressure IRR in the papilla rendered flat or concave through the increased ureteral pressure [1, 47]. Further bacterial attachment to P-fimbriae to renal tubular cells may then occur and be followed by acute renal tissue inflammation. This sequence of events would explain the fact that renal scarring can occur without demonstrable VUR [63].

In the highly susceptible host (e.g. patients with gross abnormalities, such as obstruction caused by stones, posterior urethral valves, etc.) effective adherence may not be necessary for bacteria to reach and persist in the urether or kidney. We believe that in such instances, almost any bacteria may cause UTIs [64].

Conclusions

Gross VUR and IRR – when associated with UTI – are serious risk factors for occurrence of severe renal damage. However, in many instances of clinical pyelonephritis and of renal scarring in infants and small children, VUR cannot be demonstrated by VCU either at the time of the acute UTI nor later when scarring is discovered. Therefore, the mechanistic concept of the pathogenesis of renal infection and renal scarring needs an amendment or completion.

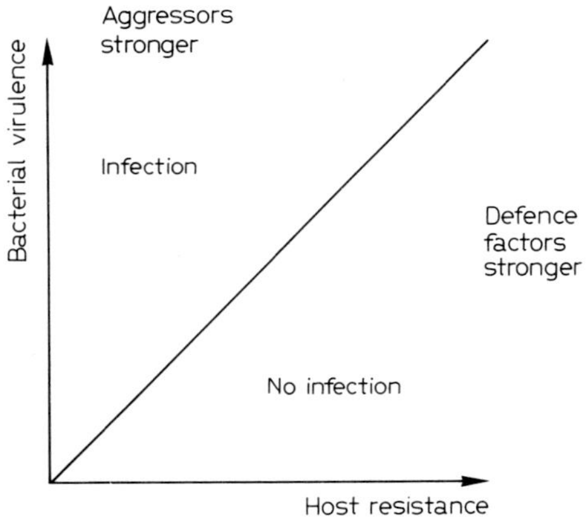

Fig. 5. Principle concept for possible interaction between host resistance and bacterial virulence (e.g. adherence). When host resistance is low (e.g. urethral valves) bacteria of low virulence (e.g. low adhesive capacity) may cause upper UTI. When host resistance is high only highly virulent bacteria (e.g. highly adhesive) will cause upper UTI.

The biologic principle of bacterial adhesion as a first step in bacterial colonization and infection of mucous membranes may be applicable to the understanding of the pathogenesis of UTI. Most pyelonephritogenic *E. coli* possess an adhesion factor – P fimbriae – which enables the bacteria to bind to specific carbohydrate receptors on the epithelial cells in the urinary tract. This P fimbriae-mediated adhesion to mucous membranes may well be the first step in the sequence of events which leads to acute pyelonephritis in patients without structural or functional abnormalities of the urinary tract. In those with gross VUR or obstruction, P fimbriae-mediated adhesion is probably not a necessary event. In other words, when host resistance is high, the bacteria have to be equipped with potent 'virulence' factors to induce infection and vice versa, according to the principal sketch shown in figure 5.

In patients with a normal urinary tract, P fimbriae-mediated bacterial adhesion is likely to promote damage of the ureteral mucosa and/or local toxic effects by the bacterial endotoxin which results in deranged ureteral motility. Studies in the monkey suggest that this causes a functional obstruction, with flattening of the renal papillae and this, in turn, may give rise to IRR of bacteria at low pressures. This situation may mimic the refluxing papillae in children with gross VUR.

If P fimbriae-mediated bacterial adhesion to specific epithelial receptors is a main factor in the initiation of pyelonephritis, it follows that among animals suited for the study of the pathogenesis of UTI and renal scarring are those possessing adequate receptors. Monkeys are one of the animals fulfilling this requirement.

Vaccination experiments in monkeys with P fimbriae protect against severe renal damage after inoculation of P-fimbriated *E. coli*. P-fimbriated *E. coli* inoculated into the ureter under normal pressure will cause pyelonephritis in the monkey while non-P-fimbriated bacteria infrequently do so. Similarly, P-fimbriated bacteria inoculated into the bladder of non-refluxing monkeys usually caused pyelonephritis; in most instances the UTI progressed to scarring; non-P-fimbriated bacteria inoculated in the same manner caused neither acute nor chronic renal infections. These findings are strong experimental evidence that gross VUR is not necessary for occurrence of acute pyelonephritis and renal scarring.

The growing understanding of the host parasite interactions on a molecular level will hopefully contribute to a deeper understanding of the delicate complexity of the pathogenesis of pyelonephritis.

References

1 Angel, J.R.; Smith, T.W., Jr.; Roberts, J.A.: The hydrodynamics of pyelorenal reflux. J. Urol. *122*: 20–26 (1979).

2 Beachy, E.J.: Bacterial adherence. Receptors and recognition; series B, vol. 6 (Chapman & Hall, London 1980).

3 Brinton, C.C., Jr.: The structure, function, synthesis and genetic control of bacterial pili and a molecular model for DNA and RNA transport in gram negative bacteria. Trans. N.Y. Acad. Sci. *27*: 1003–1054 (1965).

4 Cox, C.E.; Elkins, I.: Toxic effects of bacteria on urinary tract smooth muscle. Surg. Forum *19*: 524–525 (1968).

5 Duguid, J.P.; Smith, I.W.; Dempster, G.; Edmunds, P.N.: Non-flagellar flamentous appendages ('fimbriae') and haemagglutinating activity in Bacterium coli. J. Path. *70*: 335–348 (1955).

6 Duguid, J.P.; Gillies, R.R.: Fimbriae and adhesive properties in dysentery bacilli. J. Path. *74*: 397–411 (1957).

7 Duguid, J.P.; Anderson, E.S.; Campbell, I.: Fimbriae and adhesive properties in Salmonellae. J. Path. *92*: 107–138 (1966).

8 Duguid, J.P.; Clegg, S.; Wilson, M.I.: The fimbrial and non-fimbrial haemagglutinins of *Escherichia coli*. J. Med. Microbiol. *12*: 213–227 (1979).

9 Farmer, E.R.; Heptinstall, R.H.: Chronic non-obstructive pyelonephritis: a reappraisal; in Kincaid-Smith, Fairley, Renal infection and renal scarring, pp 233–236 (Mercedes, Melbourne 1971).

10 Fowler, J.E., Jr.; Stamey, T.A.: Studies of introital colonization in women with recurrent urinary infections. VII. The role of bacterial adherence. J. Urol. *117*: 472–476 (1977).

11 Fussel, E.N.; Roberts, J.A.: Chronic pyelonephritis. Electron-microscopic study. III. The ureter. Investve Urol. *17*: 108–119 (1979).

12 Gibbons, R.J.; Moute, J. van: Selective bacterial adherence to oral epithelial surfaces and its role as an ecological determinant. Infect. Immunity *3*: 567–573 (1971).

13 Govan, D.E.; Fair, W.R.; Filly, R.A.; Friedland, G.W.: Management of children with urinary tract infections. The Stanford Experience. Urology *6*: 273–286 (1975).

14 Herzenberg, L.; Sweet, R.; Herzenberg, L.: Fluorescence-activated cell sorting. Sci. Am. *234*: 108–117 (1975).

15 Hodson, C.J.; Edwards, D.: Chronic pyelonephritis and vesicoureteric reflux. Clin. Radiol. *11*: 219–231 (1960).

16 Hodson, C.J.; Maling, T.M.J.; McManamon, P.J.; Lewis, M.G.: The pathogenesis of reflux nephropathy (chronic atropic pyelonephritis). Br. J. Radiol. suppl. 13 (1975).

17 Hodson, C.J.; Kincaid-Smith, P.: Lesions in the pig kidney with chronic reflux nephropathy; in Hodson, Kincaid-Smith, Reflux nephropathy, pp. 197–212 (Masson, New York 1979).

18 Janson, K.L.; Roberts, J.A.: Experimental pyelonephritis. V. Functional characteritics of pyelonephritis. Investve Urol. *15*: 397–400 (1978).

19 Jones, G.W.: The attachment of bacteria to the surfaces of animal cells; in Reissig, Microbial interactions. Receptors and recognition, ser. B, vol. 3, pp. 139–176 (Chapman & Hall, London 1977).

20 Kaijser, B.; Hanson, L.A.; Jodal, U.; Lindin-Janson, G.; Robbins, J.B.: Frequency of *E. coli* K antigens in urinary tract infections in children. Lancet *i*: 663–664 (1977).

21 Kaijser, B.; Larsson, P.: Experimental acute pyelonephritis caused by enterobacteria in animals. A review. J. Urol. *127*: 786–790 (1982).

22 Källenius, G.; Winberg, J.: Bacterial adherence to periurethral epithelial cells in girls prone to urinary tract infections. Lancet *ii*: 540–543 (1978).

23 Källenius, G.; Möllby, R.: Adhesion of *Escherichia coli* to human periurethral cells correlated to mannose-resistant agglutination of human erythrocytes. FEMS Microbiol. Lett. *5*: 295–299 (1979).

24 Källenius, G.; Möllby, R.; Svenson, S.B.; Winberg, J.; Lundblad, A.; Svenson, S.; Cedergren, B.: The p^k antigen as receptor for the haemagglutinin of pyelonephritic *Escherichia coli*. FEMS Microbiol. Lett. *7*: 297–302 (1980).

25 Källenius, G.; Möllby, R.; Svenson, S.B.; Winberg, J.; Hultberg, H.: Identification of a carbohydrate receptor recognized by uropathogenic *Escherichia coli*. Infection *8*: suppl. 3, pp. 228–293 (1980).

26 Källenius, G.; Möllby, R.; Winberg, J.: In vitro adhesion of uropathogenic *Escherichia coli* to human periurethral cells. Infect. Immunol. *28*: 972–980 (1980).

27 Källenius, G.; Svenson, S.B.; Möllby, R.; Cedergren, B.; Hultberg, H.; Winberg, J.: Structure of carbohydrate part of receptor on human uroepithelial cells for pyelonephritogenic *E. coli*. Lancet *ii*: 604–606 (1981).

28 Källenius, G.; Möllby, R.; Svenson, S.B.; Helin, I.; Hultberg, H.; Cedergren, B.; Winberg, J.: Occurrence of P-fimbriated *Escherichia coli* in urinary tract infections. Lancet *ii*: 1369–1372 (1981).

29 Källenius, G.; Svenson, S.B.; Möllby, R.; Korhonen, T.K.; Winberg, J.; Cedergren,

B.; Helin, I.; Hultberg, H.: Carbohydrate receptor structures recognized by uropathogenic *E. coli*. Scand. J. infect. Dis. *33*: suppl., pp. 52–60 (1982).
30 Källenius, G.; Svenson, S.B.; Hultberg, H.; Möllby, R.; Winberg, J.; Roberts, J.: P-fimbriae of pyelonephritogenic *Escherichia coli*: significance for reflux and renal scarring. A hypothesis. Infection *11*: 73–76 (1983).
31 Köllermann, M.W.; Ludwig, H.: Über den vesico-ureteralen Reflux beim normalen Kind im Säuglings- und Kleinkindalter. Z. Kinderheilk. *100*: 185–191 (1967).
32 Korhonen, T.; Väisänen, V.; Saxén, H.; Hultberg, H.; Svenson, S.B.: P-antigen-recognizing fimbriae from human uropathogenic *Escherichia coli* strains. Infect. Immunity *37*: 286–291 (1982).
33 Leffler, H.; Svanborg-Edén, C.: Chemical identification of a glycospingolipid receptor for *Escherichia coli* attaching to human urinary tract epithelial cells and agglutinating erythrocytes. FEMS Microbiol. Lett. *8*: 127–134 (1980).
34 Long, S.; Nergårdh, A.: Autonomic receptor functions of the human ureter: an in vitro study. Scand. J. Urol. Nephrol. *12*: 23–26 (1978).
35 Naiki, M.; Kato, M.: Immunological identification of blood group p^k antigen on normal human erythrocytes and isolation of anti p^k with different affinity. Vox Sang. *37*: 30–38 (1979).
36 Nergårdh, A.: The functional role of adrenergic receptors in the outlet region of the urinary bladder. Scand. J. Urol. Nephrol. *8*: 100–107 (1974).
37 Nergårdh, A.; Boréus, L.O.; Holme, I.: The inhibitory effect of coli-endotoxin and alpha-adrenergic receptor function in the lower urinary tract. An in vitro study in cats. Scand. J. Urol. Nephrol. *11*: 219-224 (1977).
38 Ørskov, I.; Ørskov, F.: Special O:K:H serotypes among enterotoxigenic *E. coli* strains from diarrhea in adults and children. Occurrence of the CF (colonization factor) antigen and of hemagglutinating abilities. Med. Microbiol. Immunol. *163*: 99–110 (1977).
39 Ransley, P.G.; Risdon, R.: Renal papillary morphology and intrarenal reflux in the young pig. Urol. Res. *3*: 105–109 (1975).
40 Ransley, P.G.; Risdon, R.A.: Renal papillary morphology in infants and young children. Urol. Res. *3*: 111–113 (1975).
41 Ransley, P.G.; Risdon, R.A.; Godley, M.L.: High pressure sterile vesicoureteral reflux and renal scarring: an experimental study in the pig and minipig (Chapter 25, this volume).
42 Roberts, J.A.; Clayton, J.D.; Seibold, H.R.: The natural incidence of pyelonephritis in the nonhuman primate. Investve Urol. *9*: 276–281 (1972).
43 Roberts, J.A.: Experimental pyelonephritis in the monkey. III. Pathophysiology of ureteral malfunction induced by bacteria. Investve Urol. *13*: 117–120 (1975).
44 Roberts, J.A.; Domingue, G.J.: Experimental pyelonephritis in the monkey. II. The prognostic value of radionuclide evaluation of the urinary tract. Investve Urol. *12*: 374–380 (1975).
45 Roberts, J.A.; Riopelle, A.J.: Vesicoureteral reflux in the primate. II. Maturation of the ureterovesical junction. Pediatrics, Springfield *59*: 566–568 (1977).
46 Roberts, J.A.: Studies of vesicoureteral reflux: a review of work in a primate model. Sth. med. J., Nashville *71*: 28–30 (1978).
47 Roberts, J.A.; Angel, J.R.; Roth, J.K., Jr.: The hydrodynamics of pyelorenal reflux. II. The effect of chronic obstructive changes on papillary shape. Investve Urol. *18*: 296–301 (1981).

48 Roberts, J.A.; Kaack, B.; Källenius, G.; Möllby, R.; Winberg, J.; Svenson, S.B.: Receptors for pyelonephritogenic *Escherichia coli* in primates (submitted).
49 Rolleston, G.L.; Maling, T.M.J.; Hodson, C.J.: Intrarenal reflux and the scarred kidney. Archs Dis. Childh. *49*: 531–539 (1974).
50 Savage, D.: Adherence of normal flora to mucosal surfaces; in Beachey, Bacterial adherence. Receptors and recognition, ser. B, vol. 6, pp. 30–59 (Chapman & Hall, London 1980).
51 Smellie, J.M.; Normand, I.C.S.: Bacteriuria, reflux and renal scarring. Archs Dis. Childh. *50*: 581–585 (1975).
52 Söderlind, O.; Möllby, R.: Enterotoxins, 0-groups, and K88 antigen in *Escherichia coli* from neonatal piglets with and without diarrhea. Infect. Immunity *24*: 611–616 (1979).
53 Svanborg-Edén, C.; Hanson, L.A.; Jodal, U.; Lindberg, U.; Sohl-Akerlund, A.: Variable adherence to normal human urinary tract epithelial cells of *Escherichia coli* strains associated with various forms of urinary tract infections. Lancet *ii*: 490–492 (1976).
54 Svanborg-Edén, C.; Eriksson, B.; Hanson, L.A.; Jodal, V.; Kaijser, B.; Lidin-Janson, O.; Lindberg, U.; Olling, S.: Adhesion to normal human uroepithelial cells of *Escherichia coli* from children with various forms of urinary tract infection. J. Pediat. *93*: 398–403 (1978).
55 Svanborg-Edén, C.; Freter, R.; Hagberg, L.; Hull, R.; Hull, S.; Leffler, H.; Schoolnik, G.: Inhibition of experimental ascending urinary tract infection by an epithelial cell-surface receptor analogue. Nature, Lond. *298*: 560–562 (1982).
56 Svenson, S.B.; Källenius, G.; Möllby, R.; Hultberg, H.; Winberg, J.: Rapid identification of P-fimbriated *E. coli* by a receptor specific particle agglutination test. Infection *10*: 209-214 (1982).
57 Svenson, S.B.; Hultberg, H.; Källenius, G.; Korhonen, T.K.; Möllby, R.; Winberg, J.: P-fimbriae of pyelonephritogenic *E. coli*: identification and chemical characterization of receptors. Infection *11*: 61–67 (1983).
58 Svenson, S.B.; Källenius, G.: Density and localization of P-fimbriae specific receptors on mammalian cells: fluorescence-activated cell analysis. Infection *11*: 6–12 (1983).
59 Teague, N.; Boyarsky, S.: Further effect of coliform bacteria on ureteral persistalsis. J. Urol. *99*: 720 (1968).
60 Winberg, J.; Andersen, H.J.; Bergström, T.; Jacobsson, B.; Larson, H.; Lincoln, K.: Epidemiology of symptomatic urinary tract infection in childhood. Acta pediat. scand. suppl. *252*: 1–20 (1974).
61 Winberg, J.; Bergström, T.; Jacobsson, B.: Morbidity, age and sex distribution, recurrences and renal scarring in symptomatic urinary tract infection in childhood. Kidney int. *8*: suppl., pp. 101–106 (1975).
62 Winberg, J.; Bollgren, I.; Källenius, G.; Möllby, R.; Svenson, S.B.: Clinical pyelonephritis and focal renal scarring. A selected review of pathogenesis, prevention and prognosis; in Fine, Pediatric nephrology. Pediat. Clins N. Am. *29*: 801–814 (1982).
63 Winberg, J.; Bollgren, I.; Källenius, G.; Möllby, R.; Svenson, S.B.: Bacterial virulence and host defence in pathogenesis of renal infection and renal scarring. A selected review with emphasis on bacterial adherence; in Francois, Perrin, Urinary infection: insights and prospects (Butterworth, London).

Stefan B. Svenson, Department of Bacteriology, National Bacteriological Laboratory, S–105 21 Stockholm (Sweden)

Contr. Nephrol., vol. 39, pp. 273–279 (Karger, Basel 1984)

21. Comments on the Role of Bacterial Adherence in the Pathogenesis of Urinary Tract Infections

M.J. Harber, Ruth Mackenzie, A.W. Asscher

Department of Renal Medicine, Welsh National School of Medicine, K.R.U.F. Institute, Royal Infirmary, Cardiff, Wales, UK

Strains of *E. coli* [27] or *Klebsiella* sp. [3] isolated from the urine of 30 adult patients with a history of recurrent urinary tract infections (UTI) were examined for fimbriation by electron microscopy and standard haemagglutination reactions. All but one of the strains were non-fimbriate on initial isolation, although 70% expressed fimbriae after repeated subculture in nutrient broth. Periurethral cells obtained from 8 patients were found to have *E. coli* attached to their surface, but none of these organisms possessed fimbriae. These results show that fimbriae are not a virulence factor for bacteria within the lumen of the urinary tract, and neither are they required for bacterial colonization of the perineum which precedes the onset of UTI. It is not known whether pathogens associated with acute pyelonephritis express fimbriae once they have gained access to the renal parenchyma.

Our interest in the subject of bacterial adherence was stimulated by the reports of *Svanborg-Edén* et al. [10, 11] in the late 1970s that urinary pathogens showed variable adherence to normal uroepitheial cells in vitro. These workers reported that strains of *E. coli* associated with pyelonephritis were more adherent than strains isolated from patients with cystitis, which in turn were more adherent than strains associated with asymptomatic UTIs or those from the normal faecal flora. All these observations, which related the severity of symptoms to the adherence capacity of the pathogens, were made on subcultured bacteria isolated from children. We decided to test whether the same considerations applied to adult patients with recurrent UTIs and whether there might be any possibility of preventing UTI simply by inhibiting bacterial attachment to uroepithelial surfaces.

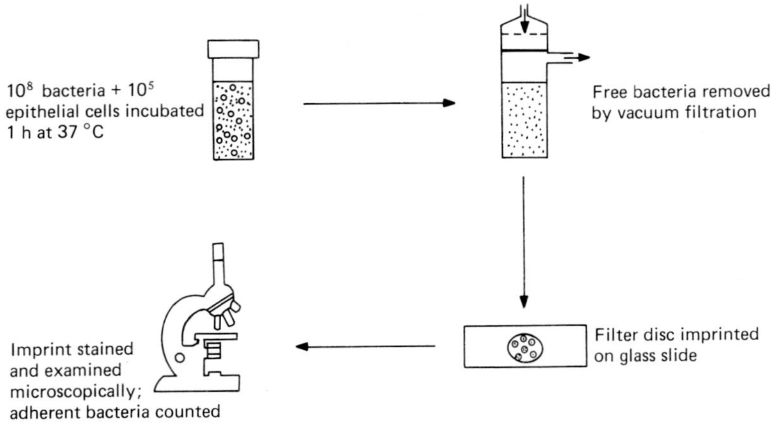

Fig. 1. Flow diagram of modified method for measuring bacterial adherence to isolated urinary epithelial cells.

During the course of our studies we encountered two problems which caused us to question the fundamental concept that adherence is an important bacterial virulence factor in UTI. The first problem concerned the methodology used by *Svanborg-Edén* et al. [10, 11] and others for testing the adherence of uropathogens to isolated uroepithelial cells. On attempting to repeat this technique we found that it was not possible to distinguish between bacterial adhesion to uroepithelial cells and adhesion to uromucoid. However, this technical difficulty was overcome by staining our epithelial cell preparations with 0.25% toluidine blue in 1% borax which rendered the mucoid visible under the microscope [2]. A scheme of our adherence testing method is presented in figure 1. Using the modified procedure it became apparent that strains of *E. coli* with type 1 (mannose-sensitive) fimbriae adhered only to uromucoid, while those with mannose-resistant fimbriae adhered predominantly to uncoated uroepithelial cells, these observations confirming a preliminary report by *Ørskov* et al. [8].

The specificity shown by different strains of *E. coli* for adhesion to uromucoid or uroepithelial cells is of great potential significance, since the uroepithelial surface of human and rodent bladders appears to be coated with a layer of mucopolysaccharide. This electronegatively charged layer has been demonstrated by electron microscopy after staining bladder preparations with colloidal iron [9] or ruthenium red [3]. Hence the initial contact between uropathogens and the bladder is not with the uroepithelial

Table I. Lack of fimbriation of freshly isolated urinary pathogens from adult patients with recurrent urinary tract infections

Clinical diagnosis	Number of strains tested	Number of strains with fimbriae on initial isolation
Acute pyelonephritis	5	1
Cystitis	15	0
Asymptomatic bacteriuria	10	0

The pathogens were strains of *E. coli* in all patients apart from 2 cases of pyelonephritis and 1 of cystitis in which the urinary isolate was a *Klebsiella* sp.

cell surface per se, but with the mucopolysaccharide cell coat. Unfortunately, desquamated bladder cells will inevitably have an incomplete coat of mucopolysaccharide. Furthermore, many sloughed-off urinary epithelial cells are likely to be dead, while the majority of epithelial cells appearing in the urine do not even originate from the uroepithelium but are squamous cells derived from the trigone. The use of epithelial cells obtained from the urine sediment in an in vitro assay for bacterial adherence is therefore of dubious relevance to bacterial pathogenecity in the urinary tract.

The second major problem we encountered was the great variability in the expression of different types of fimbriae exhibited by bacteria under different conditions of culture. Because of this variation it seemed important to look at the fimbrial characteristics of uropathogens on initial isolation from the urine. So far we have examined 30 freshly isolated uropathogens in which fimbriation was investigated by electron microscopy and by standard haemagglutination reactions. To our surprise only one of the strains was found to possess fimbriae on initial isolation (table I). In addition, cells of *E. coli* adhering to the periurethral cells of 6 patients with cystitis and 2 with acute pyelonephritis from whom a periurethral swab had been obtained were found to be non-fimbriate when examined by electron microscopy (fig. 2). These results do not indicate a fault with our methodology since 70% of our isolates were found to express fimbriae after four or more daily subcultures in nutrient broth. However, in contrast to the findings of *Svanborg-Edén* et al. [10, 11] there was no association between the adher-

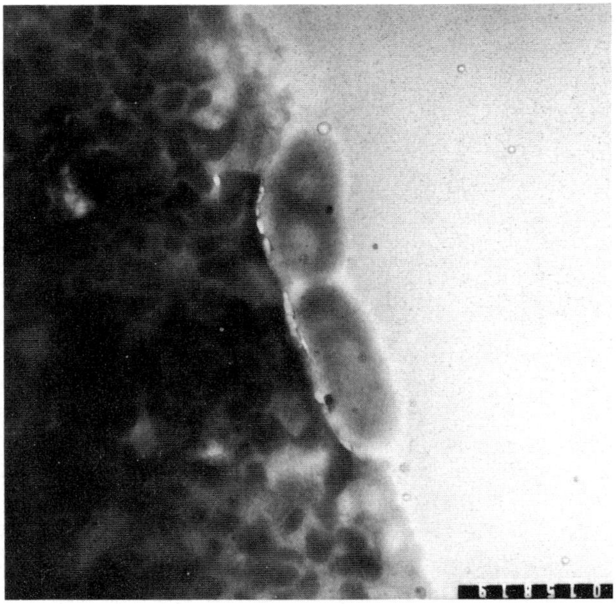

Fig. 2. Transmission electron micrograph showing non-fimbriate *E. coli* attached to the surface of a periurethral cell from a patient with acute pyelonephritis. × 8,500.

ence of our subcultured strains to epithelial cells in vitro and their pathogenicity in vivo [4]. These observations lead to the inevitable conclusions that fimbriae-mediated adherence cannot be an important virulence factor for bacteria in the bladder, and neither can it play a role in perineal colonization which precedes entry of pathogens into the urinary tract.

The reason for the lack of fimbriation of urinary pathogens on initial isolation appears to be 2-fold. Firstly, urine is a poor medium for the expression of fimbriae, as shown by the fact that only 26% of our isolates produced fimbriae after four or more daily subcultures in pooled normal urine. An independent study by *Ofek* et al. [7] has confirmed this observation. This lack of expression of fimbriae could be due either to a nutritional deficiency in urine, or to the presence of an inhibitor of fimbrial synthesis. Secondly, even when bacteria are subcultured in nutrient broth maximum expression of fimbriation does not occur until the organisms enter the stationary phase of growth, and yet bacteria growing in urine within the bladder are known to be in the exponential growth phase since the environmental conditions are analogous to those in a continuous culture vessel. Adherence assays are invariably performed with stationary phase cultures, which introduces yet another artefact into this experimental model.

A possibility arising from data by *Svenson* et al. [this volume] is that fimbriate bacteria may go undetected in urine if they are coated with antifimbrial antibody. This is unlikely to have been an important factor with our isolates, however, since the majority were from patients with infection of the lower urinary tract in which antibody coating of bacteria is negligible or absent [5, 12], while bacteria colonizing the perineum are even more likely to be free from antibody. Futhermore, antibody coating could not account for the gross differences in fimbriation observed with our strains after subculture in normal urine compared with subculture in nutrient broth. However, it will be important to take this factor into consideration when investigating fresh urinary isolates from patients with upper UTIs.

The demonstration of non-fimbriate bacteria adhering to periurethral cells (fig. 2) is particularly interesting since this dispels the popular belief that fimbrial attachment is the only mechanism by which gram-negative bacilli can adhere to cell surfaces. Fimbriae provide one means by which some bacteria can increase their surface hydrophobicity, but pathogens may also adhere to host cells through less specific hydrophobic interactions depending on such factors as their surface charge, capsular antigen content and somatic antigen type. Whether or not urinary pathogens are capable of associating hydrophobially with bladder epithelium in vivo remains to be investigated.

The term 'urinary tract infection' covers a spectrum of different conditions, and considerable misunderstanding can arise over the interpretation of published data if observations made with uropathogens isolated from selected groups of patients are extrapolated to other clinical types of UTI. A symptom-producing UTI confined to the bladder (cystitis) is quite different from an aetiological point of view to one in which bacteria gain entry to and multiply within the parenchyma of the kidney (pyelonephritis), despite the fact that the two types of infection arise via a common route. Asymptomatic UTI also deserves separate consideration since this benign condition is equally likely to involve renal infection as to be restricted to the bladder [5]. Our observations, to date, are based mainly on adult patients with a history of recurrent cystitis or symptomless UTI, and we have found no evidence that fimbriae-mediated adherence plays any role in the development or maintenance of these conditions. The report by *Källenius* et al. [6] of a low incidence of P fimbriae in subcultured strains of *E. coli* isolated from children with cystitis (19%) or symptomless UTI (14%) supports this conclusion. However, the same workers demonstrated a very high incidence of P fimbriae (91%) in subcultured strains from pyelonephritic infants. This observation complements, rather than contradicts, our work. We have shown that urine is a poor medium for the expression of fimbriae, but we readily accept that environmental conditions in the renal parenchyma are quite different to those within the lumen of the bladder, so that fimbrial synthesis is not necessarily suppressed in the kidney.

Fimbriae would not be required for pathogens to ascend the ureters to reach the kidney since bacteria are carried in films of fluid (they do not walk!), although a combination of vesico-ureteric reflux and intrarenal reflux might be expected to be required for large numbers to reach the renal tubules. It is possible that fimbriae are expressed by genetically capable bacteria which are successful in gaining access to the renal parenchyma, in which case these organelles could affect the interaction between the pathogens and host epithelial or phagocytic cells [1], and thereby influence the course and outcome of the infection. The immature kidney of infants and children may be particularly susceptible to toxic mediators released through such host-parasite interactions. These hypotheses are highly speculative at present. Time, however, and careful experimentations will be required to clarify the role of P fimbriae, and other potential bacterial virulence factors, in the pathogenesis of pyelonephritis and renal scarring.

References

1. Björkstén, B.; Wadström, T.: Interaction of *Escherichia coli* with different fimbriae and polymorphonuclear leukocytes. Infect. Immunity *38*: 298–305 (1982).
2. Chick, S.; Harber, M.J.; Mackenzie, R.; Asscher, A.W.: Modified method for studying bacterial adhesion to isolated uroepithelial cells and uromucoid. Infect. Immunity *34*: 256–261 (1981).
3. Fukushi, Y.; Orikasa, S.; Kagayama, M.: An electron microscopic study of the interaction between vesical epithelium and *Escherichia coli*. Investve Urol. *17*: 61–68 (1979).
4. Harber, M.J.; Chick, S.; Mackenzie, R.; Asscher, A.W.: Lack of adherence to epithelial cells by freshly isolated urinary pathogens. Lancet *i*: 586–588 (1982).
5. Jones, S.R.; Smith, J.W.; Sanford, J.P.: Localization of urinary tract infections by detection of antibody-coated bacteria in urine sediment. New Engl. J. Med. *290*: 591–593 (1974).
6. Källenius, G.; Möllby, R.; Svenson, S.B.; Helin, I.; Hultberg, H.; Cedergren, B.; Winberg, J.: Occurrence of P-fimbriated *Escherichia coli* in urinary tract infections. Lancet *ii*: 1369–1372 (1981).

7 Ofek, I.; Mosek, A.; Sharon, N.: Mannose-specific adherence of *Escherichia coli* freshly excreted in the urine of patients with urinary tract infections, and of isolates subcultured from the infection urine. Infect. Immunity *34*: 708–711 (1981).
8 Ørskov, I.; Ferencz, A.; Ørskov, F.: Tamm-Horsfall protein or uromucoid is the normal urinary slime that traps type 1 fimbriated *Escherichia coli* (Letter). Lancet *i*: 887 (1980).
9 Parsons, C.L.; Greenspan, C.; Moore, S.W.; Mulholland, S.G.: Role of surface mucin in primary antibacterial defense of bladder. Urology *9*: 48–52 (1977).
10 Svanborg-Edén, C.; Eriksson, B.; Hanson, L.Å.; Jodal, U.; Kaijser, B.; Lidin-Janson, G.; Lindberg, U.; Olling, S.: Adhesion to normal human uroepithelial cells of *Escherichia coli* from children with various forms of urinary tract infection. J. Pediat. *93*: 398–403 (1978).
11 Svanborg-Edén, C.; Hanson, L.Å.; Jodal, U.; Lindberg, U.; Sohl-Åkerlund, A.: Variable adherence to normal human urinary tract epithelial cells of *Escherichia coli* strains associated with various forms of urinary tract infection. Lancet *ii*: 490–492 (1976).
12 Thomas, V.; Shelokov, A.; Forland, M.: Antibody-coated bacteria in the urine and the site of urinary tract infection. New Engl. J. Med. *290*: 588–590 (1974).

M.J. Harber, Department of Renal Medicine, Welsh National School of Medicine, K.R.U.F. Institute, Royal Infirmary, GB-Cardiff (Wales)

Contr. Nephrol., vol. 39, pp. 280–284 (Karger, Basel 1984)

Discussion on Chapters 20 and 21

Dr. *J. Winberg*: There are some observations which are not accounted for by the hypothesis that all kidney damage is the result of infected or uninfected vesicoureteral reflux (VUR) into the kidney. We have long said that we see a fair amount of acute clinical pyelonephritis in babies in whom we are unable to demonstrate any VUR. When we looked at those with symptomatic urinary track infection (UTI) during the first year of life we found VUR in only about 40%. In symptomatic children over 1 year of age we found VUR in only about 25%. This is not to say that it is absent, but probably that gross VUR is absent. We considered, therefore, there must be some other way by which the bacteria reached the kidney. If children are followed from their so-called first UTI when they have normal kidneys, we find that scarring occurs in less than 30% of those with gross VUR, and although they may all have had non-refluxing kidneys, this is unlikely. On the other hand, if UTI is important, some factor relating to the organism may also be equally important.

Our hypothesis is that adherent P-fimbriated, and perhaps other fimbriated bacteria, might cause renal infection and scarring even in the absence of gross VUR. The factor that I especially want to emphasize is that we are dealing with the first year of life – one in which therapeutic delay might be of great importance in the occurrence of scarring.

Dr. *P. Kincaid-Smith*: About bacterial fimbriae; do they occur in other species than *E. coli*? Particularly what about *Streptococcus feacalis*? It doesn't have fimbriae, as far as I know.

Dr. *S. Svenson*: The P fimbriae occur exclusively in *E. coli*. Other species do not have P fimbriae, but they have other types of fimbriae.

Dr. *P. Kincaid-Smith*: So that when we are talking about what we commonly find in association with reflux nephropathy (RN), for example *Strep. faecalis*, the significance of fimbriae doesn't apply to all pathogens?

Dr. *R. Bailey*: And what about *Staphylococcus saprophyticus*?

Dr. *S. Svenson*: They do not have fimbriae, but they have a change on the outside which recognizes the receptor.

Dr. *W. Asscher*: What we are really talking about in all of this is hydrophobicity isn't it? Fimbriae increase hydrophobicity. The attachment of an organism to a surface is determined by a negative charge. The more hydrophobic an organism, the more it is likely to attach.

Dr. *S. Svenson*: Yes, hydrophobicity, but confined with specificity.

Dr. *W. Asscher*: When you talk about fimbriation it is a two-edged weapon, because if you are a bacterium and you adhere to a white cell, that is very bad news because you tend to get ingested. So let's not get away with the idea that it is all good news. Once in the kidney, presumably you also have an increased likelihood of being eaten up if you are an *E. coli*.

Dr. *S. Svenson*: Experimentally, if a non-fimbriated bacterium is attracted to either a macrophage or a T killer cell then it is eaten up. However, a P-fimbriated bacterium is less likely to get eaten up. The fimbriae protect it.

Dr. *W. Asscher*: The hypothesis you are putting forward is very interesting, Dr. *Winberg*, but its weakness lies in fimbriation being only found in cases where there is no VUR – after all, our major worry is the child with both UTI and VUR. You say that yourself. And yet this latter is the situation where the P-fimbriated organism is *not* found. Do I interpret that correctly?

Dr. *J. Winberg*: No, you do not. If one considers first UTIs in infants, some 95% of the organisms concerned have P fimbriae. On the contrary, the Göteborg group has shown that in the case of reccurent UTIs in children with gross VUR, the organisms often lack P fimbriae. So this is evidence that gross VUR can help bacteria settle in the kidney.

Dr. *W. Asscher*: What is your explanation for that? It worries me to think an *E. coli* can know whether there is gross VUR present or not.

Dr. *S. Svenson*: It doesn't know. VUR is simply an easy means of ascent up the ureter. Without it, organisms have to rely on aids like fimbriae.

Dr. *W. Asscher*: Can you explain the mechanics of this ascent by means of fimbriae to me? Here is a bacterium fixed, as you say, to its receptor site. How does it move up if it is fixed?

Dr. *J. Winberg*: It divides, and the new organism is free to move.

Dr. *W. Asscher*: It undergoes colonization.

Dr. *J. Winberg*: Yes. Once it is anchored it begins to divide and the outermost of the two subdivisions will spread across the surface of the urothelium.

Dr. *W. Asscher*: So in other words, it is a creeping phenomenon like ivy up a wall. Is there any evidence from the animal studies that a spreading sheet of *E. coli* develops and extends upwards?

Dr. *S. Svenson*: Yes, that is so.

Dr. *J. Duckett*: Clinically we see some very destructive UTIs with Klebsiella. Is that closely enough related to *E. coli* to be fimbriated?

Dr. *W. Asscher*: No.

Dr. *S. Svenson*: They do have fimbriae, but not P fimbriae.

Dr. *J. Winberg*: Was that a satisfactory answer to your question?

Dr. *J. Duckett*: No, I want to know why Klebsiella cause clinically devastating damage in the absence of P fimbriae.

Dr. *J. Winberg*: I think one must realize that bacteria have very many virulent factors. The fimbriae perhaps do only one thing, namely to fix the bacteria to their cathedral cells and so make it easier for them to deliver other virulent substances against the host. I think one sees this also in gastrointestinal infections, when enteropathogenic *E. coli*, for example, become attached to a cell and can then deliver their enterotoxins much more effectively. If they don't attach they can't deliver their toxins. Presumably something similar goes on in UTIs. I guess that Klebsiella can attach by other means and deliver their toxins to the host.

Dr. *J. Duckett*: My other question: Is the 'slime layer', which occurs normally in the bladder, as plentiful on the urothelium of the pelvis and ureter as it is in the bladder? I was under the impression that it wasn't. It is mainly on the bladder urothelium that the slime layer is present. Does that have an effect on the ability of bacteria to cling and multiply?

(Although this question was passed over, its importance is obvious. A consensus opinion is that it extends throughout the whole upper tract and into the collecting ducts. It may partly be related to, or mixed with, Tamm-Horsfall Protein [*Orskov, I.; Ferenz, A.; Orskov, F.*: Tamm-Horsfall Protein or uromucoid is the normal urinary slime that traps fimbriated *E. coli.* (Letter) Lancet: 1887 (1980)]).

Dr. *W. Asscher*: The slime layer is quite important because if you dissolve it with 0.4 normal hydrochloric acid and then you inoculate bacteria into the bladder, they attach very readily and survive much longer than otherwise. It takes about 48 h to regenerate the slime layer locally by the urothelial cells, so that the urothelium is at least in this regard a true 'mucosa'.

Dr. *M. Dillon*: Dr. *Svenson*, please enlarge on your earlier comment on trimethoprim's role with P fimbriae, and whether any other potential antiseptics have similar specific actions on P fimbriae.

Dr. *S. Svenson*: Trimethoprim is the most efficient drug so far tested in vitro in this regard. It prevents the actual development of fimbriae.

Dr. *W. Asscher*: We have looked at periurethral cells so far in 6 adults with recurrent UTIs, and we have not found fimbriae on the bacteria attached to the periurethral cells.

Dr. *R. Bailey*: We are assuming that P fimbriae do in fact exist. Dr. *Asscher*, have you lost the courage of your convictions? I understood that you considered that they were an artifact of subculturing these organisms in nutrient broth.

Dr. *W. Asscher*: P fimbriae exist. Of course they do. But when I look at fresh urine isolates, I can't find them.

Dr. *R. Bailey*: Is not that not obviously the only situation in which to look for them?

Dr. *W. Asscher*: No. P fimbriae are a very real thing, and may be very important in the kidneys of monkeys, or even in human kidneys. But in the urine they don't express themselves.

Dr. *R. Bailey*: That suggests to me that they may not be important clinically.

Dr. *W. Asscher*: I wouldn't go as far as that, because in the first place our material is very different from that at which our Swedish friends have looked.

Dr. *R. Bailey*: You mean human? Not monkeys?

Dr. *W. Asscher*: No, I meant that their human material consists of infants with their first UTIs, whereas we are looking at adult women who have recurrent UTIs. Dr. *Svenson* tells me the difference is because there is a very high titer of anti-P antibody in the urine of the adults which glues the fimbriae together. That is a possibility. We shall have to look for anti-P antibody in the urine of these women with non-fimbriated bacteria.

Dr. *J. Winberg*: I wish to make it quite clear that by this work we haven't advanced one inch the explanation as to why some people get recurrent UTIs. What we claim to have shown, with our Göteborg friends, is that P fimbriae might be important in first-time acute pyelonephritis, but not necessarily in recurrent UTIs.

Dr. *P. Kincaid-Smith*: I want to ask what percentage of people with asymptomatic UTI have P-fimbriated *E. coli*.

Dr. *S. Svenson*: 13% of infants.

Dr. *P. Kincaid-Smith*: So 13% of these infants are not producing any symptoms. Do you know what their localization is?

Dr. *J. Winberg*: We don't know. One explanation why they don't cause symptoms, al-

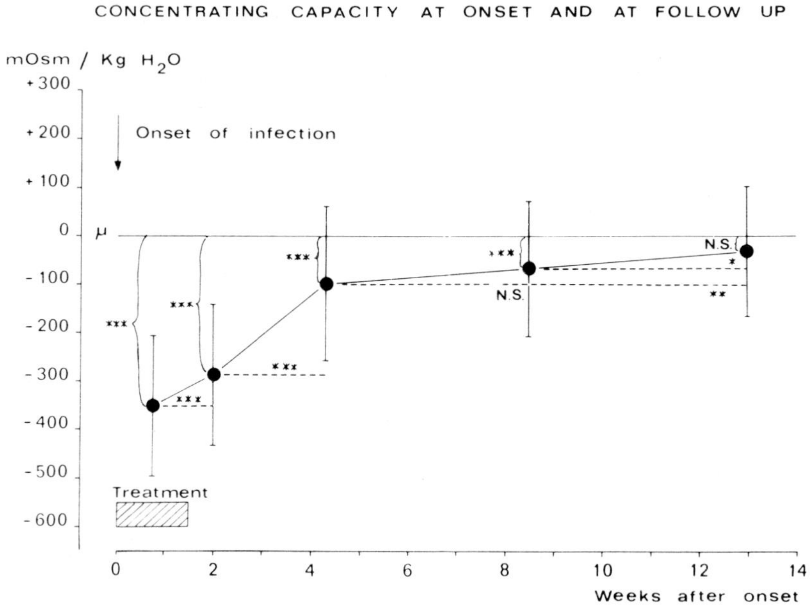

Caption to figure: Mean concentrating ability at onset and at follow-up in 95 patients with acute onset urinary tract infection with fever 38 °C and sedimentation rate 20 mm/h. The change in concentrating capacity is shown in relation to normal mean (u). Significance of difference between mean values in consecutive determinations (– – –) and between observed mean value and expected mean ([) are indicated: χ^2:p<, = or >0.05; χ^2:p<, = or >0.01; χ^2:*p*<, = or > = 0.001; n.s. = not significant.

though they have P fimbriae, might be that they lack the other kinds of virulent factors which *Hanson and Jodal* documented several years ago [*Kaijer* et al.: Frequency of *E. coli* K antigens in urinary tract infections in children. Lancet *i*: 633–664, 1977].

Dr. *J. Hodson*: Dr. *Winberg*, you maintain that 95% of acute pyelonephritides in infants were due to fimbriated *E. coli*. Are you taking that across the board and including all organisms and all first acute attacks? The retrograde pyelogram that you showed that Dr. *Roberts* produced in these monkeys, what has that got to do with the fimbriae? I never quite understood.

Dr. *J. Winberg*: He showed that some *E. coli* strains, when introduced into the ureter, regularly caused ureteral paralysis and renal infection persisting for prolonged periods of time. With the same high predictability, other *E. coli* strains never – or only rarely – caused ureteral and renal damage. Such strains were also usually eliminated spontaneously from the urinary tract. He never understood why. When he kindly sent us his strains and we examined them, we found that those causing pyelonephritis were P-fimbriated, while the others were not P-fimbriated. I think that this is central to the understanding of the whole matter of pyelonephritis and P fimbriation.

Dr. *J. Hodson*: These are presumably symptomatic attacks, as we have just been told that 13% of asymptomatic UTIs in infants also have P-fimbriated *E. coli*.

Dr. *J. Winberg*: Of those we have studied in so-called first attacks, yes. And in over 90% of these first attacks, the organism *is* an *E. coli* in our experience.

Dr. *R. White*: Pursuing the same point, I am still not clear how you diagnose acute pyelonephritis with renal parenchymal involvement. You talk about the clinical manifestations of pyelonephritis, but there is doubt here: and washout techniques don't apply in a reflux situation.

Dr. *J. Winberg*: I think there is only one way to be absolutely certain and that is to do biopsies and show that the bacteria are there. But if we disregard that, we use the following criteria: (1) The infants are really sick. (2) They have fevers of up to 41 °C. (3) Their sedimentation rates are high. (4) The CRP is high. (5) The IgM antibody response to the infecting strain goes up and then comes down. (6) They have bacteriuria. (7) They have a concentration defect that is temporary. I think that one of Dr. *Hodson*'s objections to the last criterion many years ago was that it might be due to an edema of the papilla secondary to pyelitis. As a result we subjected our studies to statistical treatment and found that it was 10–12 weeks before the concentrating capacity returned to normal after UTIs that have commenced treatment a few days after onset of symptoms (see figure). I would guess this prolonged period indicates true renal involvement more than just edema. So these have been our definitions.

Dr. *R. White*: I agree with you about the concentrating defect. All the others could be simply from bacteriuria.

Dr. *J. Winberg*: Let me add one more point relating to Dr. *Asscher*'s communication. The lack of P-fimbriated bacteria in his patients was to be expected. Adults with cystitis are infected with other types of bacteria, according to our experience.

Secondly, Dr. *Asscher* guessed that P fimbriae were not present in vivo. They are indeed present, as shown by the P fimbriae receptor-specific particle agglutination test that Dr. *Svenson* described and with which we have been able to demonstrate fimbriated bacteria in fresh urine in 50% of the cases of our first infant UTIs.

Section VII: Tamm-Horsfall Protein: An Unsettled Riddle

Contr. Nephrol., vol. 39, pp. 285–295 (Karger, Basel 1984)

22. Serum Autoantibodies to Tamm-Horsfall Protein and Their Relation to Renal Damage and Glomerular Filtration Rate in Children with Urinary Tract Malformations

Anders Fasth, Jan Bjure, Kelm Hjälmås, Bo Jacobsson, Ulf Jodal

Department of Pediatrics and Department of Immunology, Institute of Medical Microbiology, University of Göteborg, Göteborg, Sweden

Introduction

In 1975 *Hodson* et al. [13] reported that pigs with mechanically obstructed urinary tracts produced autoantibodies to a kidney protein, Tamm-Horsfall glycoprotein (THP). That report stimulated research on the role of THP in the pathogenesis of tubulointerstitial nephritis, and awoke our interest in the possibility of detecting autoantibodies to THP in humans with urinary tract infection (UTI). We later reported that all humans have such autoantibodies [8], and that the analysis of anti-THP antibodies could be used as a tool in the workup of the patient with UTI. Patients with acute pyelonephritis increased their IgG and IgA anti-THP antibody levels, but not those with acute cystitis [8, 11]. Further, in an infectious-free period, patients with renal damage had significantly lower values than both healthy controls and patients with previous pyelonephritis but no renal damage [5, 7, 11].

THP has also been shown to be an excellent marker of abnormal urinary flow and extravasation [4, 22]. In experimental obstruction of the urinary tract, THP is found within hours in Bowman's space and in the interstitium [22]. The possibility that THP autoimmunity could be part of the pathogenesis of renal damage has been studied in several experimental systems, where animals were injected with THP or urine. Rats injected with THP developed a moderate immune-complex nephritis, but no damage [14]. Rabbits, however, injected with either THP, or urine, not only developed a tubulointerstitial nephritis but also scarring related to that part of the nephron where THP is normally found and therefore focal [16], but not 'focal' in the same sense as the coarse scarring in reflux nephropathy (RN).

In the present study we report the result of the analysis of anti-THP autoantibodies in 3 groups of children with abnormalities of the urinary tract, and the relation of the antibody levels to renal damage.

Patients and Methods

79 patients treated at the Children's Hospital in Göteborg were included in the study. They were divided into 3 groups (table I):

Group A. 16 patients, 7 boys and 9 girls, 2–16 years old, with myelomeningocele (MMC) and varying degrees of neurologic handicap but all lacking control of their bladder function. 9 had renal damage on intravenous urography (IVU). All had sterile urine at the time of investigation.

Group B. 18 children, 5 boys and 13 girls, 1.5–16 years of age, who had undergone either nephrectomy or heminephrectomy. In 9 the procedure was performed because of malformation, a duplex kidney, on one side; in 3 because of obstructive damage due to posterior urethral valves; and in 2 because of pyelonephritic damage (RN). In the remaining 4 patients the etiology of the renal damage was unknown. None of the patients had had UTI for several months prior to the serum sampling, and the sampling was performed 6 months to 13 years after surgery.

Group C. 45 patients, 33 boys and 12 girls, 1.5-16 years of age with obstructive lesions of the urinary tract. 2 had posterior urethral valves, the others had ureteral stenosis either at the pelviureteral junction or in the distal part of the ureter. 37 had their obstruction surgically corrected 6 months to 12 years before the study. Radiologically demonstrable renal damage was found in 32. All were free of UTI for several months before the study.

Controls. The control material of 70 children and young adults without any urinary tract or immunologic disorders has been previously reported [8]. Serum samples were collected at the time the children underwent renal physiologic studies. The sera were stored at −20°C until analyzed.

Evaluation of Total and Unilateral Kidney Glomerular Filtration

In all patients both the total and unilateral glomerular filtration rate (GFR) was estimated, the former by ^{51}Cr-EDTA clearance, and the laterality of function by renography [10]. Single-injection ^{51}Cr-EDTA total plasma clearance determination was used for clearance

Table I. Clinical findings and serum IgG anti-THP autoantibodies

	Number (boys)	Age years	Renal damage	IgG anti-THP antibodies mean ± SD	
				renal damage	normal IVU
Group A MMC	16 (7)	2–16	9	39.1 ± 16.9[a]	128.3 ± 52.8
Group B nephrectomy	19 (5)	1.5–16	19	51.5 ± 36.4[a]	–
Group C Obstruction	45 (35)	1.5–16	29	43.3 ± 32.0[a]	141.2 ± 55.6[b]

The anti-THP antibodies are expressed as percent of the mean of a control group, i.e. 100% = mean of controls.

[a] Significantly *lower* than the control group, $p < 0.001$.
[b] Significantly *higher* than the control group, $p < 0.01$

measurements [2]. The renographic examination was performed in a standardized manner as described by *Bjure* et al. [1] and separate kidney function was thus calculated [12].

THP was prepared as earlier described [9]. For the *analysis of IgG anti-THP autoantibodies* the enzyme-linked immunosorbent assay (ELISA) was used as earlier described [8]. The tubes were coated with 10 mg/l THP. The conjugates were prepared using anti-human IgG (from Dakopatts A/S, Copenhagen, Denmark), and alkaline phosphate (from Sigma Chem. Co., St. Louis, Mo., USA). The absorbance was read at 405 nm and converted to the figure corresponding to a reaction time of 100 min. The readings were expressed as the percentage of the mean of the control group, i.e. 100% = mean of the controls.

Statistical Procedures. Student's t-test was used to compare the mean values between children with and without renal damage in the different groups, and the mean values of the groups with those of the controls. 4-fold table test was used to relate the antibody values found in group C, to the period since surgery. Spearman's coefficient of rank correlation was calculated for group B.

Results

In all three groups of children there were significant differences between the mean IgG serum anti-THP autoantibody levels of those with renal damage compared with those without, or with the controls (table I).

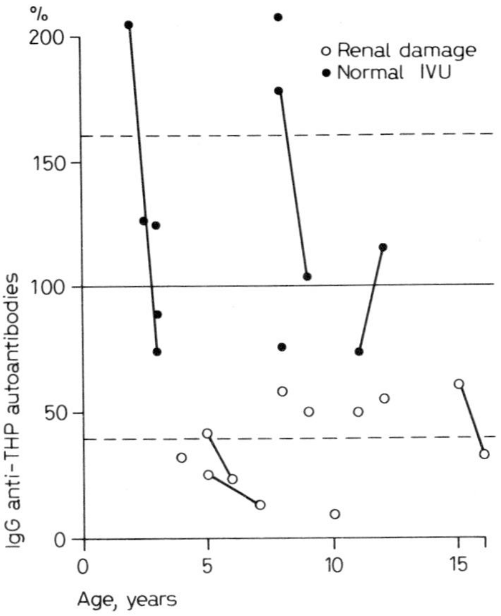

Fig. 1. IgG anti-THP antibody levels in serum from 16 children with myelomeningocele. The values connected with a line represent more than one serum sample from a single patient. The mean and ± 2 SD of the control group are indicated. The antibody levels are expressed as percent of the control group and are given as a function of age. The difference between children with and without renal damage is significant ($p < 0.001$).

In group A (children with myelomeningocele) there was no overlap between those with renal damage and those without (fig. 1). No child with renal damage had an IgG anti-THP antibody level above the mean −1 SD of the controls. In 6 of the children, 2 samples were analyzed (fig. 1) and 5 showed decreasing antibody values.

In group B (hemi-nephrectomized children) no significant difference could be found between the IgG anti-THP antibody levels in serum from individuals operated on within the previous 5 years and those operated on before that period (fig. 2). However, in 5 cases 2 or more blood samples were analyzed and all 5 showed an increased antibody level after the operation. When the IgG serum antibody levels to THP of 9 hemi-nephrectomized children were related to the GFR of the most damaged kidney a significant correlation was found ($p < 0.05$) (fig. 3). But no such relationship could be found when the GFR of the remaining kidney and the IgG anti-THP antibody levels were compared in 10 children who had undergone total nephrectomy (fig. 4). The results from group C (chidren with urinary

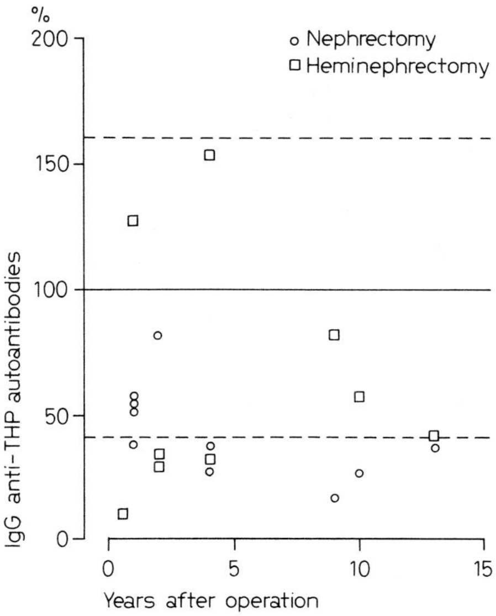

Fig. 2. IgG anti-THP antibody levels in serum from 18 children who had undergone partial or total nephrectomy in relation to time after operation. Explanations as in figure 1. The values found are significantly lower than those of the control group ($p < 0.001$).

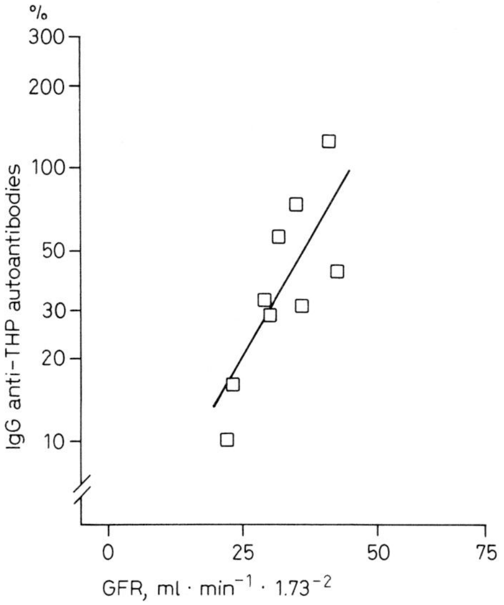

Fig. 3. IgG anti-THP antibody levels in serum from 9 heminephrectomized children in relation to glomerular filtration rate of the most damaged kidney. Explanation as in figure 1. The equation for the regression line was $x = 28.6 \log y - 12.3$, $r = 0.72$ ($p < 0.05$).

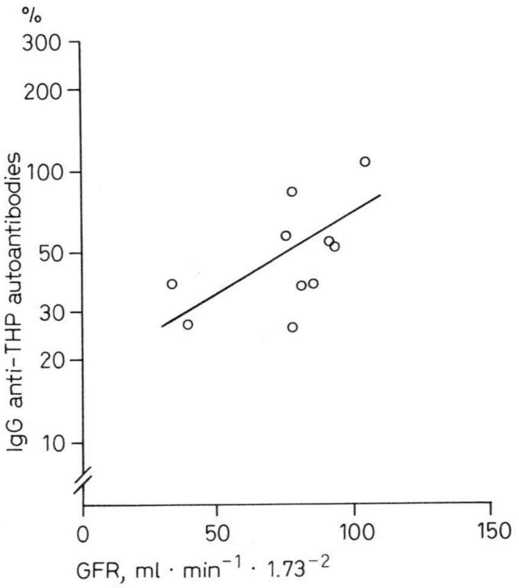

Fig. 4. IgG anti-THP antibody levels in serum from 10 nephrectomized children in relation to glomerular filtration rate. Explanation as in figure 1. The equation for the regression line was: $x = 171.4 \log y - 233.7$, $r = 0.58$ ($p < 0.1$).

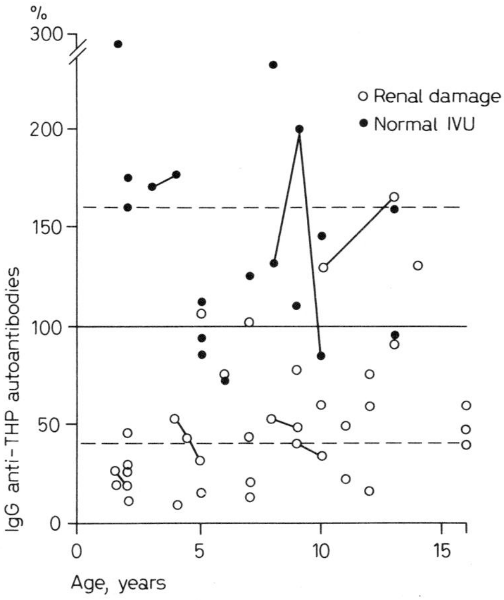

Fig. 5. IgG anti-THP antibody levels in serum from 45 children with previous obstruction of their urinary tract. Explanation as in figure 1. The values are given as function of age.

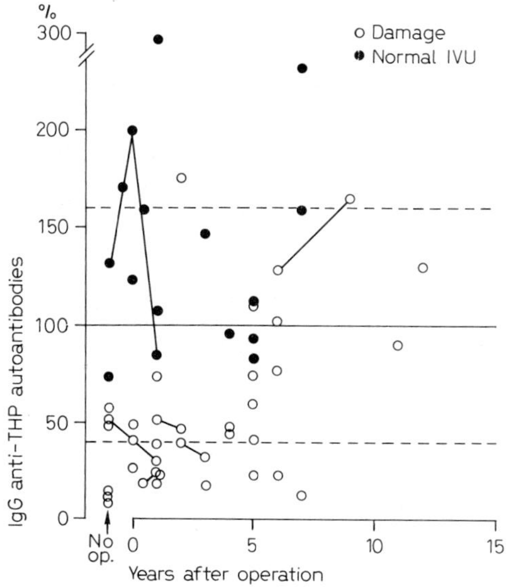

Fig. 6. IgG anti-THP antibody levels in serum from 45 children with past obstruction of their urinary tract. Explanations as in figure 1. The values are given as function of time after operation.

tract obstruction treated by surgery) are presented in figures 5–7. No correlation between IgG anti-THP antibody levels and age could be found, either before or after surgery. However, significantly more children with renal damage 5 or more years after surgery had IgG autoantibody levels above 50%, compared with those with renal damage less than 5 years after surgery (fig. 6). A strong correlation ($p < 0.001$) was found between the GFR of the most damaged kidney and the anti-THP antibody values (fig. 7). This correlation was found regardless of the time since surgery, i.e. a low filtration rate corresponded to a low antibody level and a high filtration rate corresponded to a high antibody level, regardless of whether the patient had renal damage or not.

Discussion

The present study confirms earlier reports of low levels of IgG anti-THP levels in serum from children with renal damage [5–8], and that these were found in all age groups. Previously we had also shown that the low antibody values were also not related simply to a previous history of UTI, since patients with earlier pyelonephritis, but no demonstrable renal damage 6 months after their last UTI, still had increased IgG anti-THP antibodies [7].

Children with renal damage did not have IgG anti-THP antibody values above the mean −1 SD of the control group, which is in agreement with previous reports [7, 8]. Thus, the finding of IgG anti-THP antibody levels below the mean −1 SD of the controls in a child with a history of febrile UTIs strongly indicates renal damage. THP autoantibody levels in the range of the mean of the controls, or above, were found in patients with damaged kidneys only when the diseased part had been excised, or the obstruction had been relieved or, as was shown in a previous study, when several years had elapsed since the last UTI [5].

Interestingly, in the period following surgery, the anti-THP antibodies did not increase, although the obstruction of the urinary flow was relieved. Not until 5 years later was there a significant increase of the serum antibody values in the children with renal damage, many of whom were by that time adolescents. This could support the findings of *Claësson* et al. [3] that a damaged kidney, even when the disease process was halted, did not commence to hypertrophy until puberty. And that the normal *total* GFR during childhood was usually the result of compensatory growth of the contralateral, undamaged kidney. The very clear correlation between IgG anti-THP antibody values and the GFR of the most damaged kidney supports the same conclusion.

The same correlation also suggest a role of THP in the disease process of RN; either as a marker of immunologic events of which autoimmunity to THP is only a part, or because it reflects a direct pathogenetic role of THP autoimmunity in the pathogenesis of RN. Support for the latter hypothesis can be found in the work of *Mayrer* et al. [16]. Rabbits injected with either rabbit urine or rabbit THP developed a focal tubulointerstitial nephritis with focal fibrosis. The lesions were found in those parts of the nephron where THP is normally produced and were characterized by focal mononuclear infiltrates. No immunoglobulin deposition was detected in spite of the finding that the rabbits produced anti-THP antibodies. However, a cellular immune response, cytotoxic to fibroblasts in the presence of THP, was found and concluded to be related to the cause of the nephritis rather than the THP antibodies.

In our study, the patients with urinary obstruction but no renal damage, as judged by urography, had antibody levels significantly higher than

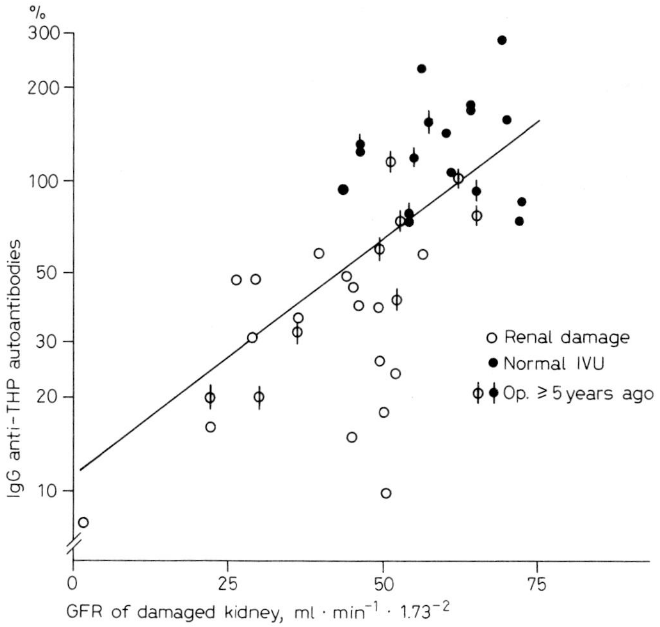

Fig. 7. IgG anti-THP antibody levels in relation to glomerular filtration rate of the most damaged kidney in 45 children with previous obstruction of their urinary tract. The equation for the regression line was: $x = 65.8 \log y - 69.1$, $r = 0.63$ ($p < 0.001$).

the controls. This increased antibody production could be due to previous UTI, as virtually all of the children had had acute pyelonephritis as their presenting symptom. Another possibility is that the obstruction had resulted in the extravasation of urine and THP interstitially and this had been the stimulus for increased anti-THP antibody production.

The latter however seems less likely, as the patients with renal damage had low antibody levels. These patients should have had more THP introduced interstitially and would, therefore, be expected to have developed even higher antibody levels. Deposits of THP interstitially have been demonstrated in a number of tubulointerstitial disorders in humans [19, 21, 23] and in experimental RN [1, 22]. One may speculate that the amount of THP introduced to the immune system regulates whether the anti-THP antibody production will be increased or not. Alternatively, in case of renal damage, other autoantigens could be released that have a general immune-suppressive effect. Such an immune suppression could be beneficial, as it would stop inflammation and further renal damage.

Activation of suppressor cell mechanisms has been demonstrated in experimental pyelonephritis [17, 20], autoimmune experimental interstitial nephritis [18], and in humans with interstitial nephritis [15]. In none of these studies was the full role of the detected immune suppressive mechanisms established; both negative [20] and positive [18] effects on the outcome of disease were discussed.

Acknowledgements

This study was given financial support by grants from the Swedish Medical Research Council (No. 215) and the Ellen, Walter and Lennart Hesselman Foundation for Scientific Research.

The author wants to thank *Monika Eriksson* for her skillful technical assistance.

References

1 Bjure, J.; Aurell, M.; Granérus, G.; Haugstvedt, S.: Methodological aspects of renography in children. Scand. J. Urol. Nephrol. *14*: 243–250 (1980).

2 Brøchner-Mortensen, J.; Haahr, J.; Christoffersen, J.: A simple method for accurate assessment of the glomerular filtration rate in children. Scand. J. clin. Lab. Invest. *33*: 139–144 (1974).

3 Claësson, I.; Jacobsson, B.; Jodal, U.; Winberg, J.: Compensatory kidney growth in children with urinary tract infection and unilateral renal scarring: an epidemiologic study. Kidney int. *20*: 759–765 (1981).

4 Cotran, R.S.; Hodson, C.J.: Reflux Nephropathy; 1st ed., pp. 213–219 (Masson, New York 1979).

5 Fasth, A.: Autoantibodies against Tamm-Horsfall glycoprotein in urinary tract infections. A new tool for diagnosing renal infections and renal damage; thesis, Göteborg (1980).

6 Fasth, A.; Bengtson, U.; Kaijser, B.; Wieslander, J.: Antibodies to Tamm-Horsfall protein associated with kidney damage and urinary tract infections in adults. Kidney int. *20*: 500–504 (1981).

7 Fasth, A.; Bjure, J.; Hellström, M.; Jacobsson, B.; Jodal, U.: Autoantibodies to Tamm-Horsfall protein in children with renal damage associated with urinary tract infection. Acta paediat. scand. *69*: 709–715 (1980).

8 Fasth, A.; Hanson, L.Å.; Jodal, U.; Peterson, H.: Autoantibodies to Tamm-Horsfall protein associated with urinary tract infection in girls. J. Pediat. *95: 54–60 (1979).*

9 Fletcher, A.P.: Glycoproteins; 2nd ed., pp. 892–908 (Elsevier, Amstedam 1972).

10 Granérus, G.; Aurell, M.; Bjure, J.; Haugstvedt, S.; Ljung, B.: Evaluation of unilateral kidney function in children. A comparison between renography and separate clearance. Scand. J. Urol. Nephrol. *14*: 263–267 (1980).

11 Hanson, L.Å.; Fasth, A.; Jodal, U.: Autoantibodies to Tamm-Horsfall protein. A tool for diagnosing the level of urinary tract infection. Lancet *i*: 226–228 (1976).
12 Haugstvedt, S.; Bjure, J.; Granérus, G.: A simple method of background subtraction in two-detector renography. Scand. J. Urol. Nephrol. *14*: 257–261 (1980).
13 Hodson, C.J.; Maling, T.M.J.; McManamon, P.J.: Reflux nephropathy. Kidney int. *8*: 50–58 (1975).
14 Hoyer, J.R.: Tubulointerstitial immune complex nephritis in rats immunized with Tamm-Horsfall protein. Kidney int. *17*: 284–292 (1980).
15 Husby, G.; Tung, K.S.K.; Williams, R.C., Jr.: Characterization of renal tissue lymphocytes in patients with interstitial nephritis. Am. J. Med. *70*: 31–38 (1981).
16 Mayrer, A.R.; Kashgarian, M.; Ruddle, N.H.; Marier, R.; Hodson, C.J.; Richards, F.F.; Andriole, V.T.: Tubulointerstitial nephritis and immunologic responses to Tamm-Horsfall protein. in rabbits challenged with homologous urine or Tamm-Horsfall protein. J. Immun. *128*: 2634–2642 (1982).
17 Miller, T.L.; Marshall, E.: Bacteriological and immunological aspects of urinary infections in children; 1st ed., pp. 163–171 (Thieme, Stuttgart 1982).
18 Neilson, E.C.; Phillips, S.M.: Cell-mediated immunity in interstitial nephritis. I. T-lymphocyte systems in nephritic guinea pigs: the natural history and diversity of the immune preresponse. J. Immun. *123*: 2373–2380 (1979).
19 Resnick, J.S.; Sisson, S.; Vernier, R.L.: Tamm-Horsfall protein. Abnormal localization in renal disease. Lab. Invest. *38*: 550–553 (1978).
20 Smith, J.W.: Clinical, bacteriological and immunological aspects of urinary tract infections in children; 1st ed., pp. 172–177 (Thieme, Stuttgart 1982).
21 Solez, K.; Heptinstall, R.H.: Intrarenal urinary extravasation with formation of venous polyps containing Tamm-Horsfall protein. J. Urol. *119*: 180–183 (1978).
22 Sterzel, R.B.; Dziukas, L.J.; Hodson, C.J.: Tamm-Horsfall protein in Bowman's space and cortical interstitium after ureteral obstruction. Proc. 8th Int. Congr. Nephrology, Athens 1981, pp. 227.
23 Zager, R.A.; Cotran, R.S.; Hoyer, J.R.: Pathologic localization of Tamm-Horsfall protein in interstitial deposits in renal disease. Lab. Invest. *38*: 52–57 (1978).

Anders Fasth, Department of Pediatrics and Department of Immunology,
Institute of Medical Microbiology, University of Göteborg, S-Göteborg (Sweden)

Contr. Nephrol., vol. 39, pp. 296–304 (Karger, Basel 1984)

23. Antibodies to Tamm-Horsfall Urinary Glycoprotein in Patients with Urinary Tract Infection, Reflux Nephropathy, Urinary Obstruction and Paraplegia

Kelvin L. Lynn[a], *Ross R. Bailey*[a], *Ann Groufsky*[b], *John S. Hunt*[b], *Allan R. Bean*[c], *A. Roy McGiven*[b]

[a]Department of Nephrology, Christchurch Hospital; [b]Department of Pathology, Christchurch Clinical School of Medicine; [c]Christchurch Spinal Injuries Unit, Burwood Hospital, Christchurch, New Zealand

Introduction

Tamm-Horsfall urinary glycoprotein (THP) is produced by, and associated with, a discrete segment of the distal renal tubule [1] and is the most abundant protein of renal origin in normal urine [2]. *Hodson et al. [3]* suggested that antibodies to THP could be formed in patients with reflux nephropathy (RN) and that their detection might prove a marker of the condition. *Fasth et al.* [4], however, did not find increased titres of anti-THP antibodies in schoolgirls with asymptomatic bacteriuria and vesico-ureteric reflux (VUR). Increased titres of anti-THP antibodies have been described in children [5] and adults [6, 7] with urinary tract infection (UTI), with or without VUR.

Interstitial deposits of THP have been found in RN, obstructive uropathy and other tubulo-interstitial disease [8, 9]. The suggestion that THP might be involved in the pathogenesis of renal diseases, such as RN, has been supported by the production of tubulo-interstitial nephritis in rats given autologous THP intradermally [10] and rabbits challenged with autologous urine or THP [11].

We have investigated the role of THP in renal disease by measuring anti-THP IgG titres in patients with UTI, RN, paraplegia, acute urinary tract obstruction and other renal parenchymal diseases.

Materials and Methods

THP Preparation. THP was extracted from pooled urine samples collected from laboratory workers by precipitation with 0.58 *M* sodium chloride [12]. This preparation gave a single protein band on polyacrylamide gel electrophoresis in sodium dodecyl sulphate.

Production and Purification of Anti-Human THP Immunoglobulin. Anti-human THP antiserum was produced in New Zealand White rabbits [13] and affinity-purified [14] as described previously.

Enzyme-Linked Immunosorbent Assay (ELISA). A modification of the method of *Fasth et al. [5]* was used. Freeze-dried THP (5 μg/ml) dissolved in phosphate-buffered saline (PBS), pH 7.3, was used to coat multiwell plates at room temperature overnight. After three washes with PBS with Tween 20 (0.05%) the wells were coated with purified human serum albumin (0.1% in PBS/Tween) for 1 h at room temperature. The serum samples (200 μl/well) to be analysed were diluted 1:10 or 1:20 in human serum albumin (0.1% in PBS/Tween) and incubated at room temperature for 3 in duplicate. After further washes with PBS/Tween, peroxidase-conjugated goat antihuman IgG (Tago Incorporated, Burlinghame, Calif.) 1:1,500 in human serum albumin (0.1% in PBS/Tween) was added and the wells incubated for 1 h at room temperature. Following further washing the enzyme substrate O′-phenylenediamine (0.4 mg/ml; Sigma Chemical Co., St. Louis, Mo.) was added and the enzymatic reaction performed at room temperature in the dark, for 30 min and then stopped by addition of 2.5 *M* H_2SO_4 to all wells. The optical densities were measured at OD_{492} on an ELISA reader. The results were expressed as a percentage of the mean of 10–12 normal adult sera included in each assay. Any titre greater than 2 SD above the normal mean was considered significantly elevated. The intra-assay coefficient of variation was 13%.

Statistical Methods. Pairwise comparison of means was effected using 2-sample t-tests, incorporating Welch's correction for unequal variances when necessary. Pairs of variances were compared using the F-ratio. Analysis of variance was used to compare the means for several groups. Levene's test for equality of variances determined whether or not some adjustment to the standard analysis of variance was necessary. All analyses were done using the BMDP statistical package.

Patients

Urinary Tract Infection. 16 patients (3 men), aged 35.9 ± 19 years, with acute pyelonephritis and a plasma creatinine concentration of 1.3 ± 1.1 mg/dl were studied from the time of presentation for periods up to 150 days (table I). 8 women, aged 25.8 ± 9.7 years, with cystitis were also studied from the time of presentation for up to 3–4 weeks. All women with cystitis had a plasma creatinine concentration of less than 1 mg/dl. The diagnosis of UTI was based on the presence of significant UTI ($\geq 10^5$ bacteria/ml) and in those with acute pyelonephritis a suprapubic aspirate of urine was usually obtained. The diagnosis of acute

Table I. Patients with acute pyelonephritis

Patient No.	Sex	Age years	IVU	Plasma creatinine concentration, mg/dl	Infecting organism	Outcome[a]
1	F	30	achalasia ureter (repaired) renal stone	0.7	*E. coli*	cured
2	F	19	RN	0.8	*Klebsiella pneumoniae*	relapsed
3	F	20	normal	0.8	*Staphylococcus* epidermidis	cured
4	F	20	normal	0.8	*E. coli*	cured
5	F	33	renal *transplant*	1.3	*Proteus*[b] *mirabilis*	*Strep. faecalis* UTI 2 days after treatment
6	M	35	normal	1.4	*E. coli*	cured
7	F	20	normal	0.8	*E. coli*	cured
8	M	50	normal	0.9	*E. coli*	relapsed[c]
9	F	23	normal	1.0	*E. coli*[b]	cured
10	F	16	single kidney reimplanted ureter	0.7	*Strep. faecalis*	cured
11	F	72	normal	1.0	*E. coli*	cured
12	F	32	bilateral staghorn calculi	2.0	*Proteus mirabilis*	cured
13	F	32	renal calculi	0.9	*E. coli*	cured
14	M	79	normal	5.2	*E. coli*	cured
15	F	27	normal	0.8	*E. coli*	cured
16	F	63	normal	2.0	*E. coli*	cured

[a] Cure – sterile urine 1 week following end of treatment.
[b] Septicaemia.
[c] Patient developed acute renal failure.

Table II. Radiological findings in patients with RN

	Grade of VUR					RN	
Group (n)	0	1	2	3	ND	unilateral	bilateral
Normal renal function (28)	7	1	6	10	4	18	10
Abnormal renal function (11)	1	0	2	5	3	3	8

ND = Not done.

pyelonephritis was made on clinical grounds and the patients received either an aminoglycoside or cephalosporin for at least 5 days.

Reflux Nephropathy. 39 patients (9 men) with RN, aged 34.4 ± 15 years, were studied on one occasion. The criteria for the diagnosis of advanced RN are described elsewhere [15]. All but 3 had sterile urine, usually obtained by suprapubic aspiration, at the time of study. Renal function was normal in 28 patients (plasma creatinine concentration, PCC, 1.0 ± 0.2 mg/dl) and abnormal in 11 patients (PCC 3.1 ± 2.0 mg/dl). The radiological findings are summarized in table II.

Acute Urinary Tract Obstruction. 15 men with benign prostatic hypertrophy, aged 67.2 ± 9.3 years, were studied at the time of admission with acute urinary retention. At presentation the mean plasma creatinine concentration was 1.4 ± 0.7 mg/dl, 1 had an *E. coli* UTI and 2 patients had radiological evidence of chronic obstructive uropathy.

Paraplegia. 34 patients (3 women) with spinal injuries, aged 40.5 ± 18 years, were studied once. They had been paraplegic for 0.5–26 years and had a mean plasma creatinine concentration of 0.9 ± 0.4 mg/dl. In 26 (76%) there was either current UTI or UTI within the preceding 6 months. In 8 (23%) there was RN and/or gross VUR. Lower urinary tract surgery had been performed in 9 of them (26%).

Other Renal Parenchymal Diseases. Blood was obtained from 21 patients (8 women), aged 41.7 ± 17 years, with either primary glomerulonephritis or tubulo-interstitial nephritis. Their mean ^{51}Cr-EDTA clearance was 58 ± 41 ml/min. None had a UTI within the preceding 6 months.

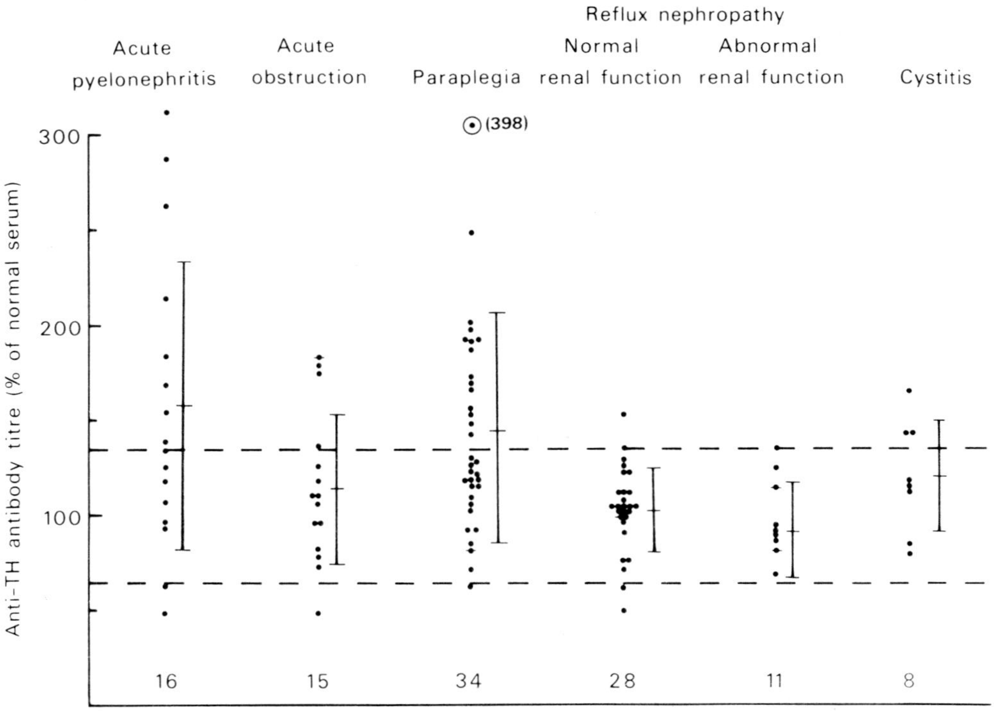

Fig. 1. Anti-THP IgG titres in different patient groups: Peak anti-THP antibody titres in 16 patients with acute pyelonephritis and 8 patients with cystitis. Anti-THP antibody titres in patients with acute urinary obstruction (15), paraplegia (34), RN with normal (28) or abnormal (11) renal function. The results are expressed as a percentage of the mean of a normal reference group and the horizontal broken lines represent ± 2 SD of the reference group. The vertical bars represent mean ± 1 SD of each study group.

Results

The peak titres of anti-THP antibodies for patients with cystitis and acute pyelonephritis are shown in figure 1. The difference in mean peak titre between those with acute pyelonephritis and those with cystitis was not significant ($p = 0.1$). The mean peak titre for the ones with acute pyelonephritis was, however, significantly greater than the normal control titre ($p < 0.01$). The changes in anti-THP antibody titre in patients with acute pyelonephritis were highly variable (fig. 2). In some (patients 2, 9, 11, 16) there was a marked increase in antibody titre which persisted for

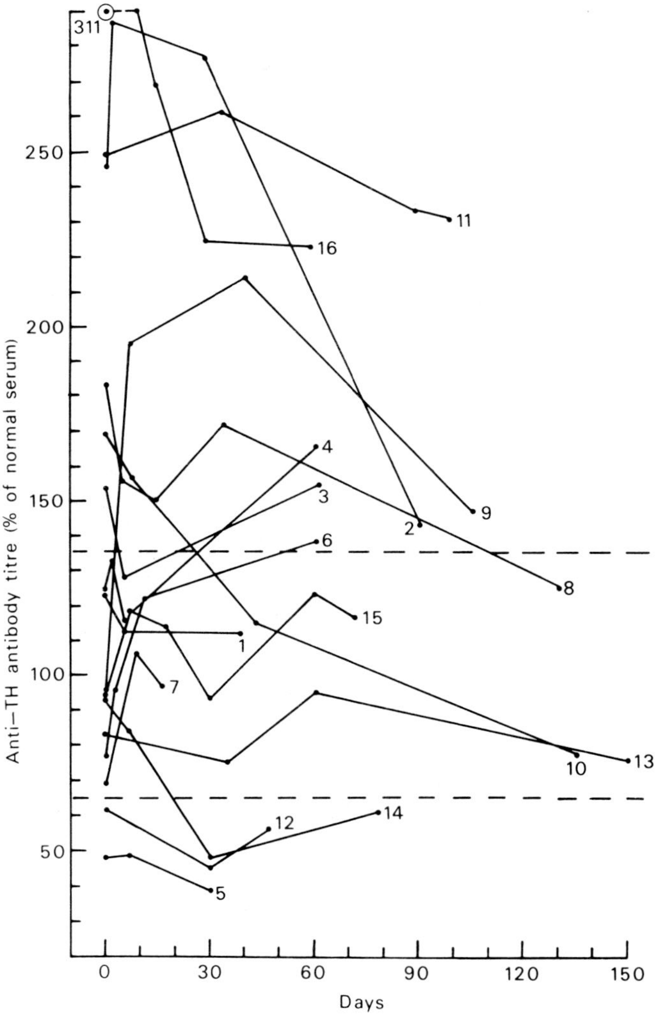

Fig. 2. Anti-THP immunoglobulin titres in 16 patients with acute pyelonephritis versus time. The horizontal broken lines represent ± 2 SD of the normal reference group. The patients' clinical details are shown in table I.

up to 90 days, in others there was no change (patients 1, 13, 15) while in some the antibody titre was depressed (patients 5, 12, 14). There was a tendency for antibody titres to be higher in patients with severe or persisting UTI.

The mean anti-THP antibody titre for patients with RN; 100 ± 23% was the same as that of the normal controls (fig. 1). There was, in fact, no correlation between anti-THP antibody titre and renal function, the severity of current VUR or the extent of RN.

3 patients with acute urinary tract obstruction had raised anti-THP antibody titres including the 1 patient with UTI (fig. 1). Nevertheless, the mean anti-THP antibody titre of 115 ± 40% was not significantly different from normal ($p > 0.1$) and there was no correlation between antibody titre and plasma creatinine concentration ($r = 0.14$; $p = $ n.s.).

The patients with glomerulonephritis or tubulo-interstitial nephritis had a mean anti-THP antibody titre of 90 ± 29% which did not differ from normal ($p > 0.1$).

15 of 34 patients (44%) with paraplegia had raised anti-THP antibody titres, including the highest (398%) observed in this study (fig. 1), the mean of 145 ± 62%, was significantly greater than normal ($p < 0.001$). Although 4 of 8 patients with VUR and/or RN had significantly raised anti-THP antibody titres there was no correlation between raised antibody titre and the presence of VUR, RN or previous lower urinary tract surgery. In addition, the antibody titre did not correlate with current or recent UTI, the duration of paraplegia or the plasma creatinine concentration.

Comparison of all the groups studied showed that patients with cystitis, RN, urinary obstruction or other renal parenchymal diseases had anti-TH antibody titres that were similar and normal with respect to means and variances. The two groups of patients that differed markedly were those with acute pyelonephritis and those with paraplegia, where not only the means but also the variances were elevated.

Discussion

We have shown elevated titres of anti-THP IgG in 50% of adults studied following acute pyelonephritis. In contrast, patients with cystitis had titres which were not significantly greater than normal. These results were in keeping with the findings of *Fasth* et al. [5, 7]. Nevertheless, the anti-THP antibody response in our patients with acute pyelonephritis was much more varied than that observed by these workers and we cannot confirm the usefulness of the measurement of anti-THP antibodies in discriminating upper from lower UTI [5]. Given the difficulties of assessing the site of UTI clinically this is hardly surprising. It appears more likely that the titre of anti-THP antibodies correlates best with the severity or persistence of UTI.

The high incidence (74%) of raised anti-THP antibody titres in patients with paraplegia is unexplained. Some, but not all, patients with VUR or a past history of surgery for high bladder pressure had raised titres and it is tempting to explain this on the basis of past or present VUR, possibly with intrarenal reflux. The low incidence of raised titres in patients with acute urinary obstruction, albeit for a much shorter duration, is of interest in this regard. In addition, it is difficult in paraplegics to dissociate the effects of UTI which is so common in these patients. Further evaluation of urodynamics and renal morphology is required in this area which provides a ready-made basis for the study of the pathogenesis of RN in the adult.

The adults with RN in this study had normal anti-THP IgG titres and there was no correlation between antibody titre and plasma creatinine concentration. These results differ from those of *Fasth* et al. [7] who found depression of these titres in adults with RN and a significant negative correlation between antibody titre and elevated plasma creatinine concentrations. The lack of correlation between the degree of VUR and antibody titre in this study agrees with the findings of others [7]. We have found no evidence of an immunological mechanism involving THP in the pathogenesis of RN.

Anti-THP antibody titres do not appear to distinguish between upper and lower UTI nor are they useful in identifying adults with RN. Further long-term studies are required to evaluate the significance of anti-THP antibodies in patients with UTI and paraplegia.

References

1 Sikri, K.L.; Foster, C.L.; Machugh, N.; Marshall, R.D.: Localization of Tamm-Horsfall glycoprotein in the human kidney using immuno-fluorescence and immuno-electron microscopical techniques. J. Anat. *132*: 597 (1981).

2 Lynn, K.L.; Shenkin, A.; Marshall, R.D.: Factors affecting excretion of human urinary Tamm-Horsfall glycoprotein. Clin. Sci. *62*: 21 (1982).

3 Hodson, C.J.; Maling, T.M.J.; McManamon, P.J.; Lewis, M.G.: Reflux nephropathy. Kidney int. *8*: suppl. 4, p. 50 (1975).

4 Fasth, A.; Hanson, L.A.; Asscher, A.W.: Autoantibodies to Tamm-Horsfall protein in detection of vesicoureteric reflux and kidney scarring. Archs, Dis. Childh. *52*: 560 (1977).

5 Fasth, A.; Hanson, L.A.; Jodal, U.; Peterson, H.: Autoantibodies to Tamm-Horsfall protein associated with urinary tract infection in girls. J. Pediat. *95*: 54 (1979).

6 Marier, R.; Fong, E.; Jansen, M.; Hodson, C.J.; Richards, F.; Andriole, V.T.: Antibody to Tamm-Horsfall protein in patients with urinary tract obstruction and vesicoureteral reflux. J. infect. Dis. *138*: 781 (1978).
7 Fasth, A.; Bengtsson, U.; Kaijser, B.; Wieslander, J.: Antibodies to Tamm-Horsfall protein associated with renal damage and urinary tract infections in adults. Kidney int. *20*: 500 (1981).
8 Resnick, J.S.; Sisson, S.; Vernier, R.L.: Tamm-Horsfall protein. Abnormal localization in renal disease. Lab. Invest. *38*: 550 (1978).
9 Zager, R.; Cotran, R.; Hoyer, J.: Pathologic localization of Tamm-Horsfall protein in interstitial deposits in renal disease. Lab. Invest. *38*: 52 (1978).
10 Hoyer, J.R.: Tubulointerstitial immune complex nephritis in rats immunized with Tamm-Horsfall protein. Kidney int. *17*: 284 (1980).
11 Mayrer, A.R.; Kashgarian, M.; Ruddle, N.H.; Marier, R.; Hodson, C.J.; Richards, F.F.; Andriole, V.T.: Tubulointerstitial nephritis and immunologic responses to Tamm-Horsfall protein in rabbits challenged with homologous urine or Tamm-Horsfall protein. J. Immun. *128*: 2634 (1982).
12 Tamm, I.; Horsfall, F.L.: A mucoprotein derived from human urine which reacts with influenza, mumps and Newcastle disease viruses. J. exp. Med. *95*: 71 (1952).
13 Hunt, J.S.; MacDonald, P.R.; Day, W.A.; McGiven, A.R.: Biochemical and mitogenic properties of Tamm-Horsfall urinary glycoprotein. Pathology *12*: 609 (1980).
14 McGiven, A,R.; Hunt, J.S.; Day, W.A.; Bailey, R.R.: Tamm-Horsfall protein in the glomerular capsular space. J. clin. Path. *31*: 620 (1978).
15 Bailey, R.R.; Lynn, K.L.: End-stage reflux nephropathy. (Chapter 9, this volume).

Kelvin L. Lynn, Department of Nephrology, Christchurch Hospital,
Christchurch (New Zealand)

Contr. Nephrol., vol. 39, pp. 305–315 (Karger, Basel 1984)

24. Autoantibodies to Tamm-Horsfall Glycoprotein – An Artifact of Technique?

P.J.G. Avis

Faculty of Medicine Memorial University of Newfoundland, St. John's, Newfoundland, Canada

Introduction

In 1981, *Fasth* et al. [1] reported that they had found autoantibodies to Tamm-Horsfall glycoprotein (THP) associated with renal damage and urinary tract infections (UTI) in adults. This paper is the latest in a series in which these authors and others [2–7] claim to have found autoantibodies to THP in infants, children and adults which various degrees of UTI and kidney disease, with or without vesicoureteral reflux (VUR). The levels of autoantibodies are given as a percentage of a normal reference serum [2] or a panel of sera from individuals who have no evidence of kidney disease or UTI [3–5]. The inference is clear, even if it were not stated [3, 5, 7], namely that all sera tested from normal individuals contain autoantibodies to THP. These autoantibodies are not limited to one class in the individual but include the classes IgG, IgA, and IgM. It is also claimed that they are present in the newborn and, although they correlate somewhat with the maternal level at birth, they assume an individual pattern at 2 months and the levels actually rise between 2 and 8 months [5].

The idea of autoantibodies being present in the serum of all adults, children and newborns is indeed a novel one and would seem to contradict the present theories of immunology, including the principal concept of recognition of self by the immune system.

The claim that autoantibodies to THP are present in normal human serum also contradicts a previous finding that THP, not antibodies to it, was present in human serum [8] and which was later confirmed by *Dawnay* et al. [9] who developed a specific radioimmunoassay for the measurement of THP in serum. The THP levels they reported (70–540 ng/ml) for a series of 95 control subjects are almost identical to a similar series studied in this laboratory. *Dawnay and Cattell* [10] also investigated the levels of THP in patients with chronic renal failure and patients receiving transplants. In an attempt further to resolve this conflict of interpretation, the following experiments were performed.

Experimental

Materials

Biogel Al.5 was obtained from BioRad Laboratories and CNBr Sepharose 4B from Pharmacia (Canada) Inc. Horseradish peroxide-conjugated goat antihuman γ-globulins (anti-IgG, IgM, IgA), affinity-purified, were purchased from Kirkegaard & Perry Laboratories. Horseradish peroxide type IV was obtained from Sigma, and Linbro EIA microtitration plates from Flow Laboratories Inc.

SDS Polyacrylamide Gel Electrophoresis

Employing a modification of the method described by *Marshall and Zamecnik* [16], gels of 7.5% were used with a 4% stacking gel in 125 *nM* Tris HCl buffer containing 0.1% sodium dodecyl Sulfate (SDS). The electrophoresis was done using a BioRad protein model 16 slab gel apparatus. Gel thickness was 2 mm. Samples were prepared in 5% sucrose 0.1% SDS, bronopherol blue was added as a marker dye. All samples were exposed to 0.1% SDS for at least 2 h before electrophoresis. Gels were fixed in a mixture of 50% isopropyl alcohol in 10% acetic acid and stained with Coomassie blue brilliant R. Results are shown in figure 1.

Tamm-Horsfall Protein

THP was prepared from a pool of urine from 8 volunteers whose sera were assayed both for THP and antibodies to it. The procedure was described in a previous paper [8]. The final product was freeze-dried.

Purification of THP

THP, as prepared from urine, is an aggregate of subunits whose molecular weights range from 76,000 to 82,000 daltons. The aggregate can have an apparent molecular weight of several million and has been shown to complicate attempts to assay it quantitatively by any method involving reactions with antibody [8, 12]. Dissociation of the aggregate by SDS has been shown not to affect its immunological properties [13, 14]. Furthermore, isolation of THP from human serum [9] by gel chromatography showed that it was eluted in the same position as the disassociated standard.

Purification of disassociated THP was carried out on a 2.5-cm diameter × 85 cm column (Pharmacia Limited), packed with Biogel Al.5m200–400 mesh, equilibrated with pH 7.2 phosphate-buffered saline (PBS) (1.6 mmol/l NaH_2PO_4 H_2O; 8.4 mmol/l Na_2HPO_4; 145 mmol/l NaCl) with SDS added to a concentration of 0.1%. The freeze-dried THP (5 mg) was dissolved in 1.5 ml of PBS containing 0.5% SDS (SDS/THP ratio w/w = 1.5:1) and left overnight before being applied to the column. The effluent was monitored on a Uvicord at 280 nm. The major peak, comprising over 90% of the applied material, was pooled and freeze-

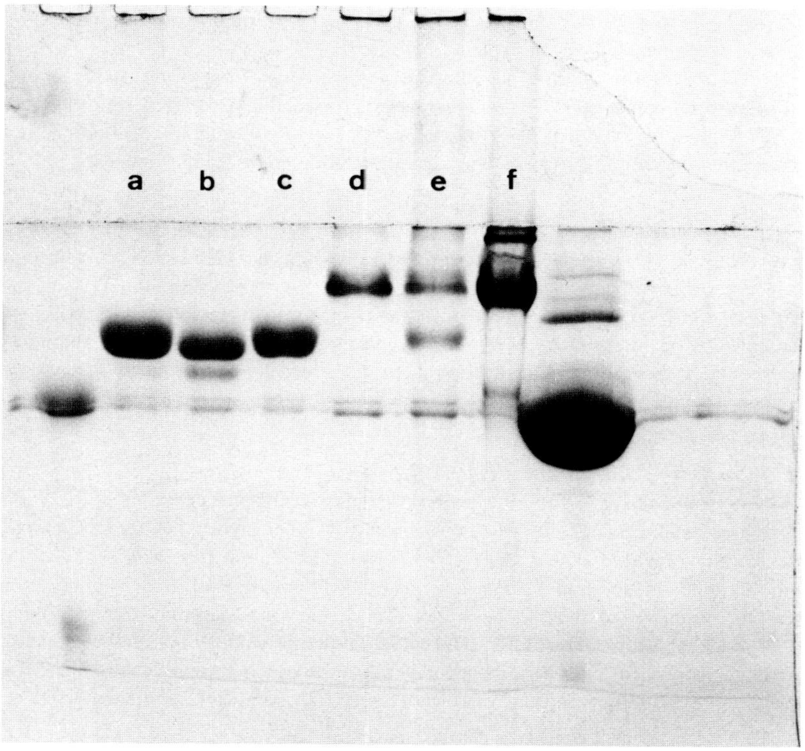

Fig. 1. a 10 μg of THP preparation 1 before purification on gel column. *b* 10 μg of THP preparation 2 before purification showing a record brand. *c* 10 μg of column-purified THP. *d* 20 μg of specific antihuman antibodies prepared by affinity chromatography. *e* A mixture of 20 μg of specific antihuman antibody and 5 μg of column-purified THP. A precipitate formed or mixing in the presence of 0.1% SDS. *f* Rabbit antihuman THG γ-globulin prepared by ammonium sulfate precipitation from the same antiserum used to prepare the specific antibody *(d)*.

dried without dialysis, since complete removal of the SDS by dialysis results in reaggregation of the THP.

The material was checked by Ouchterlony double diffusion against rabbit antihuman THP, obtained by immunizing rabbits with native THP prepared from pooled human urine, and gave one precipitin line.

Immunoabsorbent

(1) For the absorption of THP from serum, rabbit freeze-dried γ-globulin fraction, prepared by ammonium sulfate precipitation from antihuman THP serum obtained from rabbits immunized with native THP, was coupled to cyanogen bromide-activated agarose (CNBr-ac-

tivated Sepharose, W.B. Pharmacia). The conditions used and the concentrations of reagents were as recommended by *Eveleigh and Levy* [15].

(2) For the absorption of possible THP autoantibodies from serum, and the preparation of specific antibodies to THP from immune sera, purified disassociated THP was coupled to CNBr Sepharose. 2.5 mg of THP was coupled to 1 ml of gel, with other conditions as above, except that the coupling reaction was carried out in the presence of 0.1% SDS.

Antisera

Antibodies were raised to freeze-dried native human THP in rabbits by intramuscular injection of 2 ml of equal volumes of Freund's adjuvant and a solution of THP containing 1 mg of freeze-dried preparation. The dose was divided into 0.5 ml lots and given at four separate sites. After 4 weeks the rabbits were given a further injection of the same amount of THP in incomplete Freund's adjuvant. The rabbits were bled 2 weeks after the second injection. Sodium azide (0.1 mg/ml) was added as a preservative and the serum stored at 4°C until used.

Specific Antihuman THP Antibodies

A small column (12 mm diameter × 6.5 mm) was packed with 5 ml of the Sepharose-THP immunoabsorbent and washed through with 20 ml of Tris/HCl buffer (200 mmol/l) with the addition of NaCl (500 mmol/l) and 0.5% Tween 80. Rabbit antiserum to human THP (15 ml) was applied to the column. The flow rate of the column was adjusted to about 3 drops/min until the serum had passed into the column. The serum was then washed into the column with a small amount of the Tris buffer. The column flow was stopped and the serum allowed to remain in contact with the absorbent for 30 min at room temperature. The column was then washed through with the Tris/HCl Tween buffer until the monitored effluent was free of material absorbing at 280 nm.

Specific anti-THP antibody was eluted with a mixture of equal volume of glycine NaOH buffer pH 11 (200 mmol/l) in NaCL (1 mol/l) and ethylene glycol. The column could be used repeatedly provided it was stored at 4°C and azide added to the rinsing buffer.

Conjugation of Anti-THP Antibodies

The periodate method *Wilson and Nakane* [11] was used. Horseradish peroxidase (4 mg) was dissolved in 1 ml of distilled water, 2 ml of 100 mmol/l $NaI0_4$ was added. The reactants were gently stirred for 20 min at room temperature. The peroxidase-iodate solution was dialyzed overnight against 1 mmol/l sodium acetate buffer pH 4.4.

The peroxidase was transferred to a small flask and 20 μl of 200 mmol/l carbonate buffer pH 9.5 was added, followed immediately by 8 mg of specific anti-THP immunoglobulin dissolved in 1 ml of 10 mmol/l carbonate buffer pH 9.5. The reactants were gently stirred for 2 h at room temperature. A fresh solution of sodium borohydride was prepared containing 4 mg/ml in distilled water and 100 μl was added to the reaction mixture which was then allowed to stand for 2 h at room temperature.

An equal volume of saturated ammonium sulfate was added and the mixture centrifuged. The precipitate was washed twice with 50% saturated ammonium sulfate, and then dissolved in distilled water and dialyzed extensively against PBS.

The dialyzed material was centrifuged at high speed to clear any insoluble matter and bovine serum albumin added to yield a final concentration of 1%. The conjugate was finally

Table I. Results of test of THP-sepharose immunosorbent

Specific antihuman THP, μg	100	50	25	12	6.5
Protein remaining after Absorption with THP Sepharose Immunoabsorbent, μg	12	2	0	0	0

filtered through a 0.22 μM Millipore filter. For storage for several weeks at 4°C and equal amount of glycerol can be added to preserve the integrity of the conjugate. In the present instance the majority of the conjugate was divided into aliquots and stored in liquid nitrogen.

Test of THP Immunoabsorbent Used To Absorb for Anti-THP Antibodies

The immunoabsorbent used to absorb any THP antibodies from the test serum was tested against a series of dilutions of specific antihuman THP antibodies. A series of dilutions of the specific antihuman THP was prepared in a volume of 100 μl and transferred from siliconized glass tubes to tubes containing 100 μl of packed immunoabsorbent. After gentle agitation for 1 h at room temperature, the tubes were centrifuged and the antisupernatant carefully removed. The immunoabsorbent was washed twice with 200 μl of buffer and the supernatants bulked with the first. The volume was made up to 800 μl with buffer and then assigned for protein, using microassay procedure of the BioRad one-step protein assay kit, with bovine γ-globulin as a standard. The developed color was read at 595 n*M* using a microcell. The results are shown in table I. At a concentration of antibody of 100 μg in 100 μl, 88 μg was absorbed under the conditions used. At concentration of 50 μg in 100 μl and below there was no measurable amount of antibody left unabsorbed. The limit of sensitivity of the method is 2 μg.

Test of anti-THP Immunoabsorbent for THP

The procedure for the test was the same as the procedure used for absorbing THP from serum except that dilutions of a standard THP solution in the range 500–200 ng in 300 μl of PBS Tween 20 buffer were used. After treatment, 200 μl of the supernatant was removed and assayed for THP using the enzyme-linked immunosorbent assay (ELISA) described. The results before and after absorption are shown in table II.

Absorption of Test Sera

Absorption of Possible Anti-THP Autoantibodies. The immunoabsorbent Sepharose-THP that had been successfully employed to prepare specific anti-THP antibodies was used. A volume of a suspension of the immunoabsorbent, calculated to give 100 μl of packed volume of gel, was transferred to a small siliconized glass tube, and centrifuged at 1,000 *g* for 5 min and the supernatant carefully removed. An equal volume (100 μl) of the

Table II. Results of test of anti-THP-sepharose immunosorbent

THP, ng	500	250	125	50
Results of ELISA expressed as optical density units	1.4	0.74	0.38	0.15
Results after absorption with anti-THP Sepharose, optical density	0.105	0.046	0.064	0.027

test serum was pipetted into the tube and the latter then gently agitated to keep the immunoabsorbent in suspension. After 1 h at room temperature 1 ml of PBS containing 0.05% Tween 20 buffer was added and the suspension centrifuged. The supernatant was carefully removed. The immunoabsorbent was washed twice with 1 ml of PBS and the supernatants bulked with the first. The volume was then made up 10 ml (final dilution 10^{-2}) which was the dilution used in the assay.

Absorption of THP from Test Sera. The immunoabsorbent Sepharose–antihuman THP was used. The test serum (300 μl) was added to 100 μl of immunoabsorbent gel. After treatment for 1 h the samples were centrifuged, 200 μl of the supernatant carefully removed and diluted to 1 ml with PBS Tween 20; the dilution used in the assay.

Enzyme-Linked Immunosorbent Assay

Assays for THP Autoantibodies. Microplates were coated with THP with 0.1% SDS prepared as described. The THP was dissolved in bicarbonate/carbonate buffer pH 9.5 (35 mmol/l $NaHCO_3$; 15 mmol/l Na_2CO_3) at a concentration of 1 mg/dl. The wells were filled with 200 μl of this solution, or plain buffer, and allowed to stand overnight at 40°C. The plates were then washed with PBS pH 7.2 (1.6 mmol/l NaH_2PO_4; 8.4 mmol/l Na_2HPO_4; 145 mmol/l NaCL) and then filled completely with the bicarbonate/carbonate buffer containing 0.5% bovine serum albumin (BSA) and allowed to stand for 2 h at room temperature. The plates were then washed 3 times with PBS containing 0.5% v/v Tween 20. Before attempting to assay for THP autoantibodies in serum the absorption of THP onto the polyvinyl plates was checked by adding 100 μl of 1:400 dilution of horseradish peroxidase rabbit antihuman THP conjugate to the wells and incubating at room temperature for 3 h. After washing 4 times with PBS the substrate was added and the procedure followed as described below. The mean optical density for the treated wells was 1.624 compared with a control value of 0.094 for wells not treated with THP.

Sera from the 8 volunteers were divided into aliquots and kept in the gaseous phase of a liquid nitrogen storage container. Samples were thawed immediately before use. For the assays for THP autoantibodies, sera were diluted to 10^{-2} with PBS Tween 20 buffer and 200 μl pipetted into the wells of the microplates. Assays were performed in parallel with serum that had been treated with the Sepharose-THP immunoabsorbent. Controls were (1) wells untreated with THP with and without the addition of diluted serum, and (2) wells treated with THP but incubated with PBS Tween 20 instead of serum. All assays were done in triplicate. The plates were incubated at room temperature in a moist chamber for 2 h. They were then washed 3 times with PBS Tween 20, after which 100 μl of horseradish peroxidase-conjugated goat antihuman IgG, IgA, and IgM affinity-purified preparation at a dilution of 1/200 in PBS Tween 20 buffer containing 0.5% BSA, was added to all wells. The plates were then incubated at room temperature for 3 h, after which they were washed 4 times with PBS Tween 20 buffer. The enzyme substrate and indicator was made up to a concentration of 32 mmol/l H_2O_2. *O*-phenylenediamine 2.2 mmol/l, in phosphate buffer, pH 6 (8.7 mmol/l NaH_2PO_4 H_2O; 1.2 mmol/l Na_2HPO_4). 200 μl was pipetted into each well and the plate incubated at 37 °C for 30 min. The enzyme reaction was stopped and the color developed by the addition of 40 μl of 8 mol/l of sulfuric acid. The optical densities were read at 492 mm and recorded on a Dynatech Multiskan rapid microplate reader.

Assay for THP in Human Serum. Because positive results could be obtained in this assay using standard dilutions of THP corresponding to the range in human serum [10], the optimum concentrations of the reagents used were determined by checkerboard titrations (a standard procedure for this type of assay). The plates were coated with specific rabbit antihuman THP γ-globulin. The specific γ-globulin was diluted in the bicarbonate/carbonate buffer pH 9.5 at a concentration of 2.5 μg/ml and 100 μl was added to each well. Serum samples were diluted (1 vol of serum to 4 vol of PBS Tween 20 buffer); 100 μl of the dilutions being pipetted into the wells. Assays were performed in parallel with serum treated with Sepharose antihuman THP immunoabsorbent. The plates were incubated for 2 h at room temperature, washed 3 times with PBS Tween 20. 100 μl of diluted antihuman peroxidase conjugate containing 300 mg of antibody protein in PBS Tween 20 buffer containing 0.5% BSA, were then added. The plates were incubated for 2 h at room temperature, washed 4 times with PBS Tween buffer, and the substrate then added. The rest of the procedure was as described above.

Results

SDS Polyacrylamide Electrophoresis

Polyacrylamide electrophoresis in the presence of 0.1% SDS of THP prepared by salt precipitation only sometimes shows the presence of another component that migrates faster than the major band. This appears to be removed by gel chromatography. The purified THP fraction (fig. 1, c) was tested against specific anti-THP using the Ouchterlony technique and gave a single line over a range of dilutions. The specific antibody (fig. 1, d) showed no trace of THP and presumably therefore no THP was eluted with the antibody during the affinity column procedure. A mixture of specific antibody and THP in an approximate molar ratio of 2:1 in 0.1% SDS resulted in some precipitate being formed, but the presence of SDS

Table III. Results of assays for THP and autoantibodies to THP

Serum No.	Microplate Treatment: buffer only		THP			specific antihuman THP		
	no serum control (a)	serum added to well (b)	no serum control (c)	untreated serum (d)	serum absorbed with THP (e)	no serum control (f)	untreated serum (g)	serum absorbed with antihuman THP(h)
1	0.085	0.580	0.472	1.101	1.110	0.0680	0.620	0.097
2	0.077	0.528	0.385	1.179	1.172	0.063	0.612	no serum available
3	0.087	0.557	0.414	1.225	1.262	0.076	0.60	0.109
4	0.082	0.606	0.443	1.116	1.112	0.069	0.485	0.102
5	0.088	0.525	0.425	1.146	1.161	0.070	1.057	0.122
6	0.078	0.677	0.439	1.190	1.190	0.060	0.281	0.076
7	0.080	0.471	0.412	1.094	1.086	0.064	0.624	0.082
8	0.082	0.409	0.412	1.206	1.195	0.060	0.399	0.075

Columns a and b are values obtained with wells pretreated with buffer only. Column b has had human serum at a dilution of 10^{-2} added to the wells. Columns c–e have had the wells coated with THP. In columns f–h, wells have been coated with specific antihuman THP.
All wells have had either goat antihuman IgG, IgM, IgA peroxidase conjugate (columns a–e); or specific rabbit antihuman THP conjugate (columns f–h) added to the wells at the appropriate stage of the assay procedure. 'No serum control' refers to wells that were not exposed to human serum during the assay. All assays were performed in triplicate. The above results are typical of several assays that have been performed at different times.

had resulted in some dissociation. A similar mixture done in the absence of SDS resulted in the complete precipitation of the antibody.

Results of Assays for THP Autoantibodies in Human Serum

The results are shown in table III. The values in columns a–e were obtained using the procedure to assay any possible THP autoantibodies.

The values in columns f–h were obtained for the specific test for THP in human serum.

Columns a and b are values obtained for uncoated microplates. Values in column a are baseline controls and represent values that should be obtained if there were no non-specific adherence of human γ-globulins to the untreated microplate. Column b, in marked contrast, shows that the addition of the human serum at the dilution used in the assay (10^{-2}) results in appreciable amounts of IgG, IgM, and IgA being absorbed onto the wells.

Columns c–e are values obtained for microplates treated in order to coat the wells with THP as described in the experimental procedures. Column c can be compared with column a. If coating the wells with THP had no effect on the assay, the values in the two columns should be identical. It can be seen, however, that the values for the treated plate are much higher. Since no human serum has been added to these wells, the high value demonstrated that coating the wells with THP results in the binding, or absorption, of the goat antihuman IgG, IgM, IgA peroxidase conjugate to the THP-treated wells. Values in column d were obtained when the diluted human serum samples were added to the THP-treated wells. The values are nearly double those of column b, but this doubling of values over the control is not considered sufficient for an ELISA type assay, rather one would expect an increase of between 5 and 10 times the control value (compare columns f and g).

Column e shows values obtained when the serum was absorbed with Sepharose-THP immunoabsorbent. Compared with column d the values are nearly identical; therefore, after absorption with THP, the amount of antibody binding to the surface of the THP-treated wells is the same. If the values in column d were, even in part, due to autoantibodies to THP binding to the THP-treated wells, some decrease in the values should be observed after absorbing the serum with THP in the form of Sepharose THP.

Results of Assays for THP in Human Serum

Column f represents the baseline control for this series. The values were obtained from wells coated with specific antihuman THP to which no human serum had been added. The values are acceptable as a control. Values in column g represent levels of THP in the sera tested, the range of values representing that found in normal human serum [10]. Values in column h were obtained from serum treated with antihuman THP in the form of the immunoabsorbent: Sepharose-rabbit-specific antihuman THP antibodies. It can be seen that this treatment has successfully removed most of the material responsible for the values in column g.

Discussion

That THP is a normal constituent of human serum has been established by three methods in two laboratories [8, 9]. The only exception being that of anephric patients, a finding to be expected if the kidney is the sole source of THP. This finding by itself is a powerful argument against the presence of autoantibodies, since they could scarcely exist in their free state in the presence of their antigen. That they may exist as a circulating antibody-antigen complex is a possibility, but it would be extremely unlikely that they would then be able to bind to the THP which coats the plastic of the tubes or plates that are the basis of all the assays for THP autoantibodies. But even if complexes were able to bind to the THP coating the plastic then they would, by the same argument, be removed by the Sepharose-THP immunoabsorbent; that this is not so is clearly demonstrated by comparing the values obtained in columns d and e in table III.

The finding that immunoglobulins are absorbed onto the surface of the plastic at the concentration of serum used for the assay can surprise no one acquainted with the ELISA technique since the whole basis of the test is the ability of the plastic to absorb proteins onto its surface, thereby acting as a fixed support for antigens or antibody.

The enhancement of the absorbtion, or binding, of immunoglobulins by pretreatment of the microplates with THP is surprising, and may account for the reports of the presence of THP autoantibodies. However, it is clear that this is not a specific antigen-antibody reaction since column c shows a 5-fold increase over column a, the control. Indeed, the only difference between the two is that the values in column c were obtained with THP-coated wells. No human serum, only the goat antihuman (IgG, IgM, IgA) peroxidase conjugate, had been added during the procedure. To argue that this is a specific reaction one would have to conclude that the goat antiserum contained antibodies to human THP and this, after purification on an affinity column, would be unlikely.

The reported increases in autoantibodies to THP in patients with a variety of kidney diseases may reflect an increase in immunoglobulin levels in response to UTI leading an increase of non-specific binding.

The possibility that an individual, under special circumstances, could produce autoantibodies to THP is recognized, but that they are produced by all individuals, healthy or otherwise from birth, as has been claimed, seems most unlikely, particularly as THP appears to be a normal constituent of human serum.

References

1 Fasth, A.; Bengtsson, U.; Kaijser, B.; Wieslander, J.: Antibodies to Tamm-Horsfall protein associated with renal damage and urinary tract infections in adults. Kidney int. *20*: 500–504 (1981).
2 Hanson, L.A.; Fasth, A.; Jodal, V.: Auto antibodies to Tamm-Horsfall protein, a tool for diagnosing the level of urinary tract infection. Lancet *i*: 226–228 (1976).
3 Fasth, A.; Hanson, L.A.; Asscher, A.W.: Auto antibodies to Tamm-Horsfall protein in detection of vesicoureteral reflux and kidney scarring. Archs. Dis. Childh. *52*: 560–562 (1977).
4 Marier, R.; Fong, E.; Jansen, M.; Hodson, C.J.; Richards, F.; Andriole, V.T.: Antibody to Tamm-Horsfall protein in patients with urinary tract obstruction and vesicoureteral reflux. J. infect. Dis. *138*: 781–790 (1978).
5 Fasth, A.; Hanson, L.A.; Jodal, U.; Peterson, H.: Autoantibodies to Tamm-Horsfall protein associated with urinary tract infection in girls. J. Pediat. *95*: 54–60 (1979).
6 Fasth, A.; Bjune, J.; Hellstrom, M.; Jacobson, B.; Jodal, U.: Autoantibodies to Tamm-Horsfall glycoprotein in children with renal scarring associated with urinary tract infections. Acta paediat. scand. *69*: 709–715 (1980).
7 Work, J.; Andriole, V.T.: Tamm-Horsfall protein antibody in patients with end-stage kidney disease. Yale J. Biol. Med. *53*: 133–148 (1980).
8 Avis, P.J.G.: The development of radioimmunoassay procedure for the estimation of Tamm-Horsfall glycoprotein in human serum. Clin. Sci. mol. Med. *52*: 183–191 (1977).
9 Dawnay, A.; McLean, C.; Cattell, W.R.: The development of a radioimmunoassay for Tamm-Horsfall glycoprotein in serum. Biochem. J. *185*: 679–687 (1980).
10 Dawnay, A.; Cattell, W.R.: Serum Tamm-Horsfall glycoprotein levels in health and in renal disease. Clin. Neph. *15*: 5–8 (1981).
11 Wilson, M.B.; Nakane, P.K.: Immunofluorescence and related staining techniques; 1st ed., p. 215 (Elsevier, Amsterdam 1978).
12 Grant, A.M.S.; Neuberger, A.: The development of a radioimmunoassay for the measurement of urinary Tamm-Horsfall glycoprotein in the presence of sodium dodecyl sulphate. Clin. Sci. *44*: 163–179 (1973).
13 Fletcher, A.P.; Neuberger, A.; Ratcliffe, W.A.: Tamm-Horsfall urinary glycoprotein: the subunit structure. Biochem. J. *120*: 425–432 (1970).
14 Marr, A.M.S.; Neuberger, A.; Ratcliffe, W.A.: Rabbit Tamm-Horsfall urinary glycoprotein. Chemical composition and subunit structure. Biochem. J. *122*: 623–631 (1970).
15 Eveleigh, J.W.; Levy, D.E.: Immunochemical characteristics and preparative application of agrose-based immunoabsorbents. J. Solid Phase Biochem. *2*: 45–77 (1977).
16 Marshall, R.D..; Zamecnik, P.C.: Some physical properties of lysyl and arginyl-transfer RNA: Synthetases of *Escherichia coli* B. Biochem. biophys. Acta *181*: 454–464 (1969).

P.J.G. Avis, Dept. of Immunology, Faculty of Medicine, Memorial University of Newfoundland, St. John's, Newfoundland A1B 3B6 (Canada)

Contr. Nephrol., vol. 39, pp. 316–319 (Karger, Basel 1984)

Discussion on Chapters 22–24

Dr. *R. Heptinstall*: Dr. *Avis*, do you maintain then that the techniques that have been used by other people have not been detecting antibodies to Tamm-Horsfall Protein (THP) but, rather, they are detecting blood group substance?

Dr. *P. Avis*: No. My thesis is that the techniques pick up non-specific absorption of immunoglobulin, which is not necessarily directed against THP but any antibodies that just happen to be there.

Dr. *R. Heptinstall*: Then you would not go so far as to say that the results of Dr. *Fasth* and Dr. *Bailey* are invalidated by your findings.

Dr. *P. Avis*: Yes, I think they are invalidated, because they are based on the argument that the normal person has autoantibodies to THP. If this were so, one would expect from my immunoabsorption work that the assay level would be reduced to those of the zero control, say from 0.6 to something like 0.06, a 10-fold difference. And this does not happen. In fact, as a result of using immunoabsorption there is no diminution in the levels at all.

Dr. *A. Fasth*: There are several points I would like to make which convince me that we are measuring specific antibodies and not non-specific absorbed material. (1) The THP antibodies could be absorbed out from serum either by mixing THP and serum before adding the sample to the THP-coated tubes [1], or by immunoabsorption to THP linked to Sepharose beads [unpublished]. (2) The kinetic of the measured THP antibody response corresponds to that of other antibody responses. (3) The antibody response involved only IgG and IgA, but not IgM, THP specific antibodies. If the response was non-specific, one would expect an increase in all three immunoglobulin classes. (4) If the antibodies are non-specific, one would also expect them to parallel other specific antibodies known to increase in somewhat similar fashion during acute pyelonephritis, for example antibodies to the somatic antigen of *Escherichia coli*, or be the result of a polyclonal antibody response. No such evidence was found [2, 3; see references at the end of this discussion].

I have also tried to absorb out the THP antibodies with substances like albumin and the somatic antigen from *E. coli*, but without success.

Dr. P. Avis: Can I quote you? You say: 'Very low levels of IgM and IgA anti-THP were found in the newborn infants. With increasing age a significant rise in level (p 0.01) was noted up to the age of 8 months' [4]. So, after birth it can't be related to the mother's level. I think that you are stretching things a bit far to say that the newborn has IgA and IgM autoantibodies to THP.

Dr. *A. Fasth*: No measurable amounts of IgA and IgM antibodies were found in most newborns, but there was an increase in antibody level from the newborn period up to about 9 months.

Dr. *P. Avis*: Then you're not saying there are no IgM and IgA. You are just saying there are very low levels. But presumably they are measurable; otherwise you would have used the words 'there are no' IgM and IgA?

Dr. *A. Fasth*: What is 'no antibodies'. If my method cannot detect any antibodies that does not necessarily mean that there are no antibodies, just that my method might not be sensitive enough to find them. I think I used care to express that fact.

Dr. *R. Heptinstall*: Could I just intervene at this stage. You then, Dr. *Fasth*, will still stand by what you have written, will you, in spite of Dr. *Avis'* contentions that you are measuring an artifact?

Dr. *A. Fasth*: Yes, I very much do, and I would like to add a comment regarding the difference between Dr. *Bailey*'s results and mine. Part of it could be different patient groups. Dr. *Bailey* investigated adults, and we children. The clinical picture in children is often more clear-cut, making the diagnosis of acute cystitis and acute pyelonephritis easier. Dr. *Bailey* has also used only clinical criteria to differentiate between upper and lower urinary tract infections (UTIs), using fever as the distinguishing feature between the two. Whereas we have used symptoms, fever, C-reactive protein, sedimentation rate and the renal concentrating capacity to differentiate between acute cystitis and acute pyelonephritis [5]. Furthermore, we have subdivided the acute pyelonephritic group according to the findings at intravenous urography (IVU) and voiding cystourethrography (VCU). Among Dr. *Bailey*'s patients with acute cystitis there could be some with acute pyelonephritis without fever, where we would expect to see an antibody response. Among those with acute pyelonephritis there could have been some with fever from other causes and some with renal damage, patients that we do not, according to our findings, expect to have a THP antibody response. Thus, our results are not strictly comparable. But the important point is that we both find autoantibodies to THP and that they are increased in patients with acute pyelonephritis.

Dr. *R. Bailey*: I am not personally familiar with the detailed methodology that has been used. The results that I presented today are really those from a group of bright and dedicated people. But Dr. *Lynn* did ask me to mention specifically that for some time he has been concerned about what he is actually measuring; that there may be some non-specific or cross-reacting substances in the serum which he didn't measure separately and that this may have an effect on his results.

Dr. *A. Fasth*: Is Dr. *Lynn* concerned that he is measuring an antibody directed to other substances, or is he concerned that he is measuring an antigen?

Dr. *R. Bailey*: He is detecting something in serum which is cross-reacting in the same sort of way.

Dr. *P. Kincaid-Smith*: Is Dr. *Avis* saying that the immunoglobulins are binding non-specifically to THP because of some sort of chemical interaction?

Dr. *P. Avis*: Well, I'm saying that if the plates are treated with THP it does increase the binding of the antibody. But I'm sure this is non-specific because if one takes the serum and absorbs it with THP, there is no difference in the amount that's absorbed.

Dr. *R. Heptinstall*: In the two presentations, acute pyelonephritis was a condition in which high titers were found, and you both stated there is cross-reactivity with certain strains of *E. coli*, and Dr. *Fasth* found high titers in certain situations and low titers in others, particularly in chronic renal failure. The high ones, could possibly be due to cross-reactivity with bacteria. Would you go along with that?

Dr. *A. Fasth*: Yes. Our experience on this point was published in 1980 [1]. We tried to find the cross-reacting substance among the different antigens deriving from *E. coli* bacteria. We could find a weak cross-reaction using very crude preparations, but not using pure substances like various lipopolysaccharide antigens. Thus, there is a cross-reaction, but the antigen is not yet defined.

Dr. *R. Bailey*: In our findings in acute pyelonephritis the important observation is the variable response. There are some patients with raging acute pyelonephritis whose titers remain normal or even low; and others with less severe UTIs where they are raised.

Dr. *R. Heptinstall*: I consider that in the combination of vesicoureteral reflux (VUR) with UTI, it is impossible as yet to determine whether the antigen/antibody comes from THP, or some other substance resulting from renal damage due to severe VUR, or from reactivity with bacterial products.

Dr. *R. Bailey*: The same problem is found in our patients with paraplegia, neurogenic bladders and VUR on the one hand and associated UTI on the other.

Dr. *B. Asscher*: Our experience of sending the sera from the children described earlier by Dr. *Verrier Jones* (chapter 14) to Dr. *Fasth* for assessment, showed no relationship of raised THP titers to either asymptomatic UTI or VUR. As regards paraplegics it is possible, since pure THP casts are found so commonly in urinary sediment in such cases, that there may be an excessive amount of antigen produced in these patients.

Dr. *R. Heptinstall*: Dr. *Fasth*, have you any explanation as to the cause of low THP levels in cases with VUR and renal scarring?

Dr. *A. Fasth*: One possible explanation could be that the anti-THP antibodies are consumed or 'trapped' by the THP deposits found in patients with reflux nephropathy. However, you would then expect to find an inflammatory reaction around the THP deposits.

Dr. *R. Heptinstall*: Well, you sometimes do.

Dr. *A. Fasth*: Yes, we sometimes do, but not very often.

Dr. *R. Heptinstall*: What of the thesis that if the amount of functioning renal parenchyma is greatly reduced, it might only be capable of producing a diminished amount of antigen?

Dr. *A. Fasth*: It is possibility, but a diminished production of THP could not be a reason for the low anti-THP antibody levels found in the children with renal damage. Most of them have small or moderate scars, and none had creatinine values in the uraemic range. The hypothesis I personally favor is that the immune mechanisms involved in UTI include a suppression of antibody production as discussed in my presentation earlier.

Dr. *W. Asscher*: I would like to ask Dr. *Fasth* on how many subjects his normal range was based.

Dr. *A. Fasth*: It comprised about 70 children and young adults between the ages of 1 and 30 years, and about 70 newborns and infants. The values found in serum from the children and young adults were used as the normal range in this study.

Dr. *P. Avis*: I think one thing that hasn't been addressed so far is the presence of THP in the serum. Nobody has challenged the findings of myself and *Dawnay* that THP *is* present in the serum. I mean we're talking of up to 500 ng in 1 ml of serum; or 1.5 mg circulating at any one time in the bloodstream. If this is so, what are the odds that there'll be antibody present in the serum at the same time?

Dr. *A. Fasth*: I don't know if I should make a comment, maybe Dr. *Bailey* should, as he is working with Dr. *Lynn*. *Lynn and Marshall* [6] looked for THP in serum but didn't find the protein. Instead they found three cross-reactive proteins each with a mobility and molecular weight different from THP.

References

1 Fasth, A.; Ahlstedt, S.; Hanson, L.A.; Jann, B.; Jann, K.; Kaijser, B.: Cross-reactions between the Tamm-Horsfall glycoprotein and *Escherichia coli*. Int. Archs Allergy appl. Immun. *63*: 303–312 (1980).

2 Fasth, A; Bjure, J.; Hellstrom, M.; Jacobsson, B.; Jodal, U.: Autoantibodies to Tamm-Horsfall protein in children with renal damage associated with urinary tract infection. Acta paediat. scand. *69*: 709–715 (1980).

3 Ahlstedt, S.; Fasth, A.; Jodal, U.: Hapten and kidney antibodies in serum from children with urinary tract infection. Acta path. microbiol. scand. sect. C *89*: 29–36 (1981).

4 Fasth, A.; Hanson, L.A.; Jodal, U.; Peterson, H.: Autoantibodies to Tamm-Horsfall protein associated with urinary tract infection in girls. J. Pediat. *95*: 54–60 (1979).

5 Jodal, U.; Lindberg, U.; Lincoln, K.: Level diagnosis of symptomatic urinary tract infections in childhood. Acta paediat. scand. *64*: 201–205 (1975).

6 Lynn, K.L.; Marshall, R.D.: The presence of serum of proteins which are immunologically cross-reactive with Tamm-Horsfall glycoprotein. Biochem. J. *194*: 561–568 (1981).

Section VIII: Sterile Reflux Nephropathy in the Pig

Contr. Nephrol., vol. 39, pp. 320–343 (Karger, Basel 1984)

25. High Pressure Sterile Vesicoureteral Reflux and Renal Scarring: An Experimental Study in the Pig and Minipig

P.G. Ransley[a,b], *R.A. Risdon*[c], *M.L. Godley*[a]

[a]Institutes of Child Health and [b]Urology, University of London; [c]Institute of Pathology, The London Hospital Medical College, London, England

Introduction

Whilst the association between vesicoureteral reflux (VUR) and segmental renal scarring (chronic atrophic pyelonephritis or reflux nephropathy, RN) during childhood is now generally accepted [2, 3, 10], the precise mechanisms involved remain unclear. In particular, controversy remains over the question whether scarring occurs only in the presence of urinary tract infection (UTI), or whether VUR of sterile urine can in some circumstances result in segmental kidney damage.

Our previous experimental work on RN using the pig model [8, 9] indicated that UTI is of prime importance in the scarring process. We showed that when VUR is present the renal pelvis is subjected to raised pressure during detrusor contraction at micturition. This results in reversal of the normal pressure gradient between the renal parenchyma and the pelvis, allowing retrograde flow (intrarenal reflux, IRR) back into the renal tubules. Any pathogenic organisms present in the bladder urine may thus gain access to the parenchyma and initiate renal scarring. The segmental nature of the scars is related to the morphology of individual renal papillae whose shape and distribution of papillary duct orifices determine whether or not IRR occurs in a particular renal lobe [7]. Papillary shape and propensity to allow IRR can change when subjected to abnormally raised bladder pressure in a refluxing system, and in this situation the extent of IRR, and any scarring which may ensue in the presence of UTI is increased. We have corroborated that when the urine is infected, parenchymal damage and subsequent scarring may occur rapidly in the course of only 1–3 weeks and that this process is particularly extensive and devastating when urinary obstruction as well as VUR is present. Conversely when there is VUR alone, eradication of UTI after 1 week considerably limits the amount of scarring.

Previously [8, 9] we produced renal scarring only when UTI was present, and never in its absence. *Hodson* et al. [3], however, produced scars in the pig model in the absence of UTI when a ring was placed around the urethra to produce high pressure VUR.

In this study we report our own experience in a similar model. Particular attention has been made to monitor bladder pressures by serial conscious voiding cystometrograms, to observe changes in voiding patterns and to follow changes in the upper urinary tract and kidneys by ultrasonography and ^{99m}Tc-dimercaptosuccinic acid (DMSA; CIS®) scanning of the kidneys in order to correlate these parameters with the pathologic changes developing in the kidney.

Material and Methods

The pig was chosen as an experimental animal for reasons discussed before [8, 9].

Experimental Model. VUR was produced either unilaterally or bilaterally in recently weaned piglets aged between 2 and 5 weeks as described previously [8]. At the same operation a silver wire 'ring' was placed around the urethra. This 'ring' was of the form devised by *Hodson* et al. [3] and consisted of an incomplete circle with hooked ends which was closed with a silk ligature at operation (fig. 1). The ring was preformed to a known internal diameter (3–7 mm).

Following this surgical procedure all animals were maintained on prophylactic antimicrobial drugs (either Septrin® 10–30 ml pediatric suspension/day or Macrodantin® 150–300 mg/day). A cystogram was performed 2 weeks postoperatively to confirm the presence of VUR.

Routine investigations were performed as follows. Weekly urine samples for bacteriologic culture were obtained by suprapubic puncture under ultrasound control, and at the same time ultra-sonograms of both kidneys were recorded.

Voiding cystourethrograms (VCUs) were performed at approximately monthly intervals. After anesthetizing the animals with a Halothane®/N_2O_2/O_2 mixture, a Portex® epidural catheter was introduced percutaneously through a hollow needle into the bladder, and a second epidural catheter was placed similarly in the peritoneal cavity. The animals were then allowed to regain full conciousness in a restraining cage. A diuresis was induced by the intravenous infusion of 0.45% NaCl with 4.5% dextrose, and a number of voids were observed. Intravesical and intra-abdominal pressures were recorded independently using Elcomatic® 750 transducers with simultaneous recording of the two traces on a two-channel chart recorder (Elcomatic® 720) fitted with an Elcomatic® 722 preamplifier.

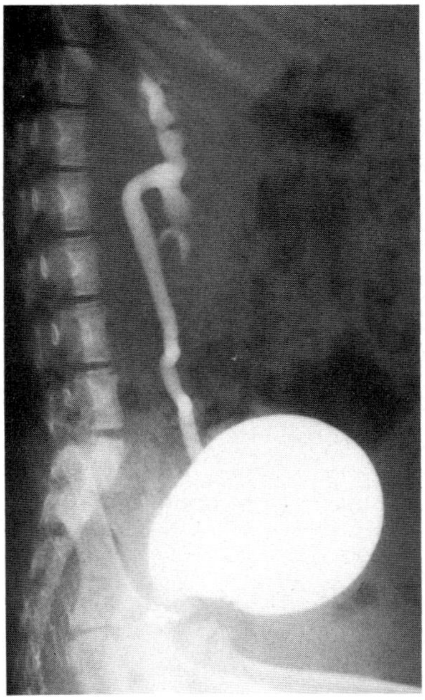

Fig. 1. R. 264; cystogram showing unilateral VUR 2 weeks following surgery. Note the position and form of the urethral ring.

All but the first 3 animals studied (R. 208, 217, and 218) had ^{99m}Tc-DMSA scans performed under general anesthesia with Halothane/N_2O_2/O_2. These were carried out at approximately monthly intervals, but in many animals were performed more frequently; at critical periods weekly scans were obtained. Between 1 and 4 mCi ^{99m}Tc-DMSA were injected intravenously and imaging performed 2–4 h later on a Nuclear Enterprises® (model NE 890C) gamma camera using high resolution and a 6 mm pin hole collimator for a total of 4×10^5 counts. Posterior and oblique views of each kidney were obtained.

At the end of the experiments the animals received a further dose of ^{99m}Tc-DMSA 2 h before sacrifice, and the isolated kidneys were scanned on a Scintag-Berthold LFOV gamma camera with high resolution collimation linked to an Informatek Sirius 3 computer. 500K anterior and posterior views of each kidney were obtained in a 64×64 matrix and the smoothed images displayed with isocontours.

A total of 17 animals have been investigated in this study. Initially 27 animals were entered, but 10 were excluded. These were 4 who died in the immediate postoperative period, 4 who developed spontaneous UTI and 2 who failed to reflux.

First studied were 7 Large White boars (group I). Having evaluated the data from these animals, a further series of 5 male (group II) and 5 female (group III) Gottingen Minipigs were investigated to ascertain if species and gender might influence the results.

Pathologic Examination. After each animal was killed the kidneys and urinary tract were removed and examined in the fresh state, the ureteric orifices particularly being examined. The whole urinary tract, the external surfaces and the cut surfaces of each kidney were photographed and close-up views of any macroscopic lesions taken. Representative blocks of parenchyma from macroscopically normal kidneys, and blocks of all lesions in those kidneys where they were present were fixed in buffered formalin (pH 7.0), processed and embedded in paraffin wax. Sections (6 μm thick) were stained by HE, van Gieson/elastic, periodic acid-Schiff (PAS) and periodic acid-methenamine silver (PAMS).

Sections of all blocks from parenchymal lesions were examined immunochemically for Tamm-Horsfall protein (THP) using the unlabelled horseradish peroxidase – antihorsradish peroxidase (PAP) method [5].

Discussion of the Experimental Model. The animal preparation employed is basically that used in our previous studies [8, 9], but with a number of additional features. Our experience with the model has confirmed that it produces reliable and reproducible VUR which can be demonstrated by cystourethrography, and the presence of an intact vesicoureteral junction on the non-operated side provides a valuable internal control.

Voiding patterns were monitored by observations of the animals in their pens, and serial VCUs were employed to record these data and to follow changes in peak voiding pressures. Placement of the catheters in the bladder and peritoneal cavity for pressure recordings necessitated anesthetizing the animals, but they were allowed to recover full consciousness in a restraining cage before the tracings were made to eliminate the effects of the anesthetic agents on detrusor and sphincter activity.

Ultrasonography was employed to aid localization of the bladder during suprapubic urine sampling for bacteriologic culture. When bladder decompensation or acute obstruction occurred the degree of bladder distension could also be assessed by sonography. This technique was also used to monitor dilatation of the upper urinary tract.

The occurrence of parenchymal lesions could be identified in the intact animal by ^{99m}Tc-DMSA scanning. The interpretation of these scans was sometimes difficult. In particular, shading of the polar regions due to respiratory excursions of the kidneys was a problem, especially if activity was low and required prolonged screening times to achieve sufficient counts. The examination of sequential scans sometimes allowed correct interpretation in retrospect of an initially equivocal abnormality, but on other occasions changes which were regarded as a possible parenchymal lesion were not confirmed at autopsy. However, the static scans obtained on the isolated kidneys after sacrifice always correlated with the presence or absence of macroscopic and microscopic abnormalities.

In 3 of the female Minipigs in which frequent ^{99m}Tc-DMSA scans were performed it was possible to pinpoint within a matter of days the precise stage at which lesions developed by observing a definite change from normal to abnormal from one scan to the next.

The emplacement of a ring loosely around the urethra in piglets aged between 2 and 5 weeks was intended to provide gradually increasing bladder outflow obstruction as the animals grew. The degree of obstruction is affected by the growth of the animal and the size of the ring. But in the male animals, both Large White, and Minipigs, the results of using a proximal urethral ring were unsatisfactory.

In most of the latter the ring was so loose that voiding pressures were only moderately elevated, or the relationship between ring size and urethral growth was such that, following a period of moderately elevated voiding pressure, sudden acute obstruction occurred without a period of bladder decompensation. In only 2 of these animals were the conditions of sustained high pressure voiding leading to a period of bladder decompensation achieved. The importance of a phase of bladder decompensation in the genesis of renal parenchymal lesions only became apparent at a late stage in the study (vide infra).

In the female Minipigs the much less muscular and relatively narrow urethra allowed the use of a smaller diameter ring. Elevation of voiding pressure occurred rapidly and progressed early into a phase of bladder decompensation.

Bladder outflow obstruction following emplacement of the urethral ring produces a progression of changes in bladder function in which 4 phases can be recognized.

Phase 1. An initial stage of acute postoperative obstruction, occurring in some animals only and lasting from 2 to 7 days. In mild cases this phase resolved without intervention becoming necessary. 4 animals were lost from the study of this stage with bladder rupture. Subsequently, the institution of daily, or sometimes twice daily suprapubic aspiration to empty the bladder allowed those animals developing this state to survive and, following this, normal micturition was reestablished.

Phase 2. A phase in which peak voiding pressure rose, but the voiding pattern in terms of the frequency and duration of micturition remained essentially normal. Some animals (from the groups of male Large White and Minipigs) did not progress beyond this stage. They developed moderately raised voiding pressures, with normal micturition which remained static even after many weeks.

Phase 3. A period in which peak voiding pressure continued to rise slowly or remained stable at an elevated level, while voiding gradually became increasingly prolonged and more frequent, so that eventually an animal might be seen to void for 3 min about every 15 min.

Phase 4. A final stage, observed in only the female Minipigs and 2 of the Large White male pigs, in which sustained bladder decompensation occurred. This was characterized by gross bladder distension with dribbling micturition, often virtually continuous. Detrusor activity was sometimes completely absent and expulsion of urine occurred only by abdominal straining (fig. 2). In some animals the detrusor continued to contract to produce high intravesical pressure for long periods. These contractions were completely ineffective and urine was only expelled with superimposed abdominal strains (fig. 3). In 2 of the male Minipigs (R. 247 and 248) *acute* bladder decompensation occurred following a period of sustained high pressure voiding with abnormal micturition (phase 3). It occurred abruptly and was associated with complete obstruction, so that the experiment had to be terminated.

It is apparent from our observations in these animals, together with those from our previous study [8], that the urodynamic consequences of placing a ring around the urethra are varied, complex and change with time; they differ subtly in individual animals apparently prepared in a similar fashion. As we will describe, renal damage in the presence of sterile VUR occurs only under clearly defined conditions for which the term 'high pressure reflux' is clearly an oversimple description.

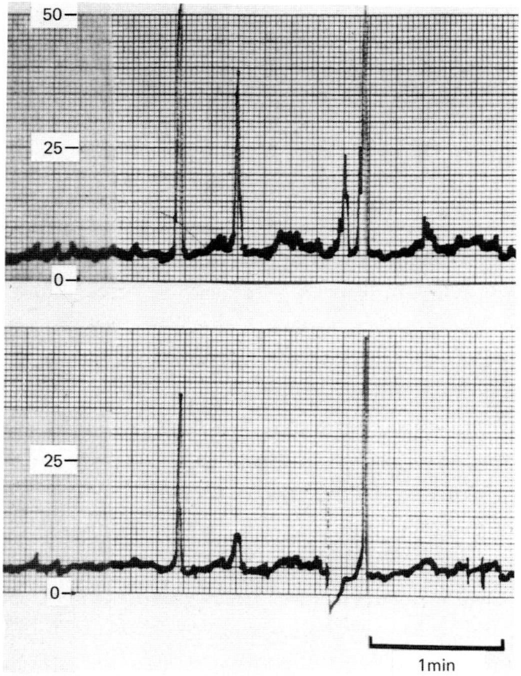

2

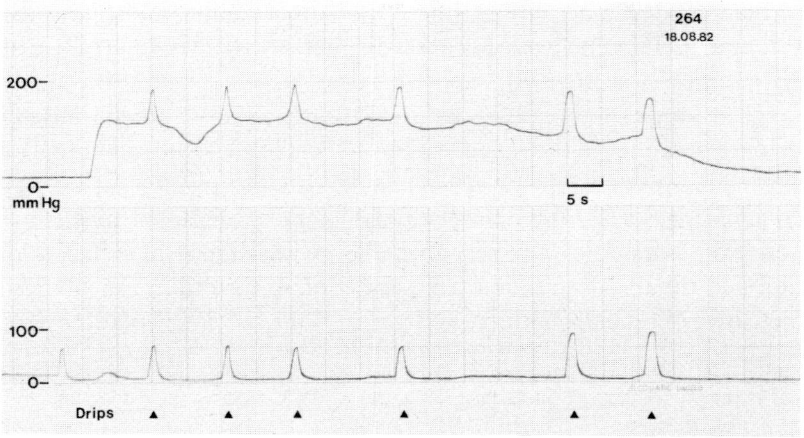

3

Fig. 2. Cystometrogram on female Minipig (R. 246) during phase 4 (bladder decompensation see text). The upper trace shows bladder pressure and the lower trace intra-abdominal pressure. Detrusor contractions are absent and expulsion of urine occurred only during abdominal strains. Scale in mm Hg.

Fig. 3. Cystometrogram on female Minipig (R. 264) during phase 4. The traces are as in figure 2. There is sustained detrusor contraction, but despite high intravesical pressure, urine is expelled only with superimposed abdominal strains.

Results

The urodynamic and gross pathologic findings in all the animals included in the study are summarized in table I. Animals R. 217–240 were Large White Male pigs (group I), R. 243–250 (except 246) were male minipigs (group II) and R. 246 and 261–264 were female Minipigs (group III). Representative VCUs and photomicrographs of the gross and microscopic pathologic findings from the animals in each group, together with illustrative sonograms are depicted in figures 4–11.

Significant segmental changes developed in the kidneys subjected to VUR in 6 animals (R. 208, 240, 246, 261 and 264) and minor abnormalities in 2 others (R. 218 and 223). The pathologic findings, including the examination for THP in these animals are summarized in table II. Kidneys from all the other animals in the study showed no pathologic abnormalities and THP was confined to its normal site in the distal tubules.

In 3 of the female Minipigs (R. 246, 261 and 264) unequivocal differences in consecutive ^{99m}Tc-DMSA scans were observed in short periods of time allowing precise definition of the circumstances existing at the time of development of parenchymal lesions. These scans are shown in figure 12. In each case the first scan was performed at or near the onset of the phase of bladder decompensation (phase 4). Abnormalities indicating the development of parenchymal lesions were then noted after 7 days (R. 261 and 264) and 14 days (R. 246).

The study shows that in the presence of sterile VUR with raised peak voiding pressures in the range of 41 to 177 cm H_2O, significant renal parenchymal lesions develop only when bladder decompensation occurs. In these circumstances acute tubulointerstitial damage ensues after only a few days and progresses quickly to scar formation with interstitial collagen formation and tubular destruction. Extravasation of THP into the interstitium, indicative of tubular rupture was noted in many but not all of these lesions.

Discussion

The primary object of this study has been to discover whether VUR of sterile urine in the pig model can initiate renal scarring, and to determine the precise urodynamic conditions under which such lesions might develop. Our difficulties in achieving this aim have been discussed above (see Discussion of Experimental Model) and we have shown that the model has to

Table I. Summary of urodynamic and pathologic changes in all the animals in the study. The center columns illustrate the evolution of bladder dysfunction (see text)

Pig No.	Sex	Type	Max PVP cm H_2O	Post op. obstruction phase 1	phase 2	phase 3	Decompensation + duration (days) phase 4	Upper tract dilatation	Refluxing side	Parenchymal changes	Duration of experiment, weeks
Group I											
217	M	LW	41		——→			no	R	none	11
218	M	LW	54		——	——→		no	R	puckering ±	17
225	M	LW	88	——	——	——→		no	R + L	none	21
226	M	LW	48		——→			no	R + L	none	30
208	M	LW	68		——	——	——→ 7+	R	R	scarring + + R	17
223	M	LW	61	——	——	——→		R + L	R	puckering + R	14
240	M	LW	98	——	——	——	——→ 7	R + L	R + L	scarring + + L & R	15
Group II											
243	M	MP	82	——	——→			no	R + L	none	26
247	M	MP	68	——	——	→		L	L	none	12
248	M	MP	61	——	——	→		R	R	none	18
249	M	MP	68	——	——→			no	L	none	18
250	M	MP	60	——	——→			no	R + L	none	22
Group III											
246	F	MP	–	——	——	——	——→ 8	R + L	L	scarring + + L	6
261	F	MP	98		——	——	——→ 6	R < L	R + L	acute lesions L+ R+	4
262	F	MP	54	——	——	——→ 2		L	L	acute lesions L±	3½
263	F	MP	109	——	——	→ 1		L	L	none	6
264	F	MP	177	——	——	——	——→ 6	L	L	acute lesions L+ +	3

LW = Large Whites; MP = Minipigs.

a

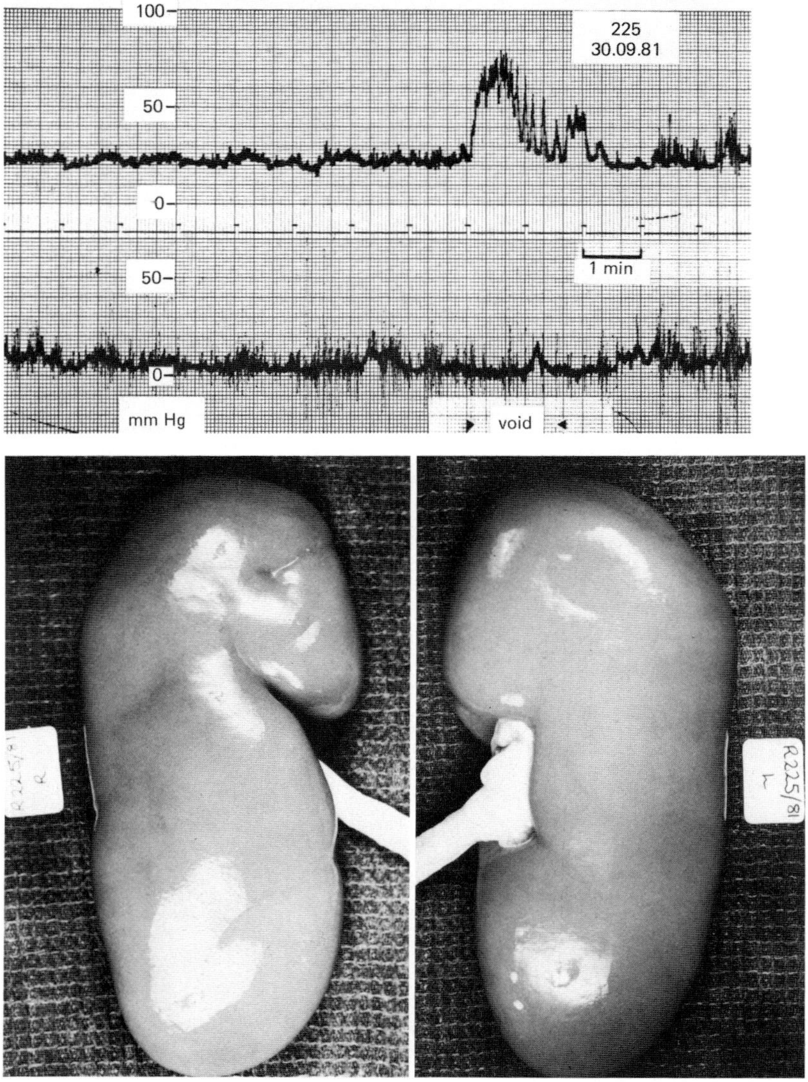

Fig. 4. Male Large White (R. 225; group 1). *a* Cystometrogram 19 weeks after surgery (traces as in fig. 2). *b* Kidneys from the same animal showing the absence of parenchymal lesions which was confirmed histologically.

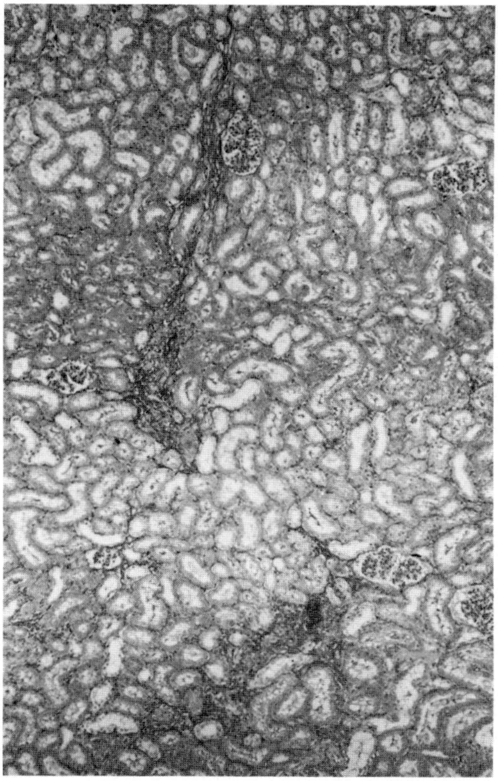

Fig. 5. Male Large White (R. 218; group 1). Histological appearances of the minor and insubstantial scarring evident in the right kidney. VG. × 40.

be manipulated to provide sustained bladder decompensation before parenchymal lesions will develop in the kidney. However, once persistent bladder decompensation is established ^{99m}Tc-DMSA scanning indicates that segmental renal damage can develop quickly in the course of a few days. Conversely, prolonged periods of high pressure voiding without decompensation (that is, where bladder pressures return to normal resting levels between voids and effective bladder emptying occurs – 'compensated bladder outflow obstruction') does not give rise to parenchymal damage. This remained true even for the 2 animals (R. 247 and 248) which progressed to acute obstruction after long periods of high pressure voiding but in which sustained bladder decompensation did not occur.

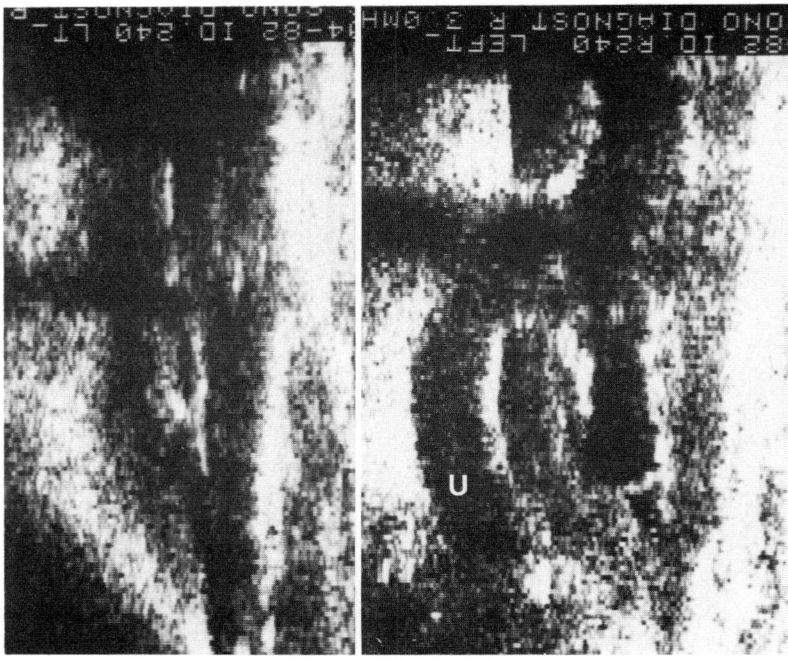

a *b*

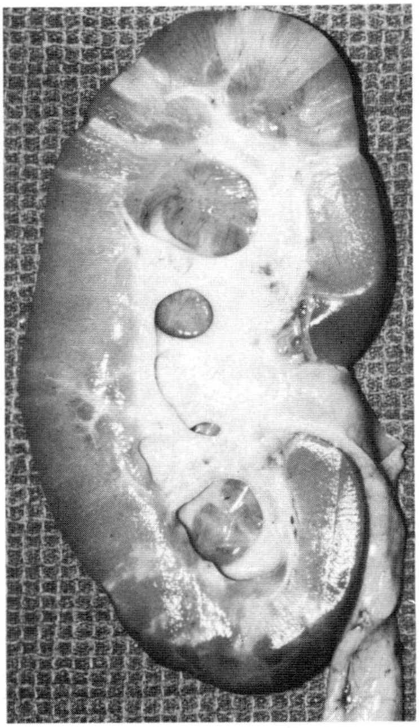

c

Fig. 6. Male Large White (R. 240; group 1) which progressed to bladder decompensation (phase 4). Sonograms of the left kidney *(a)* before and *(b)* after bladder decompensation showing the development of severe upper tract dilatation when decompensation occurs. U = Ureter. *c* View of the cut surface of the right kidney showing radiating bars of fibrosis with intervening unscarred parenchyma; note the degree of calyceal dilatation. *d* Histology of a scar showing advanced tubular loss, interstitial fibrosis, scanty inflammation and dilatation of collecting ducts. HE. × 25.

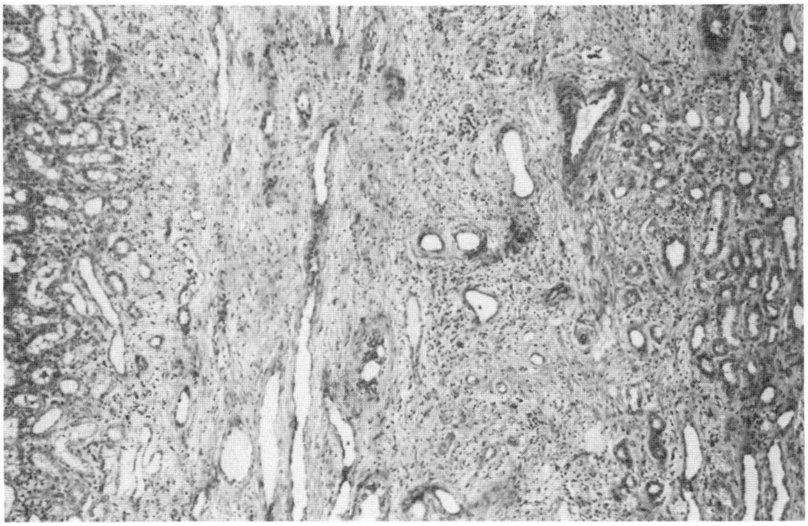
d

Acute lesions were observed in 3 of the female Minipigs (R. 261, 262 and 264) and were characterized by areas of parenchymal pallor radiating from the centers of the renal papillae into the overlying cortex. Microscopically, changes were essentially tubulointerstitial and consisted of tubular dilatation and separation with flattening of the lining epithelial cells. The edematous interstitium contained scattered fibroblasts and a generally scanty infiltrate of inflammatory cells – mostly lymphocytes. In some of the lesions deposits of THP were demonstrated, and a proportion of these deposits were associated with localized collections of lymphocytes and plasma cells.

More advanced lesions were seen in 3 animals. 2 were male Large Whites (R. 208 and 240) and 1 a female Minipig (R. 246). In these animals tubular damage was more extensive and interstitial collagen formation was an added feature. Interstitial THP deposits were frequent in the lesions from the female Minipig but were absent in those of the male Large Whites.

In comparison with the infected lesions produced in earlier studies a number of differences were noted. The sterile lesions tended to be smaller and less diffuse; they often consisted of aggregates of linear streaks or bars with bands of uninvolved parenchyma between them. The infected scars, by contrast, tended to be more confluent and usually wedge-shaped. Microscopically the infected lesions were associated with a much more intense interstitial inflammatory infiltrate, frequently with lymphoid follicle formation, and neutrophil polymorphs were seen in some tubules. Interstitial

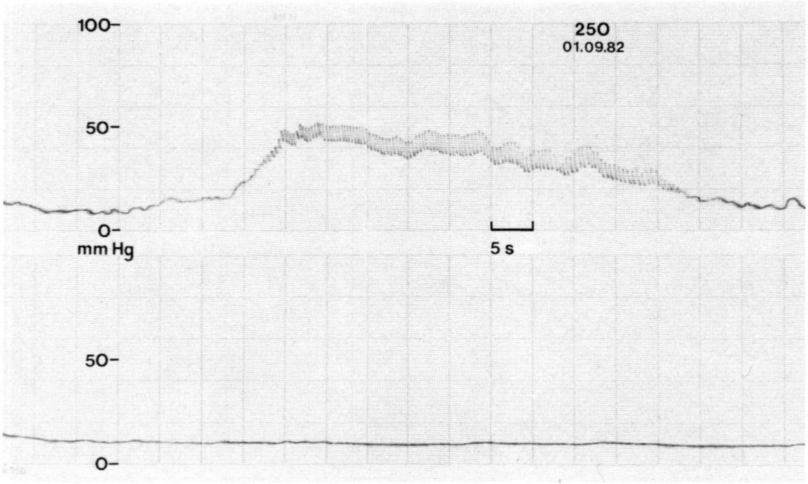

a

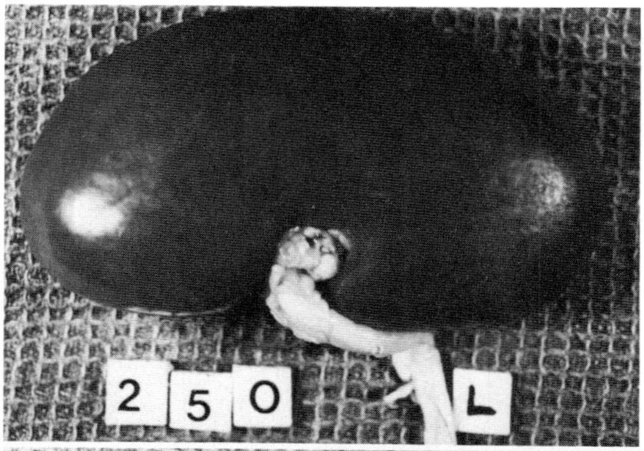

b

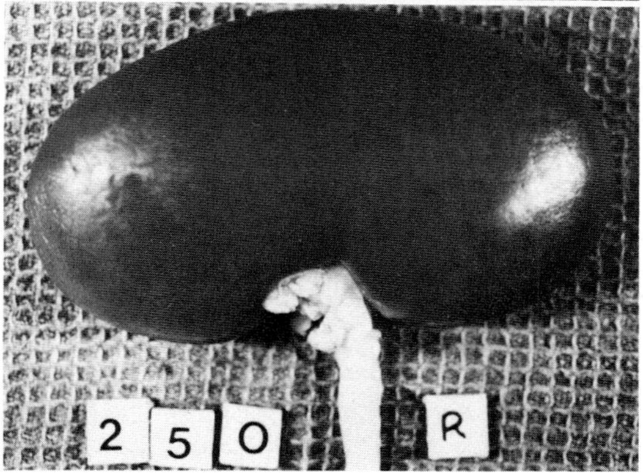

c

Fig. 7. Male Minipig (R. 250; group 2). *a* Cystometrogram after 15 weeks in phase 2 (see text). The traces are as in figure 2. *b, c* The kidneys from the same animal showing no macroscopic, nor subsequent microscopic abnormality.

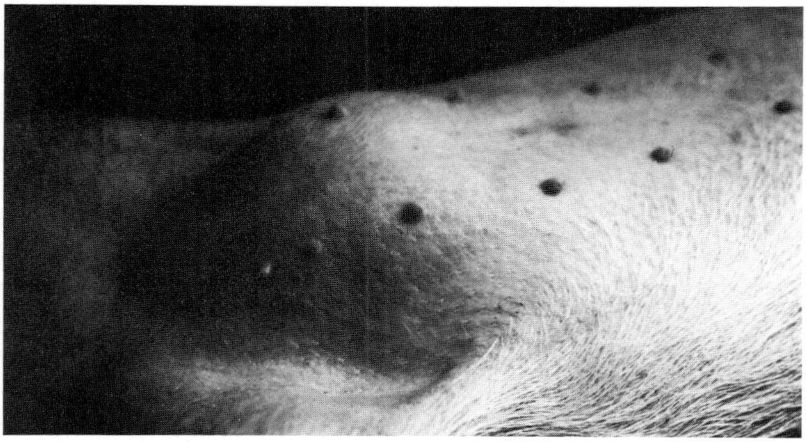

Fig. 8. Female Minipig (R. 263; group 3). Abdomen to show the degree of distension of a decompensated bladder.

THP deposits, seen in some of the sterile lesions, were never encountered in infected scars.

The status of the insubstantial scars seen in 2 additional male Large Whites (R. 218 and 223) in the present study is difficult to assess. In 1 of these animals bladder decompensation did not occur. The fine linear scarring and puckering of the surface of the kidneys in these 2 animals is identical to that we have encountered previously in animals treated with antimicrobial agents after a short period of infected VUR [9]. The possibility that both these animals sustained very short periods of UTI undetected by our bacteriologic screening has to be admitted.

Although individual sterile lesions tended to be less extensive than the infected ones, they were distributed more uniformly and occurred in both the polar regions and the midzones of affected kidneys. We have demonstrated previously how in infected lesions access of the organisms which initiate parenchymal scars is mediated by IRR. The predominantly polar distribution of infected scars occurring with VUR at normal voiding pressures is due to the fact that compound papillae which allow free IRR under these conditions are found mainly at the renal poles. When, however, voiding pressure is raised, or an elevated intrapelvic pressure is sustained, deformation of some simple papillae in the midzone of the kidney ensues and IRR then occurs up these normally resistant papillae, and any resulting scar formation becomes more generalized. Clearly, in the present series, in animals in whom parenchymal lesions developed, intrapelvic pressures were high and diffuse IRR would have occurred. The distribution of individual lesions directly over renal papillae is strong presumptive evidence that IRR is central to the development of sterile as well as infected scars. Under the conditions of bladder decompensation with upper tract dilatation in which the sterile lesions formed, the collecting ducts and tubules where IRR was occurring would be subjected to sustained high intraluminal pressures. Over and above this, there would be transmission of additional peaks of pressure during frequently repeated attempts at voiding. Three possible sequelae are suggested. Firstly the hydrodynamic effects might directly damage the epithelial cells lining the dilated tubules. Secondly tubular distension might inhibit blood flow through adjacent peritubular capillaries, adding an element of ischemic damage. Thirdly, and perhaps during phases of peak pressure transmission into an already maximally dilated system, actual rupture of tubular basement membranes could occur, allowing egress of urine into the interstitium. The demonstration of interstitial THP in at least some of the lesions during the acute phase is evidence in favor of this possibility. Whether THP itself or other urinary constituents, either directly or as a result of humoral [4] or cellular immune mechanisms [6] they may elicit, are responsible for at least some of the parenchymal damage sustained remains to be elucidated.

Comparison of the macroscopic appearances of our sterile lesions with the illustrations of those produced by *Hodson et al.* [3] is of considerable interest. *Hodson* [1] has drawn attention to the flat polar and deep cleft-like midzonal scars occurring directly over flattened papillae which he regards as characteristic of RN. We were struck by the fact that *Hodson et al.* [3] often removed the urethral ring in the course of their experiments. Judging by our own experience this would be essential, since the state of bladder decompensation necessary to initiate scar formation would be incompatible with continued survival. If, however, the ring were removed, contraction of the scarred area coupled with growth of the adjacent unaffected parenchyma would ultimately result in the deep cleft scars that *Hodson et al.* [3]

Fig. 9. Female Minipig (R. 246; group 3). The cystometrogram from this animal during phase 4 is shown in figure 2. *a*, *b* Macroscopic appearances of the left kidney showing multiple bar-like parenchymal lesions (see also fig. 12). *c* Histologic appearances of a scarred area showing interstitial lymphocytic and plasmacytic infiltration and a deposit of THP (arrowed). HE. × 250. *d* A large interstitial deposit of THP with associated interstitial inflammation and adjacent fibrous scarring. PAP technic for THP. × 250.

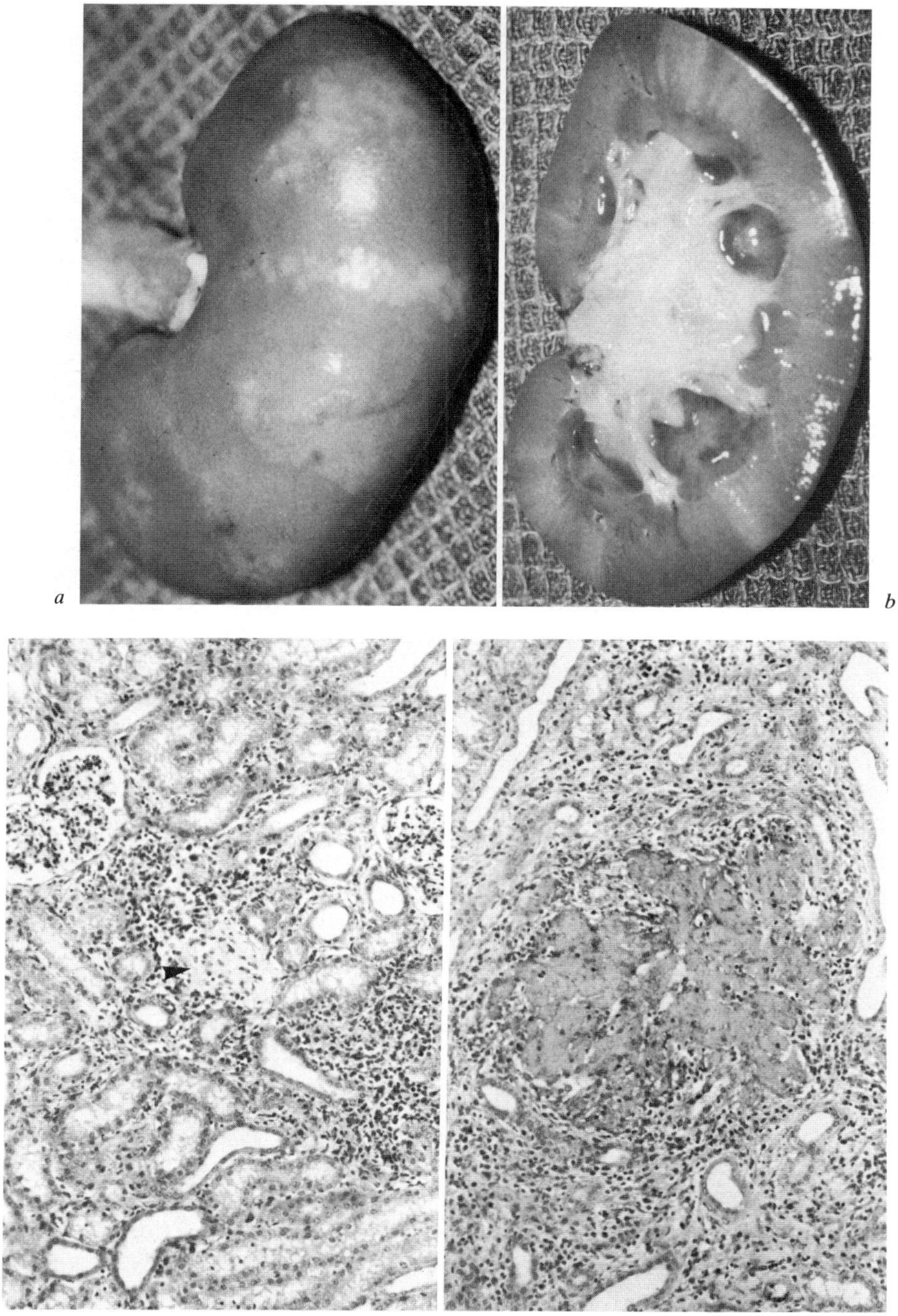

a *b*

c *d*

a 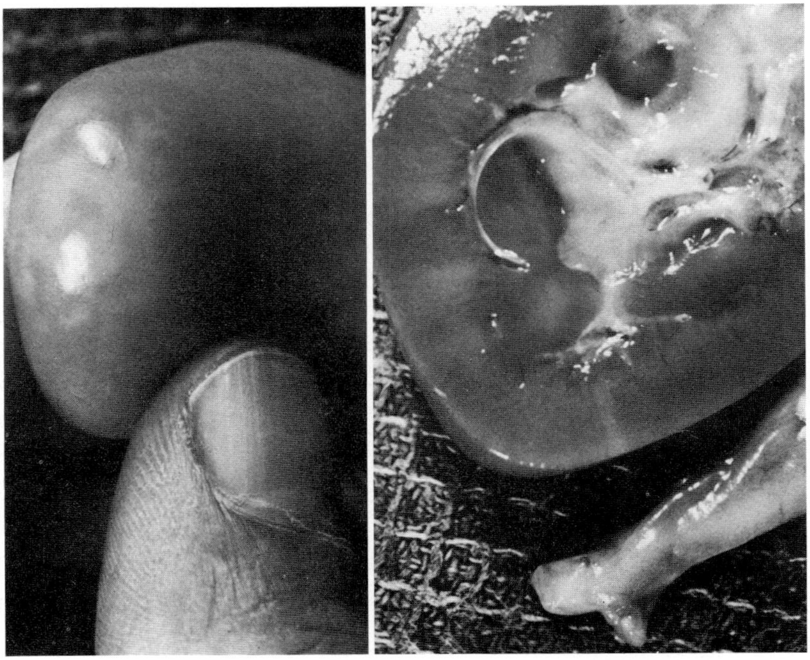 b

Fig. 10. Female Minipig (R. 261; group 3). *a*, *b* Views of the right kidney showing very early parenchymal lesions after 6 days of bladder decompensation (see also fig. 12). *c* Histologic appearances showing tubular dilatation and separation with interstitial fibroblastic proliferation but little inflammation. HE. × 100.

demonstrated. However, it is likely that the parenchymal damage leading to this scarring occurred in the period before the ring was removed. Their work, as well as our study reported here, demonstrates that in the pig model of VUR under conditions of sustained bladder decompensation and upper tract dilatation it is possible to produce segmental renal parenchymal lesions in the absence of UTI. We are, however, unwilling to ascribe great clinical significance to this observation. Our work indicates that sustained bladder decompensation with VUR rather than high pressure VUR per se is the essential prerequisite for the development of sterile scars and clinical parallels for this are few. It is possible that such a mechanism might operate, for example, in some infant boys with obstructive posterior urethral valves, or in some children with a neuropathic bladder. However, complicating factors cloud the issue, even in these situations. Firstly, UTI is

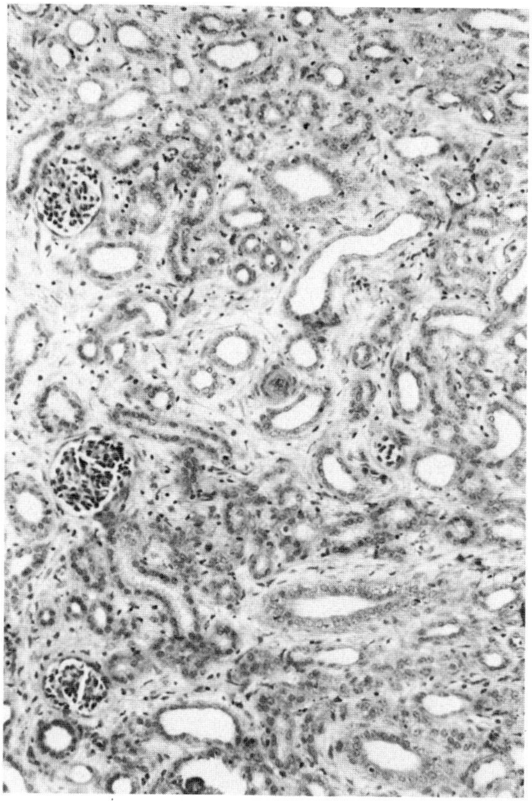

c

extremely common under these circumstances, and all workers using this model have demonstrated that the combination of infected VUR with bladder outflow obstruction produces devastating and rapid destruction of the kidney even in the absence of bladder decompensation [9]. Secondly, it is very difficult to ascertain in many of the clinical examples cited whether the renal abnormalities observed are due to maldifferentiation of the kidney during intrauterine life or lesions acquired after birth. Not uncommonly the kidneys of children with obstructive posterior urethral valves show histologic evidence of renal dysplasia, giving an unequivocal indication of maldifferentiation. It is also true that occasional examples of severe bilateral renal dysplasia associated with widely dilated refluxing ureters and narrowing of the posterior urethra are encountered. It may be possible to distinguish whether the lesions present in these kidneys are due to anomalous

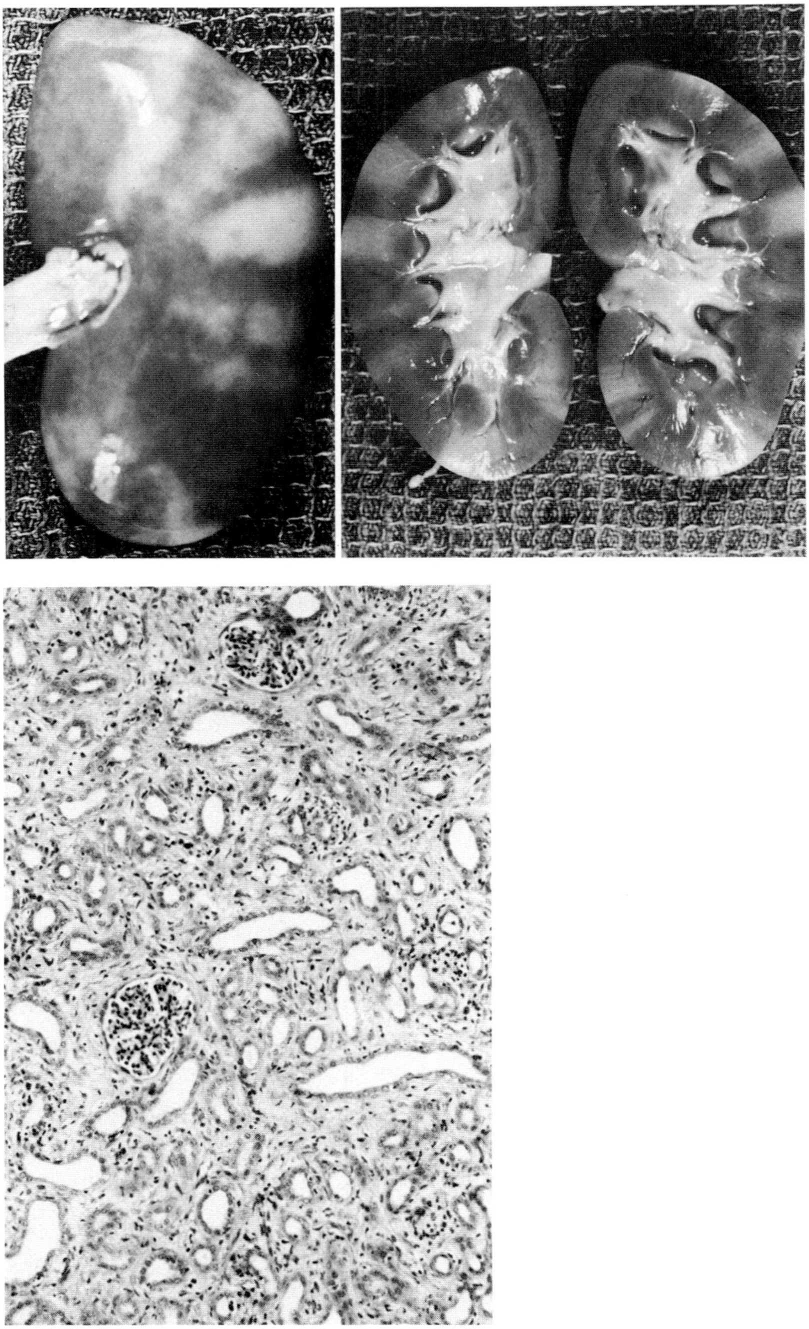

a b c

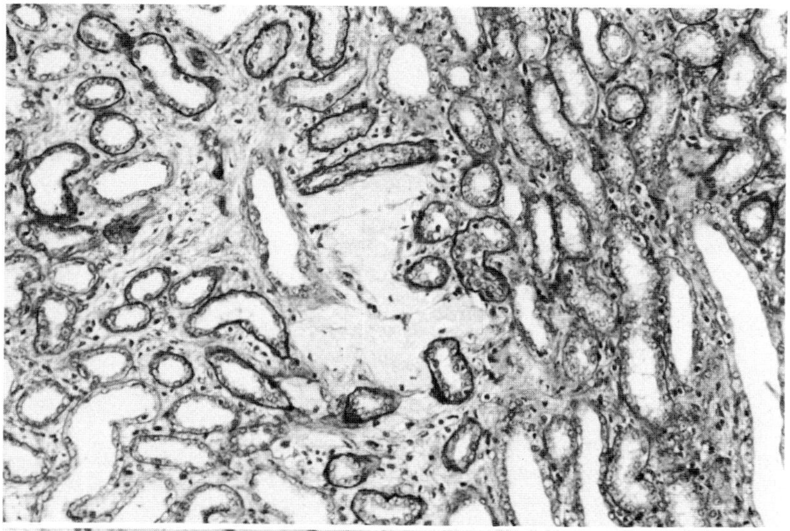

d

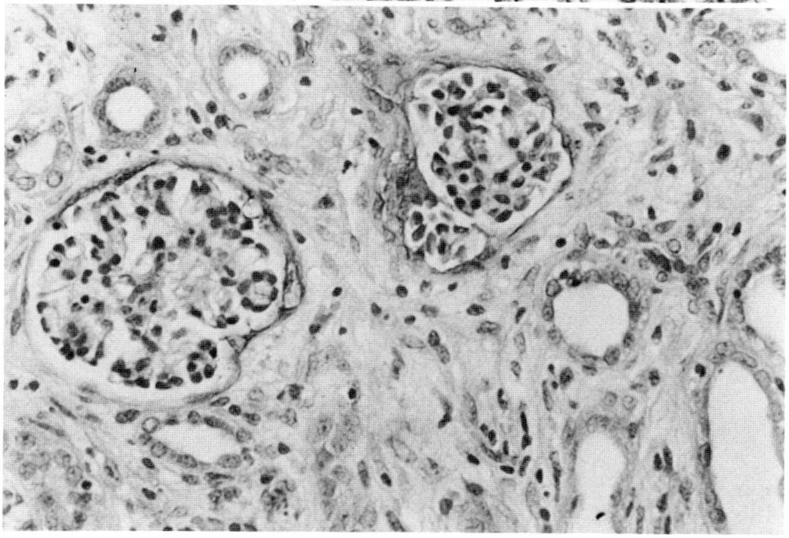

e

Fig. 11. Female Minipig (R. 264; group 3). The cystometrogram from this animal during phase 4 is shown in figure 3. *a, b* Macroscopic appearances of the left kidney showing prominent bar-like lesions (see also fig. 12). *c* Histologically these are similar to those in R. 261 (see fig. 10c). HE. × 100. *d* An interstitial deposit of THP with no associated inflammation. PAMS. × 100. *e* Deposition of THP in the glomerular urinary space along Bowman's capsule. PAP technic for THP. × 400.

Table II. Summary of parenchymal lesions in the kidney

Animal	Reflux	Affected side(s)	Pathologic lesions		Localization of THP in lesions	
			macroscopic	microscopic	in glomerular urinary spaces	deposits in interstitium
Group I						
208	R	R	coalescent contracted scars over papillae throughout kidney	dense interstitial fibrosis and widespread tubular loss; sparse interstitial inflammation	P	A
240	R + L	R + L	linear and bar-like scars with intervening bands of unaffected parenchyma over papillae throughout the kidney	dense interstitial fibrosis with tubular loss; focal interstitial inflammation; dilatation of residual tubules; generalized tubular and glomerular dilatation in unscarred parenchyma	P	A
218	R	R	focal pitting and puckering of kidney surface at poles; very fine linear cortical scarring	small foci of fine linear fibrosis with localized tubular loss and glomerular scarring	A	A
223	R + L	R	focal pitting and puckering of kidney surface at poles; very fine linear cortical scarring	small foci of fine linear fibrosis with localized tubular loss and glomerular scarring	A	A

metanephric differentiation, or to acquired UTI, or sterile scarring, particularly by radiologic or other imaging techniques alone.

It could be argued that any parenchymal maldevelopment is itself due to VUR and/or obstruction operating in utero, but equally, as suggested by *Stephens* [11], the association of grossly dilated ureters, renal dysplasia and VUR may together reflect a common developmental abnormality of the ureteric bud. It seems probable that a whole spectrum of possible

Table II. (continued)

Animal	Reflux	Affected side(s)	Pathologic lesions		Localization of THP in lesions	
			macroscopic	microscopic	in glomerular urinary spaces	deposits in interstitium
Group III						
261	R + L	R + L	focal streaks and bars of parenchymal pallor most marked at poles, radiating from papillae	focal areas of tubular dilatation and separation; interstitial edema with fibroblastic proliferation and sparse interstitial inflammation	P	P (single deposit in one lesion)
262	L	L	focal streaks and bars of parenchymal pallor most marked at poles, radiating from papillae	focal areas of tubular dilatation and separation; interstitial edema with fibroblastic proliferation and sparse interstitial inflammation	P	P in many one lesion)
264	L	L	bars of parenchymal pallor and swelling over papillae throughout the kidney	focal areas of tubular dilatation and separation; interstitial edema with fibroblastic proliferation and sparse interstitial inflammation	P	P (in some lesions)
246	L	L	bars of parenchymal pallor and swelling over papillae throughout the kidney	interstitial edema with some fibrosis; some tubular destruction; interstitial lymphocytic and plasma cell infiltration often associated with deposits of THP	P	P (in all lesions)

pathogenic mechanisms may account for the renal parenchymal lesions seen in association with VUR.

We would restate our view that the majority of parenchymal scars acquired postnatally in children with VUR are wholly or predominantly initiated by parenchymal infection. A mechanism for sterile scarring has been demonstrated and could explain at least some of the renal damage occurring in children with a combination of VUR and bladder outflow obstruc-

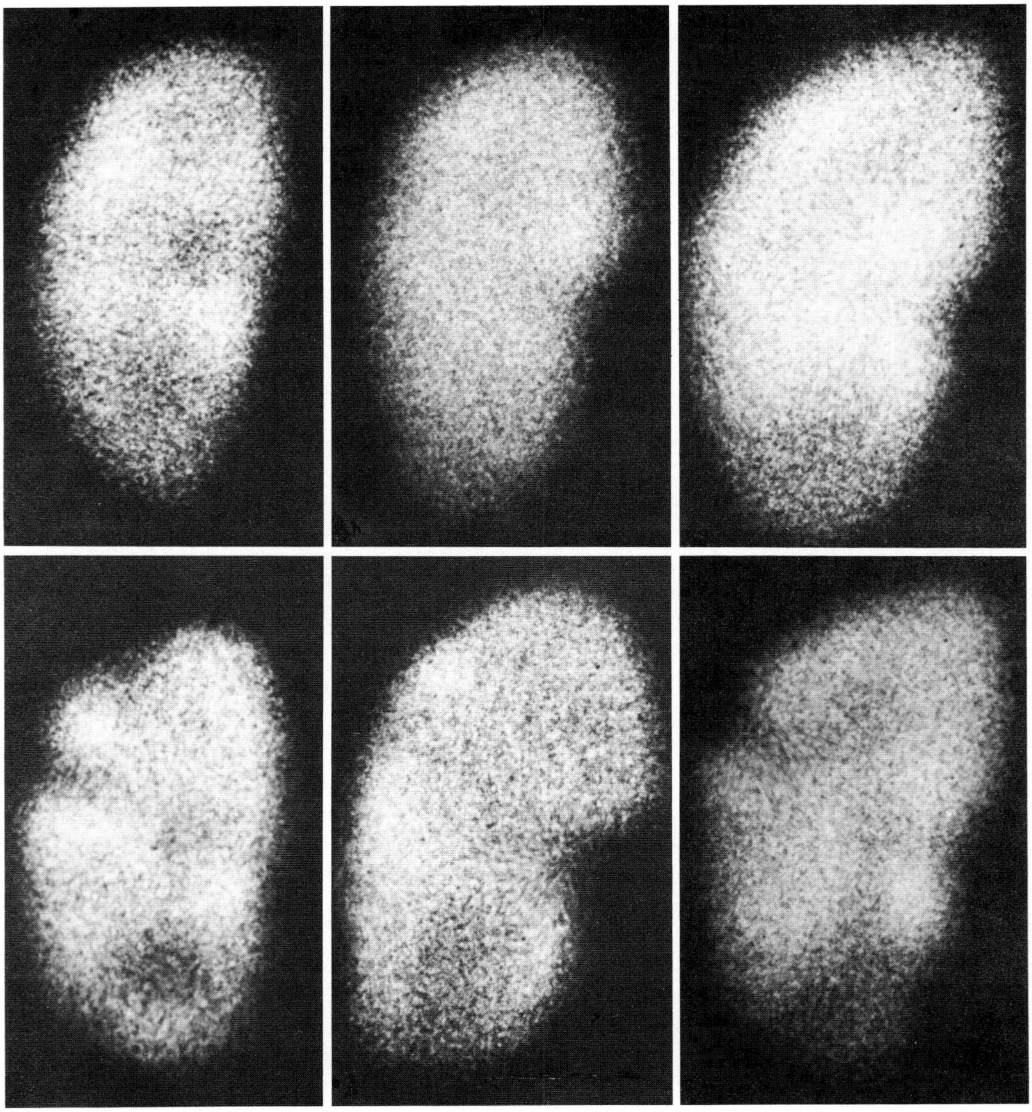

Fig. 12. Pairs of ^{99m}Tc-DMSA scans in which unequivocal parenchymal changes from normal (1) to abnormal (2) occurred with bladder decompensation (see text). These are from the female Minipigs depicted in figures 9–11. *a1, 2* R. 246 (interval between scans 14 days). *b1, 2* R. 261 (7 days). *c1, 2* R. 264 (7 days). In R. 246 calyceal dilatation without parenchymal lesions is evident. Lower pole shading (see text) is seen in some extent in all three preliminary scans.

tion. Even in these cases, however, intrauterine renal maldevelopment or coexistent UTI are probably more important factors.

Acknowledgements

This work has been supported by a grant from the Stiftung Volkswagenwerk. We wish to thank Drs. *I. Gordon* and *G. Vivian* and Mrs. *C. Haskell* of the Department of Diagnostic Imaging, The Hospital for Sick Children; Dr. *M.W. Turner*, Department of Immunology, Institute of Child Health; Mr. *R.E. Bartholomew* and the staff of the Department of Medical Illustration, Institute of Urology; Miss *Carole Nichols*, Department of Morbid Anatomy, The London Hospital Medical College and Mr. *B. Gregory* and the staff of the Animal House, Institute of Child Health for their generous help throughout the project.

References

1 Hodson, C.J.: Formation of renal scars with special reference to reflux nephropathy; in Kuhn, Brod, Contributions to nephrology, vol. 16, pp. 83–89 (Karger, Basel 1979).
2 Hodson, C.J.; Edwards, D.: Chronic pyelonephritis and vesicoureteric reflux. Clin. Radiol. *11*: 219–231 (1960).
3 Hodson, C.J.; Maling, T.M.J.; McManamon, P.J.; Lewis, M.G.: The pathogenesis of reflux nephropathy (chronic atrophic pyelonephritis). Br. J. Radiol. *48*: suppl. 13, pp. 1–26 (1975).
4 Hoyer, J.R.: Tubulointerstitial immune complex nephritis in rate immunized with Tamm-Horsfall Protein. Kidney int. *17*: 284–292 (1980).
5 Kovacs, K.; Corenblum, B.; Sirek, A.M.T.; Penz, G.; Ezrin, C.: Localisation of prolactin in chromophobe pituitary adenomas: study of human necropsy material by immunoperoxidase technique. J. clin. Path. *29*: 250–258 (1976).
6 Mayrer, A.R.; Kashgarian, M.; Ruddle, N.H.; Marier, R.; Hodson, C.J.; Richards, F.F.; Andriole, V.T.: Tubulointerstitial nephritis and immunological responses to Tamm-Horsfall protein in rabbits challenged with homologous urine or Tamm-Horsfall protein. J. Immun. *128*: 2634–2642 (1982).
7 Ransley, P.G.; Risdon, R.A.: Renal papillary morphology and intrarenal reflux in the young pig. Urol. Res. *3*: 105–109 (1975).
8 Ransley, P.G.; Risdon, R.A.: Reflux and renal scarring. Br. J. Radiol. *51*: suppl. 14, pp. 1–35 (1978).
9 Ransley, P.G.; Risdon, R.A.: Reflux nephropathy: effects of antimicrobial therapy on the evolution of the early pyelonephritic scar. Kidney int. *20*: 733–742 (1981).
10 Rolleston, G.L.; Maling, T.M.J.; Hodson, C.J.: Intrarenal reflux and the scarred kidney. Archs. Dis Childh. *49*: 531–539 (1974).
11 Stephens, F.D.: Cystoscopic appearances of the ureteric orifices associated with reflux nephropathy, pp. 119–125 (Masson, New York 1979).

P.G. Ransley, Institutes of Child Health and Urology, University of London, GB-London (England)

Contr. Nephrol., vol. 39, pp. 344–357 (Karger, Basel 1984)

26. Pathology of Sterile Reflux in the Pig

Robert H. Heptinstall[a], *C. John Hodson*[b]

[a]Department of Pathology, The Johns Hopkins University School of Medicine, Baltimore, Md.; [b]Department of Diagnostic Radiology, Yale University School of Medicine, New Haven, Conn., USA

Introduction

It is now generally accepted that the discrete parenchymal scars found in chronic non-obstructive pyelonephritis are caused by vesicoureteral reflux (VUR) of *infected* urine from the bladder into the kidney, and there is good experimental evidence to support this [1–3]. However, the idea proposed many years ago by *Hodson and Edwards* [4] that VUR of sterile urine alone could cause similar discrete scars has not been so universally accepted. One of the principal difficulties is that in clinical practice it is impossible to monitor the urine for sterility on a continuous basis, thus leaving the experimental approach as the only one available to study the problem.

In their experiments on the production of renal scars in pigs with unilateral or bilateral VUR, *Hodson* et al. [1] observed that certain animals whose urine was never infected developed discrete renal parenchymal scars. These animals all had high-pressure VUR (45–55 mm Hg) and the discrete scars were accompanied by a generalized but very variable degree of dilatation of the pelvis and calyces. The scars were associated with intrarenal reflux (IRR) and situated in exactly the same highly characteristic distribution as those resulting from infected VUR and IRR. In a comparable type of study but involving lower bladder pressures, *Ransley and Risdon* [3] were unable to produce discrete renal scars in the setting of sterile VUR, but at a later time succeeded in doing so [5, and chapter 25, this volume]. The apparent explanation for the different experience in their two studies was that in the second one the pigs showed a combination of high voiding pressure, prolonged voiding, and elevated resting pressures within the bladder. They considered that scar formation with sterile VUR could occur only under extreme urodynamic conditions in man.

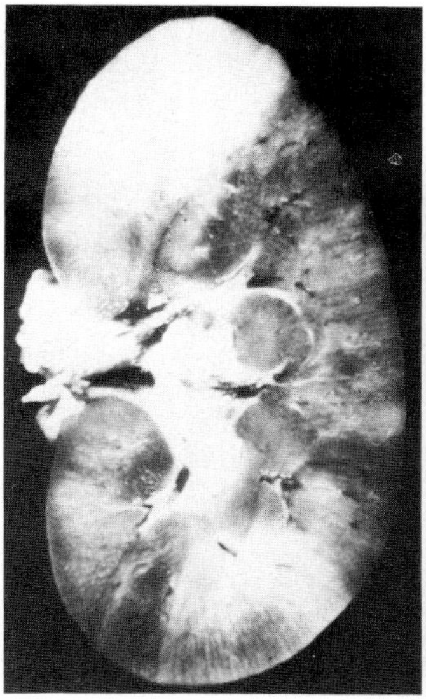

1

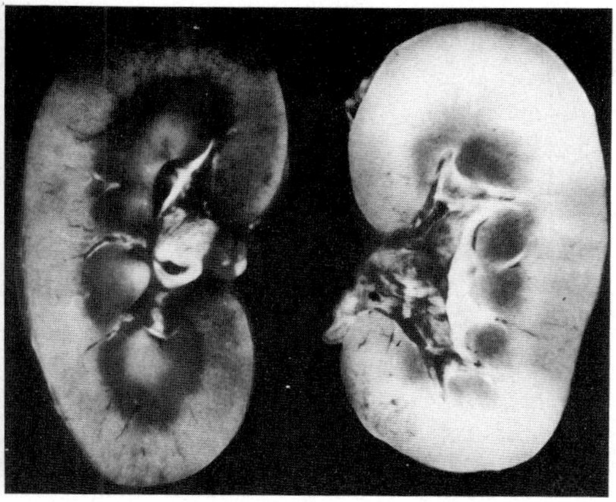

2

Fig. 1. Cut surface of kidney to show swelling (white areas) in parts where IRR is occurring. (Estimated age of lesion given in parentheses for all figures: 10 days.)

Fig. 2. Cut surface of left and right kidneys to show large white areas of swelling in most of right kidney. Left kidney is little affected. (7 days.)

Experimental Design and Methods Employed

In order to explore more fully the mechanism of discrete scar formation caused by sterile VUR, it was decided to produce high-pressure sterile VUR in miniature pigs as before – progressive urethral obstruction produced by a constrictive device placed around the proximal urethra of sows, aged 6–8 weeks, with simultaneous incision of the anterior wall of one intravesical ureter [1] – and to study the lesions occurring in the kidneys at various subsequent time periods. A number of procedures were performed at intervals up to the time of autopsy; these included regular monitoring by means of excretion urography (IVU), repeated culture of the urine, and isotope parenchymal studies in certain animals. The clinical condition of the pigs was followed by noting such features as general well-being, alertness, appetite, and ease or difficulty of voiding. In addition the abdomen was regularly examined for bladder enlargement and resistance to palpation, as this is easily defined in young pigs.

All animals were placed on continuous prophylactic antimicrobial therapy, as was the majority of the 'sterile' group in the first series, either for the duration of the experiment, or until long after the release of urethral constriction and the reestablishment of free bladder drainage.

Pigs were killed at intervals which varied from 3 weeks to 5 months after the initial surgical procedure used to produce VUR. These intervals, however, do not accurately reflect the duration of the scarring process, and a more precise estimate is given by the interval between the onset of a sudden increase in the size of the kidney – as detected by excretion urography – and the date of autopsy. On this basis the age of the scarring process ranged from 7 to 124 days. Animals developing urinary tract infection (UTI) of the bladder urine were excluded, as were those in which evidence of renal infection was detected by histologic techniques.

12 animals satisfying the criteria for sterile VUR were available for study. Kidneys obtained at autopsy were examined by gross inspection, light microscopy and immunohistology. In 2 a barium sulfate (Micropaque, Damancy) cystogram was carried out just before autopsy. Both fluorescent antibody and immunoperoxidase techniques for the demonstration of Tamm-Horsfall protein (THP) were utilized. Fluorescent antibody methods have been described in a previous communication [6] and immunoperoxidase techniques using formol-fixed renal tissue were performed according to standard procedures [7]. Slides were treated with rabbit anti-swine THP (kindly supplied by Dr. *Peter Avis*), followed by the application of swine antirabbit immunoglobulin and rabbit antiperoxidase-peroxidase complex. Hematoxylin was used as a counterstain.

Results

The early stages consisted of a swelling of the full parenchyma confined to the area of IRR (fig. 1, 2) and corresponding in time with the acute increase in size of the kidney detected by excretion urography. Two apparently distinct types of lesion were seen microscopically. In the first, the parenchyma subjected to IRR showed edema of the interstitium, separation of the tubules one from another, and dilatation of tubules, particularly the collecting ducts and ascending limbs (fig. 3). The interstitium contained scattered lymphoid and other mononuclear cells, but in one particular pig (J34) there were extremely large collections of these cells (fig. 4), often related to the presence of conspicuous deposits of THP in the interstitium and to disrupted tubules. THP was also present in the capsular spaces of the glomeruli (fig. 5) – indicative of backflow of urine within the tubular system – and sandwiched between layers of collagen in the thickened capsule. The latter was interpreted as indicative of a lymphatic run-off via the subcapsular plexus of lymphatics. Immunoperoxidase techniques enable small inapparent collections of THP to be detected in the interstitium in relation to collections of lymphoid and mononuclear cells in addition to larger collections of THP (fig. 6). Immunofluorescence studies revealed that some of the interstitial cells were producing IgG, but the majority were not. In this particular animal (J34) it was found *that the non-refluxing parts* of the kidney contained only small scattered collections of chronic inflammatory cells in the interstititium (fig. 7), together with very occasional minute deposits of THP. Similar small collections were seen in the opposite kidney.

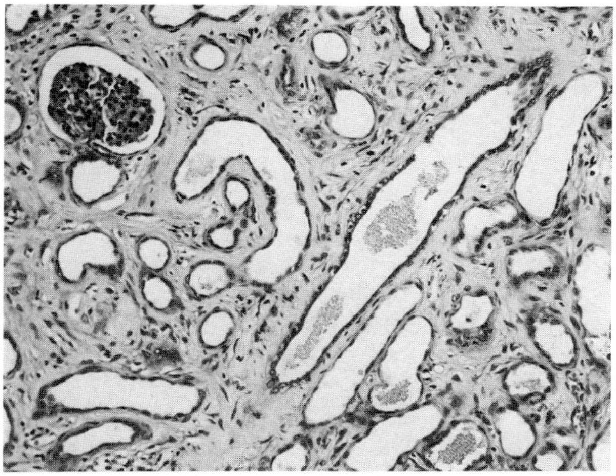

Fig. 3. Interstitial edema and very early fibrosis with tubular atrophy and dilatation. Granular material in large tubules in center is barium sulfate resulting from a pre-autopsy cystogram; it demonstrates free IRR. H&E. × 80. (16 days.)

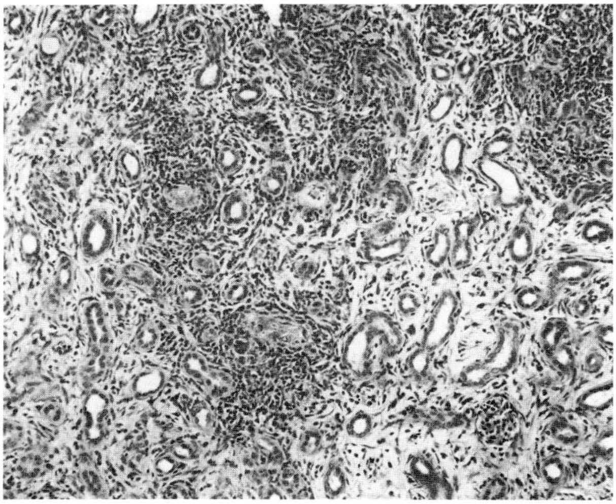

Fig. 4. Photomicrograph to show interstitial edema and considerable interstitial cellular reaction in parenchyma subjected to IRR. Most of the cells are of lymphoid type. H&E. × 130. (7 days.)

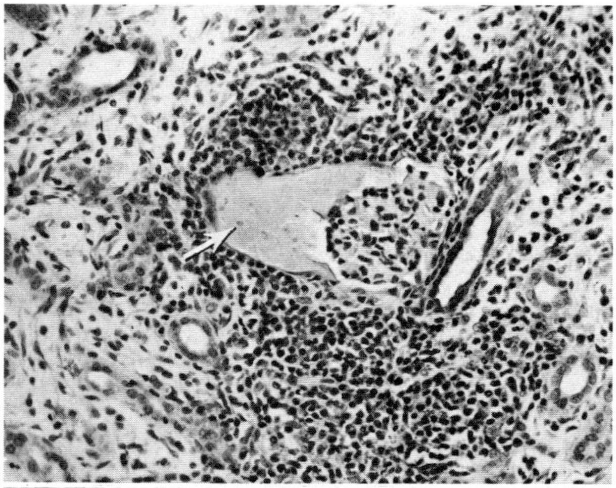

5

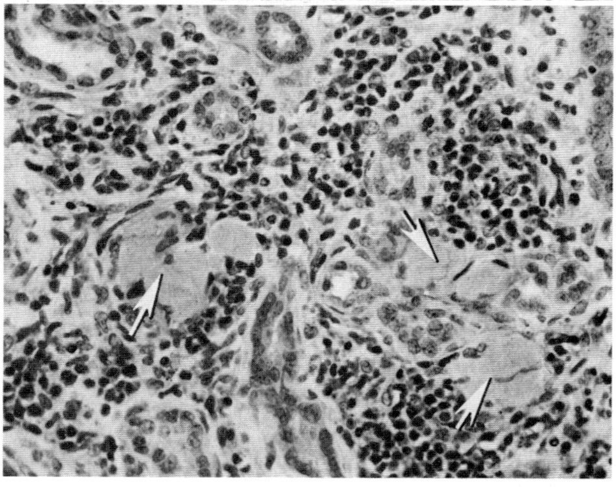

6

Fig. 5. Glomerulus from part of kidney with IRR showing dilated capsular space containing THP (arrow). There is adjacent focus of lymphoid cells in interstitium. Immunoperoxidase technique, counterstained with hematoxylin. × 190. (7 days.)

Fig. 6. Collection of THP (arrows) in relation to interstitial lymphoid cells in refluxing part of parenchyma. Immunoperoxidase technique, counterstained with hematoxylin. × 200. (7 days.)

A second and apparently distinct type of early change was provided by animals which, in the regions of IRR, showed successive dilatation and atrophy of tubules in the medullary rays, a change reminiscent of the changes in obstructive atrophy [8, 9]. Interstitial edema was not such a con-

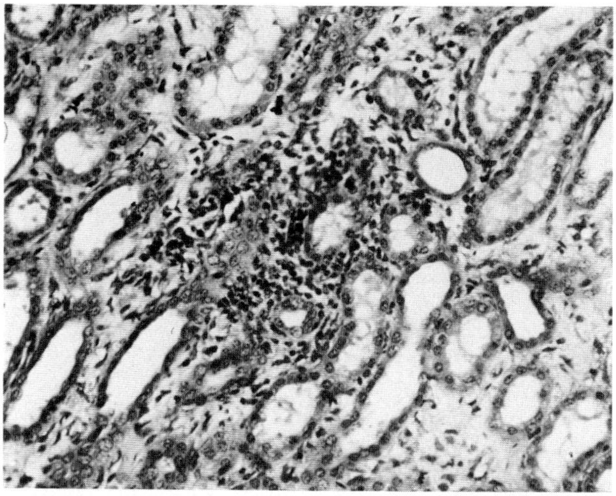

7

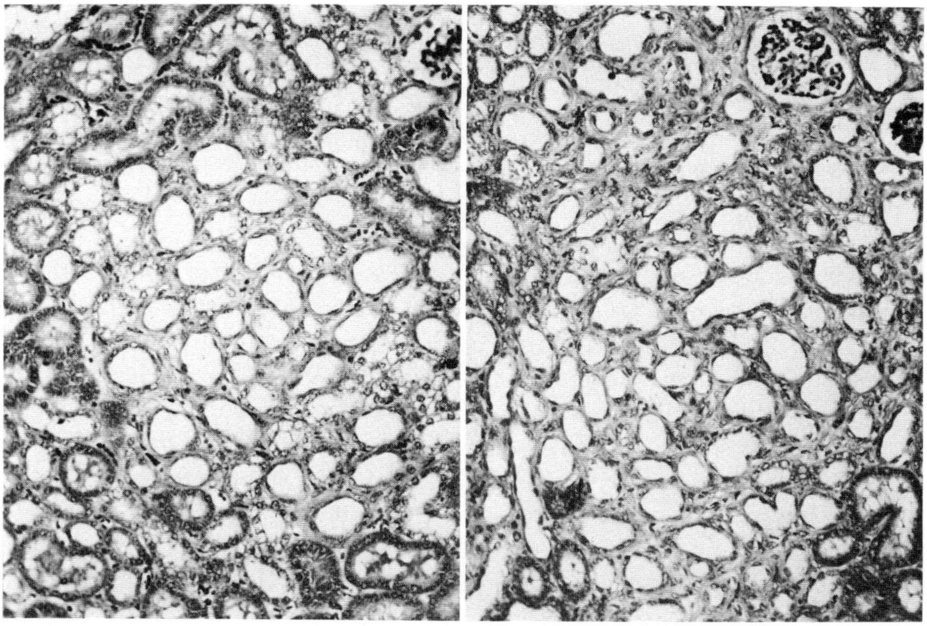

8a b

Fig. 7. Small collection of lymphoid cells in non-refluxing part of kidney. Such areas were very patchy. H&E. × 175. (7 days.)

Fig. 8. a Cross-section through medullary ray to show dilatation of central tubules with early atrophy of proximal convoluted tubules at the periphery. *b* Similar cross section to show increased atrophy of peripheral proximal convoluted tubules. Both sections stained by Masson's connective tissue method. × 150. (14 days.) These changes are identical to those seen in developing obstructive atrophy.

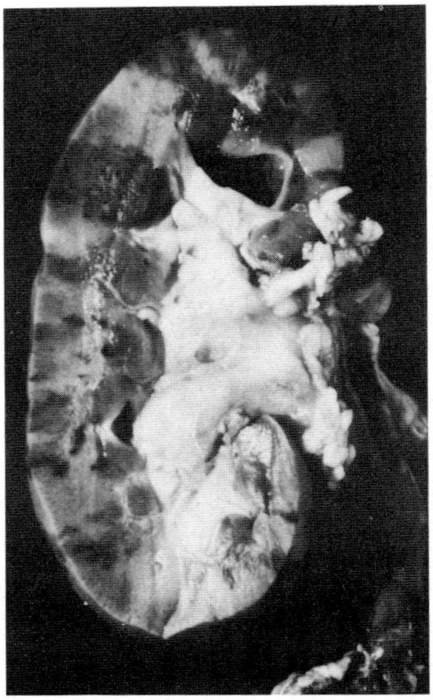

Fig. 9. Bivalved kidney to show developing scars – whitish areas – in areas of intrarenal reflux. There is early generalized calyceal dilatation seen particularly well at the upper pole. (21 days.)

spicuous feature in this type of change. The atrophic tubular changes in the medullary rays were followed by atrophy of proximal convoluted tubules at the periphery of the rays (fig. 8a, b). Fine interstitial fibrosis accompanied these changes. The non-refluxing areas showed little abnormality, although mild tubular dilatation was found in some instances.

A further stage in the evolution of the lesion was found in pigs which showed pale areas (corresponding to zones of IRR) that were either level with, or slightly depressed below, the subcapsular surface compared with the intervening normal tissue where IRR had not taken place (fig. 9). Histologically there was now considerable atrophy and/or loss of tubules, with the appearance of variable amounts of fine fibrosis in the interstitium (fig. 10). Some animals revealed areas with interstitial collections of THP (fig. 11) and a lymphoid cellular reaction which tended to be most marked at the edges of the fibrotic zones. The peripheral distribution of the inflammatory cells raises the question of a progressive lesion in parenchyma surrounding that originally involved by the first effects of IRR. Kidneys from other animals did not show interstitial THP deposits, and had only scat-

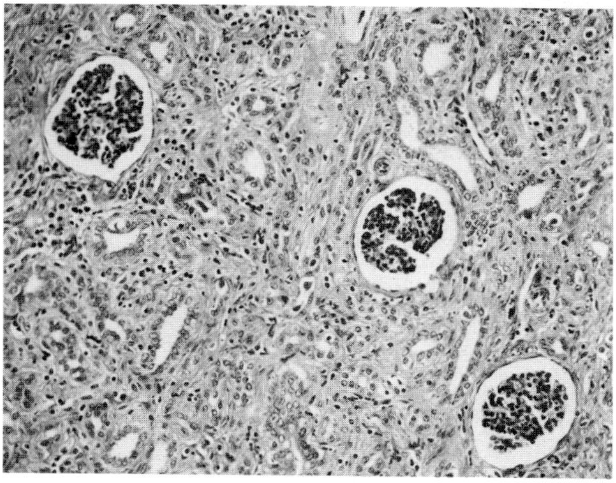

Fig. 10. Cortex from one of pale areas from pig kidney with gross appearance comparable to figure 9. Glomeruli show no change, but the tubules show loss and atrophy of those that remain. Masson. × 155. (21 days.)

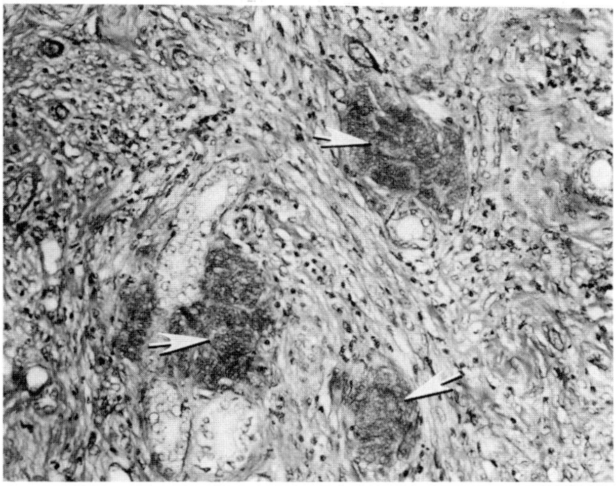

Fig. 11. Collections of THP (arrows) and increased fibrous tissue in developing scar. There is a paucity of chronic inflammatory cells. Gross appearance was similar to that of figure 9. PAS technique. × 160. (21 days.)

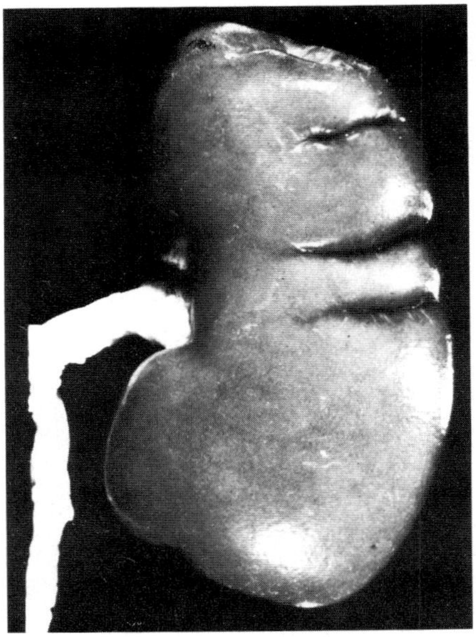

Fig. 12. Kidney which has been subjected to sterile VUR with flat scar at upper pole and 3 slit scars below it. (125 days.)

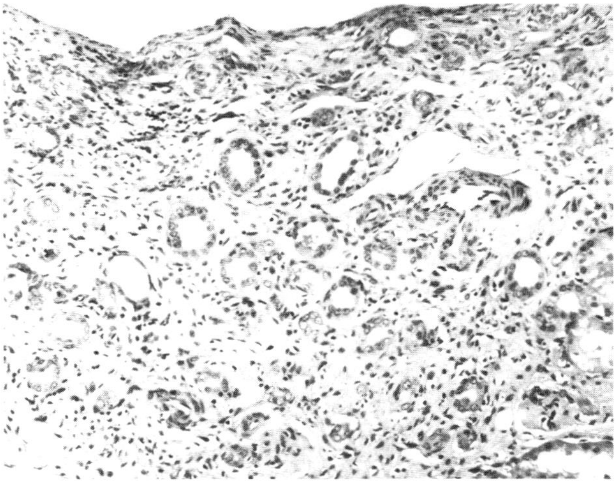

Fig. 13. Flat scar from kidney shown in figure 12. There is glomerular and tubular loss with presence of some atrophic tubules and arteries. Subcapsular surface is at top of picture. H&E. × 135. (125 days.)

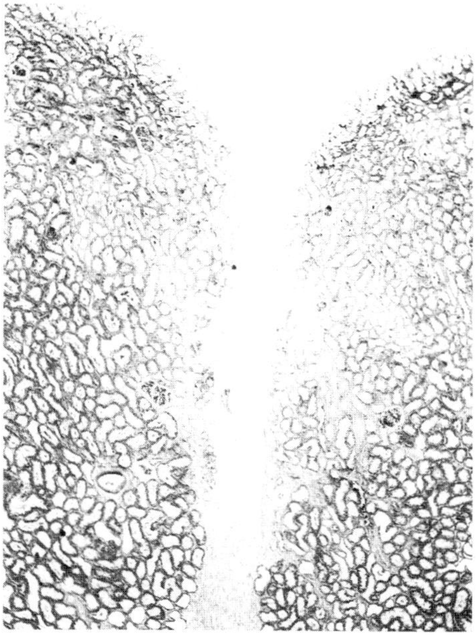

Fig. 14. Section to demonstrate tremendous depth of slit scar. Dense fibrous tissue is present at the bottom of the picture and the scar extends into the kidney substance. Masson. × 28. (125 days.)

tered chronic inflammatory cells in the interstitium. In pigs with more advanced lesions, depressed 'flat' scars were present in the cortex, predominantly at the poles (fig. 12), reminiscent of those in pigs with IRR of infected urine. Tubules and glomeruli had very largely disappeared, interstitial fibrosis was present, and chronic inflammatory cells were scanty or absent (fig. 13). Polymorphonuclear leukocytes were never seen in tubular lumina and it is important to note that this absence was a feature at *all* stages in the development of the sterile scars. THP could still be seen in the interstitium in advanced scar formation, although this was inconstant and the individual collections tended to be smaller than in younger scars. Parenchyma between the scars was usually normal, but in some instances there was dilatation of the tubules, particularly of the collecting ducts, with early tubular atrophy. It is likely that these changes in the non-refluxing areas were brought about by obstruction, because there were varying degrees of dilatation of the pelvis and calyces in all specimens, presumably a consequence of the urethral obstruction.

In addition to the large shallow flat polar scars, elongated slit scars – which were deep and very narrow – were seen in a number of the older specimens (fig. 12, 14). Histologically they were made up of dense fibrous tissue and often contained remnants of glomeruli. They could invariably be traced back to large arcuate and interlobar arteriovenous bundles, where the tail of the scar was continuous with dense fibrous tissue surrounding the artery and vein (fig. 15). In turn, this dense fibrous tissue could sometimes be followed into the renal sinus (fig. 16), where it joined a thick layer of fibrous tissue beneath the urothelium. The slit scars were therefore quite often in continuity with the renal sinus, a point that will be taken up in the Discussion.

The degree of gross papillary damage varied with the period after surgery and, to some extent, on the degree of pelvic and ureteric dilatation. In the most severe acute cases, the papillae were diminished in size but were in no way flattened or retracted. In the chronic cases there was papillary retraction in the scarred areas. This was severe in relation to flat polar scars and confined to the center of the papilla in the case of slit scars.

Discussion

Clearly there are several factors concerned in the production of discrete scars due to VUR of sterile urine in this model. First there is evidence that changes take place comparable to those accompanying urinary obstruction. It is entirely conceivable that repeated episodes of high pressure IRR with a background of chronic obstruction could produce such changes, although the exact pathogenetic mechanism cannot be defined with certainty. Interference with the blood circulation is a possibility, as it is in obstructive uropathy. The tremendous interstitial edema in the early stages of high pressure IRR must have some compressive effect on the intertubular capillaries, and 'splaying' of afferent arterioles by dilated tubules [8] would contribute to the impaired blood supply. Second, the part played by THP or some other constituent of urine from disrupted tubular cells must be considered, because extravasation of THP is a prominent feature in so many of the scars, and because in animal J34 there was a tremendous cellular reaction wherever THP was found it is tempting to invoke an immunologic reaction of either humoral or cell-mediated type. The former of these appears unlikely in light of the inability to demonstrate immunoglobulins, or C3, in relation to the deposits in both this and previous studies

15
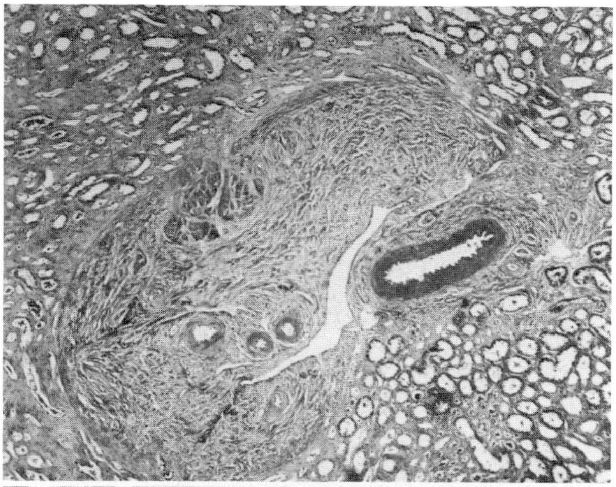

16
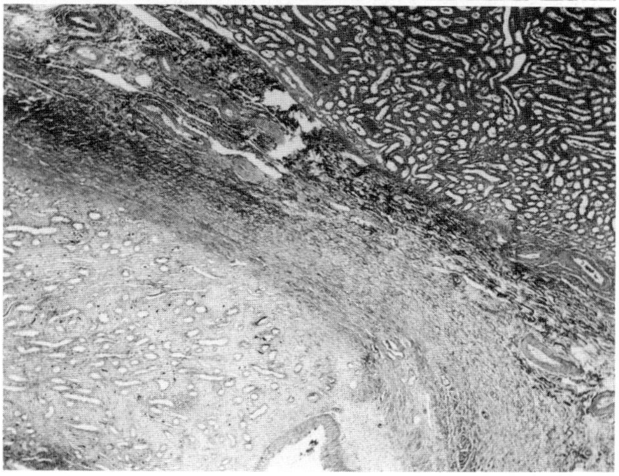

Fig. 15. Dense fibrous tissue surrounding artery and vein. This fibrotic arteriovenous bundle was in continuity with the fibrous tail of a slit scar. Masson. × 45. (90 days.)

Fig. 16. Dense fibrous tissue courses from the renal sinus (bottom right) alongside blood vessels gaining access to the kidney. Septum of Bertin can be seen at top right and part of papilla with calyceal epithelium at bottom left. Masson. × 28. (90 days.)

[10, 11]. In the present investigation IgG was not demonstrated in relation to the deposits although it was present in some of the interstitial inflammatory cells. The other possibility is that cellular immunity is playing a role, and this receives support from the studies of *Mayrer* et al. [12] in the rabbit. There is nothing in the present study that conflicts with this idea, and in pig

J34 the minimal, although definite, cellular reaction in the adjacent, non-refluxing areas of kidney and in the contralateral kidney are quite consistent with it. Its contralateral kidney, as judged by the urographic appearances, was almost certainly subjected to VUR as well as to severe obstruction. The difference in the intensity of change between the zones subjected to IRR and those protected from it is explicable on the grounds of increased pressure projected through the papilla by IRR. It is not clear from this study how commonly such a cell-mediated immunologic mechanism is likely to occur, and how important a contribution it makes to the renal damage.

Lastly, note should be taken of the slit scars and their relation to dense fibrosis around arteries and veins entering and leaving the kidney from the renal sinus. It is insufficiently appreciated that arteries entering the renal substance carry with them a connective tissue sheath derived from the lining of the renal sinus, and that it is within this sheath that the dense leashes of lymphatics course toward the hilus. This provides a route by which urine, forced into the kidney during high pressure VUR, can gain access to the interstitial space [13] and from there to the renal lymphatics going to the hilus in one direction, and to the subcapsular lymphatics in the other. It is of great interest in this context that in J34 and other animals with a less severe cellular reaction, the appearance of the focal interstitial cellular reaction was often first noted in the neighborhood of blood vessels and was followed by an increasingly dense fibrotic reaction. It is thus tempting to suggest that some strongly immunogenic substance is entering the interstitial space and then being borne away by the lymphatic system which it eventually enmeshes and obliterates. The resulting perivascular fibrosis is likely to have a significant effect on the blood supply to surviving areas attempting to undergo hypertrophy.

In conclusion, the sterile focal scarring in this pig model is in the same distribution as the scarring resulting from IRR of infected urine in pigs. In some animals there is an acute lesion which occurs as the result of IRR, lasts as a focal swelling for 10–15 days, and then undergoes increasing contraction until few parenchymal elements remain, apart from arteries of varying sizes. In other animals in the early stages, a mechanism akin to obstructive atrophy appears to be at work in the areas of subjected to IRR; interference with the blood supply is the probable pathogenetic mechanism in these. There is evidence to suggest that diffuse fibrous encasement of the arterial system in the affected zones may be a major factor in the pathogenesis of the subsidiary scarring, i.e. slit scars. The role of possible immunologic mechanism in the genesis of sterile scarring is yet to be clarified.

References

1 Hodson, C.J.; Maling, T.M.J.; McManamon, P.J.; Lewis, M.G.: The pathogenesis of reflux nephropathy (chronic atrophic pyelonephritis). Br. J. Radiol. *13*: suppl., p. 1 (1975).
2 Hodson, C.J.; Maling, T.M.J.; McManamon, P.J.; Lewis, M.G.: Reflux nephropathy. Kidney int. *8*: suppl. 4, pp. S50–S58 (1975).
3 Ransley, P.G.; Risdon, R.A.: Reflux and renal scarring. Br. J. Radiol. *14*: suppl., p. 1 (1978).
4 Hodson, C.J.; Edwards, D.: Chronic pyelonephritis and vesicoureteric reflux. Clin. Radiol. *11*: 21 (1960).
5 Ransley, P.G.: The renal papilla. Intrarenal Reflux and Chronic Pyelonephritis. Zurukzoglu, Papadimitrious, Pypasopolulus, Simon, Zamboulis, Proc. 8th Int. Congr. of Nephrology, p. 363 (Karger, Basel 1981).
6 Cotran, R.S.; Hodson, C.J.: Reflux nephropathy, p. 213 (Masson, New York 1979).
7 Sternberger, L.A.; Hardy, P.H.; Cuculis, J.J.; Meyer, H.G.: The unlabeled antibody enzyme method of immunohistochemistry: preparation and properties of soluble antigen-antibody complex (horseradish peroxidase-antihorseradish peroxidase) and its use in identification of spirochetes. J. Histochem. Cytochem. *18*: 315 (1970).
8 Rao, N.R.; Heptinstall, R.H.: Experimental hydronephrosis. A microangiographic study. Investve Urol. *6*: 183 (1968).
9 Hodson, C.J.; Craven, J.D.; Lewis, D.G.; Matz, L.R.; Clarke, R.J.; Ross, E.J.: Experimental obstructive nephropathy in the pig. Br. J. Urol. *41*: 5 (1969).
10 Resnick, J.S.; Sisson, S.; Vernier, R.L.: Tamm-Horsfall protein: abnormal localization in renal disease. Lab. Invest. *38*: 550 (1978).
11 Zager, R.A.; Cotran, R.S.; Hoyer, J.R.: Pathologic localization of Tamm-Horsfall protein in interstitial deposits in renal disease. Lab. Invest. *38*: 52 (1978).
12 Mayrer, A.R.; Kashgarian, M.; Ruddle, N.H.; Marier, R.; Hodson, C.J.; Richards, F.F.; Andriole, V.T.: Tubulointerstitial nephritis and immunologic responses to Tamm-Horsfall protein in rabbits challenged with homologous urine or Tamm-Horsfall protein. J. Immun. *128*: 2634 (1982).
13 Bhagavan, S.B.; Wenk, R.E.; Dutta, D.: Pathways of urinary backflow in obstructive uropathy: demonstration by pigmented gelatin injection and Tamm-Horsfall uromucoprotein markers. Human Pathol. *10*: 669 (1979).

Robert H. Heptinstall, MD, Department of Pathology, The Johns Hopkins University School of Medicine, Baltimore, MD (USA)

Contr. Nephrol., vol. 39, pp. 358–369 (Karger, Basel 1984)

27. The Time Factor in the Development of Sterile Renal Scarring following High-Pressure Vesicoureteral Reflux

C. John Hodson, Susan A. Twohill

Yale University School of Medicine, Department of Diagnostic Radiology, New Haven, Conn., USA

Introduction

Kidney Size Changes – Focal and General

The observations outlined below are based on the radiographic identification of changes in kidney size, both focal and generalized in distribution. Their definition depends on the renal contours being made visible by a dense nephrogram – resulting from the rapid i.v. injection of a large 'bolus' of contrast medium (0.5 ml/kg of 50% contrast) together with a 4-day bowel preparation of nourishing fluids to get rid of 'background' gas and faeces.

The normal 'elasticity' of the kidney allows of a 15–20% increase in size during diuresis [1] and a decrease, as much as 40%, following a drop (80–100 mm) in blood pressure [2]. These are acute changes which occur over a period of minutes. The slower changes resulting from normal growth, hypertrophy, scarring, etc., occur over periods of months or years, and have been minutely documented [3–7]. The miniature pig used in this study shows a normal renal growth rate in the region of 2–3 mm/week during the first 6 months of life. The effect of contrast-induced diuresis may be as much as a 3–4 mm in kidney length. Frequent monitoring by serial intravenous urograms (IVUs) provides a realistic means of assessing kidney size. The normal nephrogram is seen uniformly throughout the kidney (fig. 1), and zones of diminished function can be identified by a 'negative' nephrogram (fig. 2, 3).

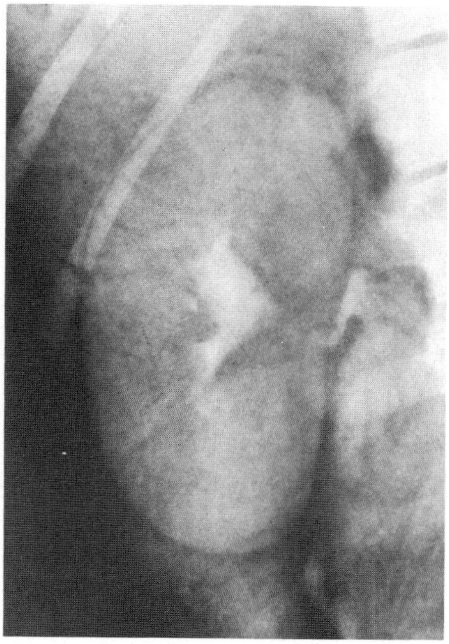

1

Fig. 1. Example of normal nephrogram in miniature sow. 10 min film of right kidney 34 days after surgery.

Fig. 2. a IVU 40 days after surgery. Arrows point to two bulges from kidney surface with negative nephrogram (NN) in mid-zone. No hydronephrosis. *b* Same animal 29 days later. The two NN zones are now recessed. (Note shrinkage also of upper pole [overlain by gas in *a*]). See also figure 4a.

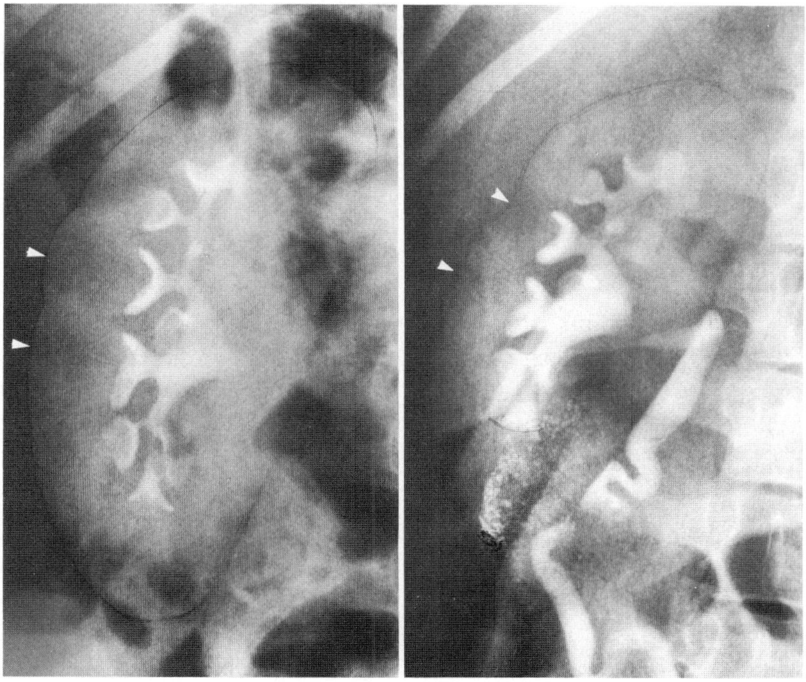

2 *a* *b*

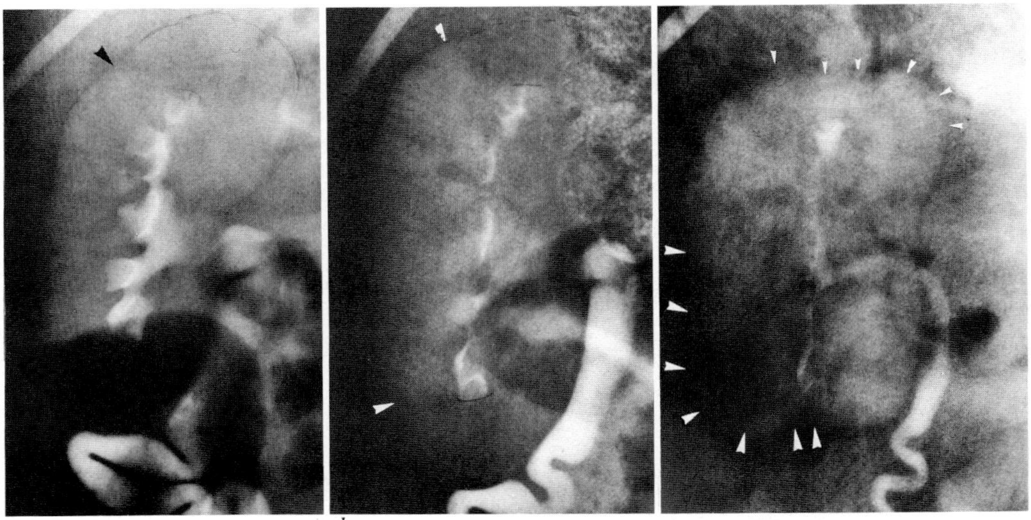

a b c

Fig. 3. Another example of focal absence of nephrogram with affected zones progressing to severe scar formation. *a* Nephrogram lost in upper pole (arrow shows edge of lesion) 39 days after surgery. *b* IVU 14 days later shows early shrinkage of both poles (arrows show zone edges). *c* Advanced bipolar scarring 2 weeks later – 9.5 weeks after surgery. See also figure 4b.

Experimental Model

The 3 programs from which the following observations are derived employed the same basic model [8]. In a Hormel miniature swine piglet (sow), 4–6 weeks old, one or both ureteral orifices are rendered incompetent by incising their anterior intravesical wall over a distance of 5–8 mm through a small anterior cystotomy opening. After bladder closure, a silver wire, omega-shaped, device ('ring') is placed around the proximal urethra, its internal diameter (3–3.5 mm) making it a loose 'fit' in sows of this age. As the animal grows the ring becomes increasingly obstructive, the bladder wall hypertrophies, voiding pressure increases and later bladder capacity increases also, until these compensatory propulsive forces fail, and the whole system dilates. Meanwhile, immediately following surgery or within

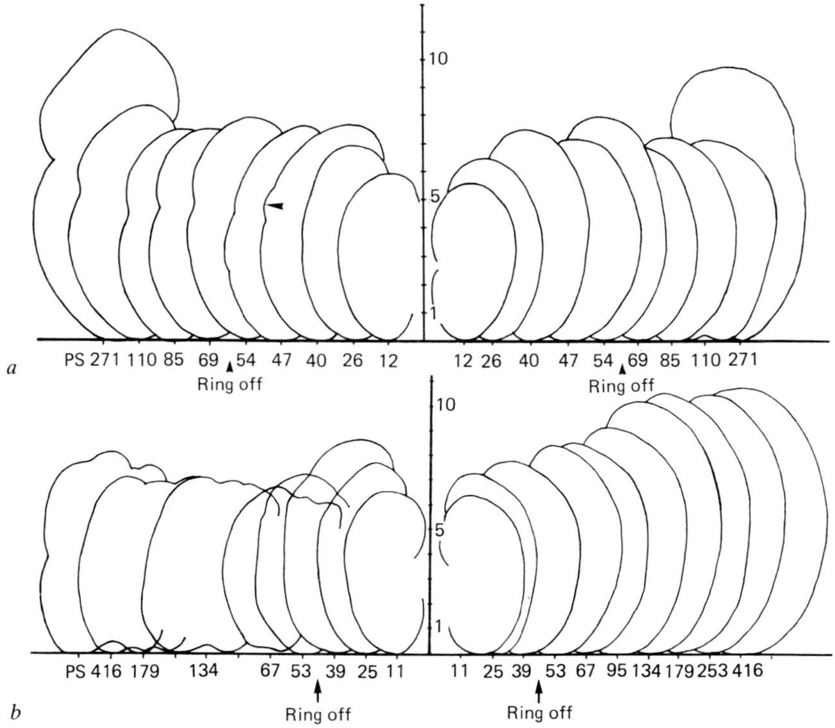

Fig. 4. *a* Tracings of serial IVUs of sow (fig. 1) showing size increases with age and onset of acute lesion (arrow head) with subsequent course of events. Autopsy showed slit scars in both poles and mid-zone of right kidney. *b* Tracings of IVUs of same sow as figure 3 showing size increase at time of acute lesion 39 days after surgery and subsequent severe bipolar scarring. PS = Days after surgery. Length in cm.

a few days, vesicoureteral reflux (VUR) occurs and, together with the bladder background pressure, gives rise to ureteral dilatation and tortuosity. Later still (1–4 weeks), intrarenal reflux (IRR) occurs and, finally, the renal pelvis commences to dilate and the parenchyma to become thinner. It is commonly at this stage that the focal lesions with which this article is concerned appear, together, usually, with a sudden overall increase in the size of one or both kidneys. Serial IVUs (with the 4-day fluid preparation mentioned above) every 2 weeks, and every week after the bladder enlarges and projects from the lower abdomen, monitor the march of events. In the last 2 programs and in some animals in the first, maintenance antibiotics were continued until autopsy, or until after the 'ring' had been removed and free urethral flow reestablished.

In the last one, cystography and cystometry were omitted because (a) they added no further information than was already known about this model, (b) they involved a very real risk of introducing infection, (c) once a high-pressure situation develops any bladder puncture can give rise to leaking into either the peritoneal or retroperitoneal 'spaces' (fig. 5b).

After a period following initial surgery, a sudden dramatic increase in kidney size was documented in most animals and is illustrated by the tracings in figure 4. One or both organs are involved in this swelling (often the untouched ureter may be refluxing by this time) and if a dense enough nephrogram is obtained and the abdominal preparation good enough, focal, bulging, zones with negative 'nephrograms' may be seen, usually on the right (operated) side. These are commonly in the two polar regions, but may sometimes be in the mid-zone. They, therefore, correspond to the classical areas of IRR and on three occasions have been shown to be the sites of IRR. After an interval, the swollen areas shrink back to, and later become recessed in relation to, the kidney border. They are still without contrast on IVU and eventually turn into scars, of the same distribution as uninfected cases (fig. 2, 3).

These acute lesions admittedly were thought at first to represent the onset of infection ('acute lobar nephronia') as focal negative nephrograms are common to both [9, 10] but, as in consecutive animals scheduled for a long-term follow-up, the urine remained sterile and their general condition good, they were used as an indication for ring removal, and no kidney specimen was obtained until much later when advanced scarring was already present. So we went back to the radiographs and records of our previous series, where several sterile kidney specimens with different ages of scarring were available, and in 5 were able to match these up with radiographs of satisfactory quality.

Finally, 1 animal died during anesthesia for an IVU, and autopsy showed sterile urine and large acute lesions mainly in both poles of the right kidney (fig. 5a). Its general condition had been good, its blood chemistry was normal (BUN 7 mg/100 ml, creatinine 0.7 mg/100 ml), and its last IVU, 2 days before, (fig. 5b) showed moderate ureteral dilatation and tortuosity with minimal, if any, pelvicalycine changes (scarcely a gross situation by any stretch of the imagination!). Histology of the specimen showed none of the very obvious stigmata associated with infection in this model. We therefore set out to obtain more specimens of this lesion, and to document their natural history, using both past and future data.

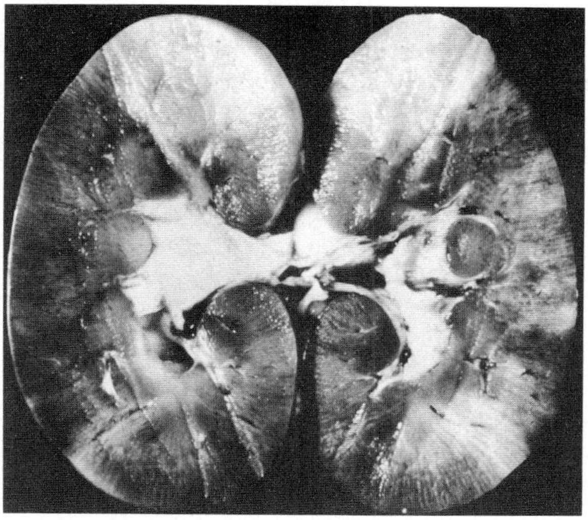

5a

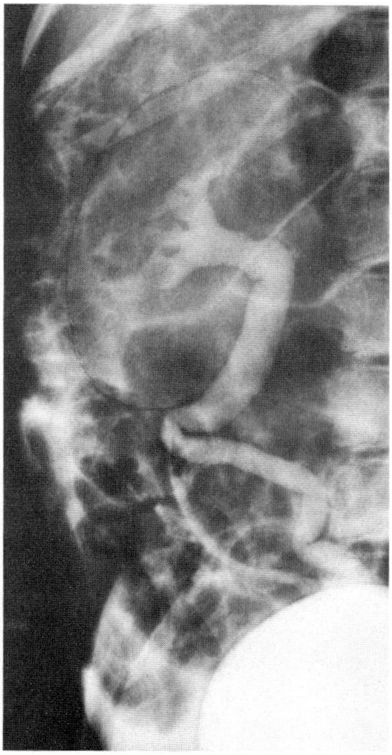

b

Fig. 5. *a* Acute sterile reflux nephropathy (23 days after surgery) showing distribution. Urine specimen sterile. Note distribution is mainly polar but scattered in other zones and minimal, if any, papillary flattening. Lesion less than 1 week old. *b* IVU of fig. 5a, 2 days before death, shows degree of ureteral and pelvic dilatation and extensive intraperitoneal extravasation of contrast medium due to leaking from bladder puncture to obtain urine specimen for culture. Such leakage occasionally occurs in high-pressure situations.

Table I. Estimate of time factors of radiographic evidence of kidney damage

Pig No.	Age at surgery days	Ring size	Ring off days post-surgery	Estimate age of radiographic evidence					
				A	B	C	D	E	necropsy
B-2	39	tape (12F) RUO	–	15–20	–	38	66	46	66
B-5	51	tape (12F) RUO	–	?	?	28	–	–	43
C-29	56	4 mm, RUO	123	109	–	119	145	36	197
C-35	33	3.5 mm, RUO	74	35	–	73	110	38	198
C-41	45	3.25 mm, RUO	–	55	–	–	–	–	79
C-49	138	4 mm, bilat.	47	–	–	46	–	–	48
C-51	145	4 mm, bilat.	–	36	–	–	–	–	45
J-5	51	3 mm, RUO	–	6	–	–	–	–	77
J-6	51	4 mm, RUO	–	14	–	–	–	–	23
J-22	61	3 mm, RUO	56	26	40	47	85	45	957
J-23	70	3 mm, RUO	39	25	39	48	53	14	–
J-24	73	4 mm, RUO	45	25	39	53	67	28	–
J-26	70	3 mm, RUO	32	32	43	69	92	49	954
J-34	53	3 mm, RUO	–	77	–	–	–	–	77
J-36	44	3 mm, RUO	–	59	78	–	–	–	88
J-37	44	3 mm, RUO	–	51	–	–	–	–	51
J-38	58	3 mm, RUO	–	64	–	–	–	–	73

A = Sudden size increase; B = focal nephrogram defect with bulge; C = focal nephrogram with early recession; D = focal nephrogram with moderate recession; E = age of established scars, i.e. D–A or B; necropsy = days after initial surgery; RUO = right ureteric orifice incised.

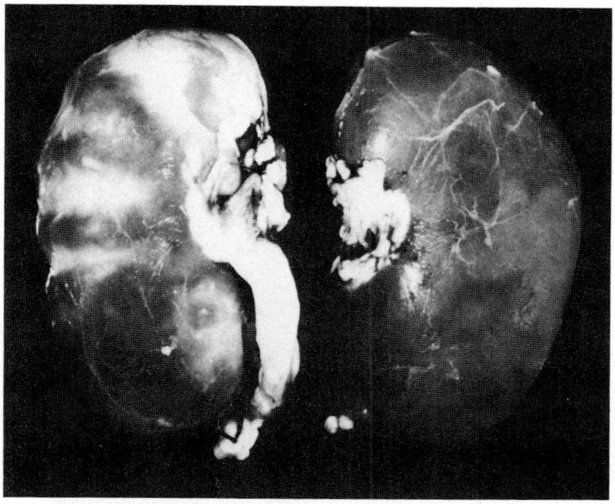

6a

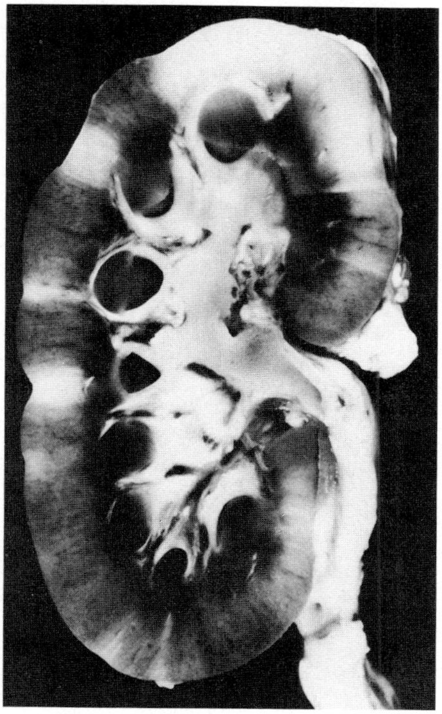

b

Fig. 6. a Sterile RN. Specimens of right and left kidneys showing early shrinkage of multiple scars of right kidney 77 days after surgery, but scars only 3 weeks old. *b* Cut surface of same specimen shows early hydronephrosis and damage (pale areas) to some papillary tips.

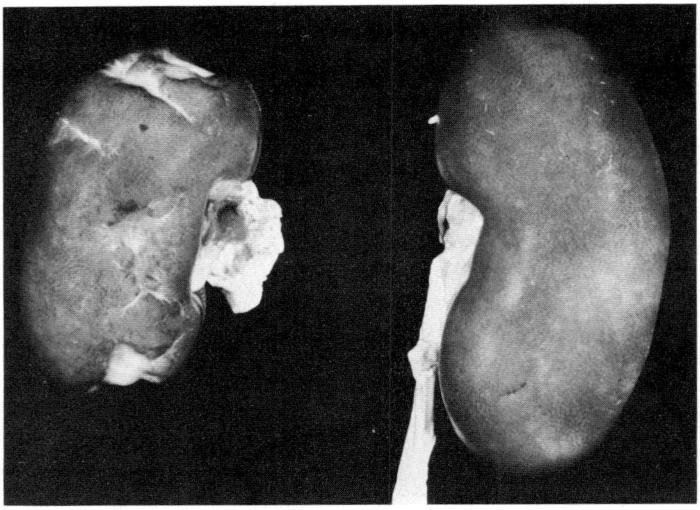

Fig. 7. Sterile RN. 'Classical' bipolar 'flat' and mid-zone 'slit' scars in right kidney 398 days after surgery. Left kidney macroscopically normal.

Materials

From our original program, 5 kidney specimens were obtained within 80 days of surgery. All of these came from animals in which the urethra was still obstructed at autopsy. 2 further animals had their ring removed and provided late scar specimens, the estimated ages of which were 88 and 124 days.

In the present program 2 animals were terminated with their rings still on. 4 others showed good radiographic changes, had their rings removed, and could then also be followed until scarring was advanced. In the final 4 animals, rings were again left on until autopsy (or the day before it, in one instance).

Results

These are from 17 animals. They are partly illustrated in table I and figures 2–8. These include (1) progress up to a sudden size change (Nos. J5, J6, J22, J24, J34), (2) acute focal lesion onset, (3) acute lesion subsiding, (4) early scarring data, and (5) late (3 months or more) scars.

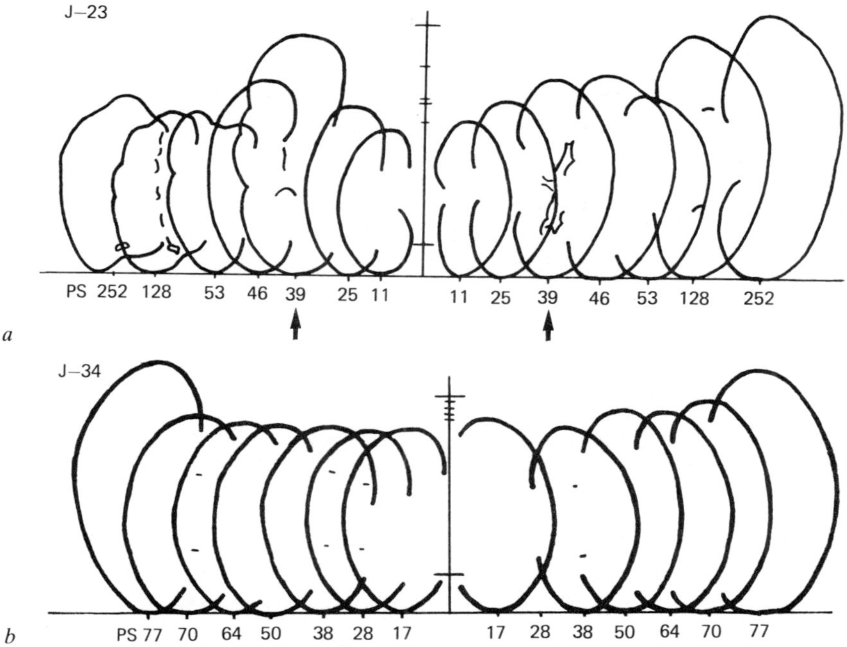

Fig. 8. Further IVU serial tracings. *a* Shows dramatic size increase of right (operated) kidneys 39 days after surgery, followed by severe bipolar scarring. *b* IVU tracings of J-34, a sow with a marked cellular reaction. Both kidneys grew normally until the 10th week after surgery, then suddenly increased in size. Minimal cellular reaction in left side (non-operated). Arrows indicate when ring was removed.

Discussion

If sterile renal damage results from severe VUR in early infancy and early childhood, it presupposes a high-pressure situation commencing either in utero or within the first few days, weeks or months of life. At the time of writing there is, however, very little clinical evidence in support of this idea. But, it is a fact that few people are presently interesting themselves in this particular facet of the clinical problem in this age group and, so far, those that are, are still largely involved in methodology, and are only just commencing to achieve any data. Whereas, in the experimental field, there seems to be a reluctance to aim for really high pressure states, as they are thought to be unrealistic. Nevertheless, what clinical data are already available in this age group no longer rule out the concept of very high bladder pressures indeed (> 200 cm H_2O) due to non-organic obstruction. It is argued that these could only represent a very small fraction of children with VUR but, even if this is so, they are the worst of the spectrum, with a very poor prognosis, and this is no reason why they should be disregarded. So much attention is being paid presently to rare disease in childhood it seems irrational that this group, or even this possibility, be neglected. One has only to review how many chapters in this book terminate, to appreciate that there is a general realization among most of those concerned with this disease that the age category in which the real problems present is early infancy – say the first 6 months of life.

And to what does the experience outlined in our pigs add up? Firstly it reflects a hydrodynamic situation which is a mixture of obstruction and VUR; one in which bladder pressure, once the bladder wall has lost some of its compliance (mainly due to fibrosis of its musculature), does not return to a normal baseline between voiding acts. Instead it maintains an increased pressure which is continuously reflected back up into the upper tract. If strong bladder contractions are superimposed on this background (and peak pressures of over 70 cm H_2O were recorded in 2 of these animals, both before and after ring removal [8] then the situation becomes very similar to that in boys with posterior urethral valves, or neurogenic bladders.

Furthermore, once the ureteral propulsive mechanism is overcome and similar fibrotic changes occur in the ureteral walls, dilatation and incomplete (and therefore inefficient) contraction of peristaltic waves result, and these high pressures are transferred directly to the now unprotected kidney tissue.

It is under these conditions, which can develop within a month of the onset of the obstructive situation in this model, that the acute lesions may develop. A month later they are well on the way to advanced scarring, without any functioning tissue left within them, and only a future of further scarring. If this state of affairs is comparable with what happens in the human infant it may be only a matter of 3 months from the onset of a serious bladder detrusor muscle-external urethral sphincter dysfunction until severe permanent renal damage could result.

The time factor is, in fact, of the utmost importance because, as we showed in our original publication on this subject in 1975 [8], gross *generalized* damage of this type (not of obstructive nephropathy, which is a very much milder disease by comparison [11]) may occur in a matter of weeks, and may affect all papillae, simple or compound, with IRR and lead to what we recognize as the generalized or 'obstructive' form of reflux nephropathy.

References

1 Dorph, S.; Pigaard, A.: Variations in renal size in the diagnosis of renovascular hypertension. Br. J. Radiol. *46*: 181–190 (1973).

2 Hodson, C.J.: Physiological changes in size of the human kidney. Clin. Radiol. *12*: 91–94 (1961).

3 Effman, E.L.; Ablow, R.C.; Siegel, N.J.: Renal growth. Radiol. Clins N. Am. *15*: 3–17 (1971).

4 Claesson, I.; Jacobsson, B.; Olsson, T.; Ringertz, H.: Assessment of renal parenchymal thickness in normal children. Acta radiol. (Diagn.) *22*: 305–314 (1981).

5 Claesson, I.; Jacobsson, B.; Jodal, U.; Winberg, J.: Early detection of nephropathy in childhood urinary tract infection and unilateral renal scarring: an epidemiological study. Acta radiol. (Diagn.) *22*: 315–320 (1981).

6 Eklof, O.; Ringertz, S.: A method of kidney size measurement in children. Acta radiol. (Diagn.) *17*: 617–625 (1976).

7 Hodson, C.J.; Davies, Z.; Prescod, A.: Renal parenchymal radiographic measurement in infants and children. Pediatr. Radiol. *3*: 16–19 (1975).

8 Hodson, C.J.; Maling, T.M.J.; McManamon, P.J.; Lewis, M.G.: The pathogenesis of reflux nephropathy (chronic atrophic pyelonephritis). Br. J. Radiol. suppl. 13 (1975).

9 Rosenfield, A.T.; Glickman, M.G.; Taylor, K.J.: Acute focal bacterial nephritis (acute lobar nephronia). Radiology *132*: 553–561 (1979).

10 Hodson, C.J.: Neuhauser lecture. Reflux nephropathy: a personal historical review. Am. J. Roent. 137: 451–462 (1981).

11 Hodson, C.J.; Craven, J.D.: Experimental obstructive nephropathy in the pig. Br. J. Urol. *14*: suppl. 6, pp. 3–57 (1969).

C. John Hodson, Yale University School of Medicine, Department of Diagnostic Radiology, 333 Cedar Street, New Haven, CT 06510 (USA)

Contr. Nephrol., vol. 39, pp. 370–375 (Karger, Basel 1984)

Discussion on Chapters 25–27

Dr. *P. Kincaid-Smith*: One of the statements made in these papers was that sterile scars have little clinical relevance. It seems to me, with my preconfirmed ideas about reflux nephropathy (RN) in the male, that in fact these sterile scars might be very relevant, because many of our male patients who progress to end-stage renal failure in the late teens or early twenties have never had urinary tract infection (UTI), or at least none that we can document. Perhaps we can start out with the question of whether sterile scarring has clinical relevance?

Dr. *J. Hodson*: Well, I have always been the first to admit that our pig model has one weakness and that is that it is the product of a single progressive state which has to be terminated or else the pig will go into bladder failure and expire. One can remove and later try and reapply urethral constriction, but this doesn't work too well.

The difference between this situation and that which obtains in the child – assuming we are talking about children – is that this progressive state only faithfully imitates boys with severe posterior urethral valves. But most recent research (chapters 16–19) into the pressures found in children below the age of 5 appears increasingly to indicate that there are functional disturbances which are much more common than hitherto suspected, and which achieve just as high bladder pressures. And as it seems to be pressure which is the factor that is driving sterile urine into the kidney, then any high-pressure situation, e.g. the neurogenic bladder, will have the same effect. So I completely discount this idea that there is no clinical relevance and will go on discounting it, because I've actually seen it happen twice following spinal cord trauma in the absence of documented infection in adult patients on continuous chemotherapy.

I have also seen at least 5 children with the radiologic criteria of generalized damage and severe vesicoureteral reflux who had never had a history or the symptoms of UTI; and remember, it is mainly children with symptomatic UTI who have been shown to develop RN. Thus, I believe this pig model is highly relevant to certain prescribed clinical situations.

Dr. *P. Ransley*: I must disagree with you. I think that if we are considering RN in its proper context, namely children with either dysfunctional voiding or primary VUR, which is an enormous pool of patients, that the sterile lesions are in no way relevant to this population. I believe there are only two clinical situations in children to which it they relate. The first is posterior urethral valves with the associated complication of dysplastic renal development, where any renal changes and any ultimate renal failure are properly a reflection of that primary dysplasia. VUR occurring after birth is of little relevance once you remove the obstructive lesion. It behaves just like the pigs do when you remove the urethral obstruction.

The other situation is the neuropathic bladder. It could possibly simulate the bladder decompensation type of situation. The problem here, in clinical practice, is that 99% of these children get UTIs.

Dr. *P. Kincaid-Smith*: Do children with urethral valves always have what you call dysplastic kidneys? Don't they sometimes just have an obstructive-looking picture? Presumably, if they are operated on they might end up with kidneys that look very much like these pig kidneys because they have already developed sterile RN.

Dr. *P. Ransley*: Not all babies with urethral valves have VUR. Some only reflux on one side. When this occurs the bad kidney is on that side. The general tendency of these kidneys, after removal of the urethral valves is either to stay the same or to improve. If one removes a kidney in early childhood one only does so if it is severely damaged and, in general, these kidneys show renal dysplasia. If one leaves the kidneys, bilateral VUR will occur and the patient end up in chronic renal failure in his early twenties. He does so, probably not as a consequence of continuing VUR in childhood, but because the natural history of the few nephrons he has left which, by the time he reaches the age of 15, develop nephron hyperperfusion and, probably, proteinuria from secondary glomerulopathy.

Dr. *P. Kincaid-Smith*: But presumably the lesions he had originally were like the acute lesions in the pig model, they are thus the basic problem.

Dr. *P. Ransley*: But they commence in utero. We musn't get confused between the cause of dysplasia and the consequence of high pressure VUR.

Dr. *J. Winberg*: Shouldn't we discriminate between the two things, the experimental model that these two groups have used and its underlying pathology? It may be that the circumstances of the model occur very rarely in childhood, but the effects, namely the forcing of urine into the parenchyma, might perhaps occur in other situations. I would like to ask, do these findings mimic any other clinical situation? The only thing I can think of clinically that would compare to this would be the Ask-Upmark kidney. I would like to ask if these lesions are similar to those found in the pig.

Dr. *J. Hodson*: This very point was discussed extensively at our previous workshop. The answer is, 'yes'. Lesions exactly identical to the Ask-Upmark one are commonly found in the advanced state.

Unless they are infected no pus casts are found in the tubules in the pig model. That is perhaps the most notable feature, but there are several others which enable a distinction to be made between the infected and the uninfected lesions. To emphasize something that was said before, and which came through more and more clearly as one looked at the progressive picture that Dr. *Risdon* was describing, and that is that it is only in the more advanced stages of the acute scars that one begins to see the peculiar histological cellular reaction. This fits in with both Dr. *Heptinstall*'s and my conception of the delayed hypersensitivity reaction. Inflammatory cells are not a feature of the early stages of 'scarring'. It is only when a certain stage in the progress of events is reached that the cells appear. We believe this represents a delayed hypersensitivity reaction and once this stage has been reached events proceed inevitably to total necrosis of the affected tissue, the results being either the 'flat' polar or 'slit' mid-zone scar.

Dr. *T. Risdon*: I'm not prepared to accept an immunological basis for this lesion without some concrete evidence in favor. I mean the cellular reaction doesn't impress me at all. I regard this as a marker of urinary extravasation. There are a large number of other things in urine that might elicit an inflammatory response other than Tamm-Horsfall protein (THP).

Dr. *J. Hodson*: But I'm not talking about THP, I'm talking about the cellular reaction.

Dr. *T. Risdon*: Well, what about it?

Dr. *J. Hodson*: I pointed out that it only developed in your sterile pigs in the older scars.

Dr. *T. Risdon*: It was only a marked feature in one, the change in which was perhaps a couple of weeks old. It wasn't a big feature in the others.

Dr. *J. Hodson*: So can I pin you down now? You do not believe that this is a delayed sensitivity reaction?

Dr. *T. Risdon*: I don't have an opinion about it. I don't think there is anything like enough evidence one way or the other. I'm not an immunologist but it seems to me that if there is either a cellular or a humoral antibody reaction directed against THP, why doesn't it attack THP in the other distal tubules as well?

Dr. *J. Hodson*: Perhaps I should once more attempt to clarify our viewpoint in this matter. We are not claiming that THP is necessarily the chief antigen responsible for what we believe to be an immunologic reaction, although a number of workers have shown it to have antigenic potenial. We regard its presence outside the nephron as a reliable sign of recent tubular disruption and interstitial spillage. I have always been at pains to point this out. In fact, in the animal in which the cellular reaction was most marked, there are interstitial THP deposits surrounded by large aggregates of cells in some areas. In others THP deposits occur without any such cells, and yet again large aggregates of cells are present without evidence of THP. Finally, there is no sign of cellular aggregates around those parts of the nephron where THP normally occurs in any part of either kidney, such as was demonstrated by *Mayrer* et al. [Tubulointerstitial nephritis and immunologic responses to Tamm-Horsfall protein in rabbits challenged with homologous urine or Tamm-Horsfall protein. J. Immun. *128*: 2634–2642, 1982] in their rabbits inoculated with rabbit urine. So that the accumulated evidence is against the concept of THP being a major factor in the causation of the inflammatory reaction at this stage.

Dr. *P. Avis*: About the question of delayed hypersensitivity, I wish we could settle this issue. It does seem to be a type of inflammatory reaction, as Dr. *Hodson* has said, and not necessarily associated with THP at all, but possibly with other sorts of debris that have accumulated as a result of the destruction of the tubular cells. The intracellular material alone could quite well elicit an inflammatory response.

Dr. *P. Kincaid-Smith*: Can I just get back to this question of the timing of it. The implication from your slides was that there was a sudden increase in the size of the kidneys; and if you looked at them, at that time, they showed the reaction. That's correct, isn't it?

Dr. *J. Hodson*: That's correct, two of them did, once they had been swollen for 2–3 weeks. Three others, swollen for only 1–2 weeks, did not show any cells. So that one does not yet know what part the time factor plays, or whether the commonly occurring period of obstruction following original surgery is needed to 'prime' the animal for an immune response, or whether other factors are needed. It becomes obvious to everybody who works with these animals that there is no means of predicting almost any of the events which follow surgery. If one fits urethral constricting devices of exactly the same size on 2 pigs from the same litter, and the operation appears to be a technical success in both instances, one of them may start quickly to show the effects of VUR; and the other may take a much longer time. It is impossible to say, unless one makes use of some means of monitoring such as the elevation of serum THP to say exactly when this whole process of renal damage is to be expected.

Dr. *P. Ransley*: I must disagree. That was the importance of the 3 animals we described in whom there was unequivocal change in the dimercaptosuccinic acid (DMSA) scan in the course of a week, from normal to abnormal. The DMSA scan does indeed give us the ability to tell when an area of renal parenchyma stops working.

Dr. *J. Hodson*: Well, we have similarly demonstrated bipolar avascular lesions in pigs using glucoheptonate which, on microscopy show only oedema and no cellular reaction. In no way could these lesions be predicted or called 'scars', although they may later develop into what I demonstrated. Personally, I don't believe true scarring can develop in 3 weeks in a sterile situation, on simple pathological grounds. But I was speaking about prediction at the start of an experimental series.

Dr. *P. Kincaid-Smith*: It seems to me to favor an immunological reaction.

Dr. *R. Bailey*: I would like to reiterate a comment made by Dr. *Kincaid-Smith*, namely that in those patients who progress to end-stage renal failure from RN one of the notable features, both in our own experience and in the literature is the absence of UTI as a major clinical problem.

In the pig in which there was a florid cellular reaction to sterile internal renal disruption sesondary to intrarenal reflux (IRR) and just an oedematous acellular swelling in the other kidney, why couldn't that just be a straight immunological effect without VUR or obstruction? Secondly, what do you feel is the aetiology of the slit scar?

Dr. *R. Heptinstall*: I think the reason, Dr. *Bailey*, why you probably need reflux into the contralateral kidney, is that you have to have a target against which the sensitized T cells can be directed. As for the slit scars I cannot be absolutely certain, but it is apparent that something is happening in the connective tissue framework which accompanies arteries and veins as they enter in or leave the kidney. It is possible that the fibrosis present in relation to arteries and veins could be due to extravasation of urine with an attending reaction. The continuity of a slit scar all the way down to the fibrosis in the renal sinus is a very conspicuous feature.

Dr. *P. Kincaid-Smith*: This is essentially the same explanation we proferred in Bermuda in 1978 [*Kincaid-Smith and Hodson*, Reflux nephropathy, Masson, New York 1979]. I can only say that to me the more recent work only tends to make the idea of a 'toxic' substance more plausible – something in the nature of an antigen of some sort.

Dr. *R. Heptinstall*: This may be how the slit scars form, but how do you explain this continuity of extremely dense fibrous tissue from the base of the scar out into the renal sinus?

Dr. *P. Kincaid-Smith*: We used to refer to this as the 'concrete' fibrosis, it was so hard to cut. Well, I also have ideas about it, but I don't think we can say any more yet. From my study of the pig kidneys it looks as though the drainage pathways from these areas of IRR (which later form the scars) was out through the capsular lymphatics, giving rise to a lot of fibrosis there, and also down the perivascular lymphatics where there is another lot of fibrosis. These two amount to the main lymphatic run-off pathways. I also assume this is a reaction to whatever the substance is that causes the collagen, as it drains away from the damaged kidney.

Dr. *P. Ransley*: In the pig model one usually only sees sterile scars in a decompensated urinary tract which is dilated throughout. So one now has to define the role VUR plays in this situation. I believe sterile urine under certain circumstances can result in scarring. I just don't think it is terribly relevant to the clinical situation.

Dr. P. Kincaid-Smith: Apart from urethral valves, which you obviously don't think much of, what about paraplegics with spastic bladders which have been mentioned?

Dr. *P. Ransley*: I think that condition is certainly a possibility, where these data are relevant.

Dr. *S. Koff*: I was puzzled by the fact that in the pig model the kidney damage didn't appear to occur when the voiding pressures were high but rather only after they were lowered as the result of bladder decompensation. I think that the answer may be that measurement of *bladder* pressure may be very misleading as a reflection of *renal pelvic* pressure during VUR in a normal non-dilated system. Actually, VUR in these circumstances does not transmit pressure directly, it only transmits volume. Not until the upper urinary tract becomes distended will bladder pressure be transmitted to the renal parenchyma. Consequently, in a dilated or distensible system, such as would occur in the pigs who are voiding normally but under high pressure, the latter may not be directly transmitted to the kidneys during VUR. But, at a later date, when the bladder decompensates and the upper tract remains overly distended, the bladder pressure will be continually transmitted to the kidneys and produce damaging effects.

The relationship between bladder pressure and renal pressure during reflux is very similar to the discussion held yesterday regarding bladder pressure during voiding cystourethrograms. At that time we indicated that the pressure in the bladder is independent of the height of the infusion reservoir during bladder filling. The pressure in the bladder is simply a function of the volume in the bladder at any point in time, and determined by a characteristic pressure volume curve. Changes in the height of the reservoir do not directly affect the bladder pressure, they simply change the rate at which fluid is transmitted to the bladder. Only when the flow stops are the reservoir and bladder pressures identical. Since the renal pelvis is a hollow viscus entirely analogous to the bladder, the pressure representations in the two systems are similar, and it is easy to see why renal pelvic pressure does not always equate with bladder pressure during VUR. Consequently that may make the model clinically relevant since, as the bladder commences to decompensate and the ureteral capacity increases and stays increased, the distensibility is lost and high pressure or higher pressures will be transmitted.

Dr. *J. van Gool:* I would also like to make a similar comment. We have all assumed that bladder pressure can be transmitted to the kidney pelvis when there is VUR. That is not necessarily so. One condition for such transmission is that there must not be any flow down the ureter. If the refluxing urine meets urine flowing into the bladder then there is no pressure increase in the ureter. When on the other hand, the ureter is widely dilated, pressure would be readily transmitted from the bladder to the renal pelvis because the compliance of a wide dilated system is very large and any pressure change will be accommodated by a volume change in that system.

Another thing that I didn't understand from Dr. *Ransley's* paper was how a decompensated bladder could still generate a high pressure. In my experience a decompensated bladder is one that is totally incapable of generating pressure anymore.

Dr. *M. Dillon:* As partially representing Dr. *Smellie*, I think she would want me to say at this moment that in her large experience of sterile refluxing children over many years, sterile VUR has in general *not* been associated with progressive scar development, or with impaired renal growth, and in only those children in which UTIs have been documented has scarring developed.

Dr. *W. Asscher:* Another clinical situation in which sterile scarring has happened in the past – and it doesn't now so often – is following retrograde pyelography. When that is performed by the inexpert, too forcibly, a sterile scar can sometimes develop later.

As regards Dr. *Smellie's* cases, it must be remembered that all her children initially presented with infection, although for years most of them remained uninfected. This brings me to the infected scar and how quickly absolute commitment to the formation of a scar occurs. Drs. *Ransley and Risdon* showed that they could prevent scarring in pigs if they started antimicrobial chemotherapy after 7 days of the onset of infected VUR. That surprised me a little because in our rat model we showed that *E. coli* are injected into the rat cortex, antimicrobial chemotherapy has to be commenced within 16 h in order to prevent scar formation, and this corresponds exactly to the appearance of monocytes on the scene. There is some evidence now of the interactions of *E. coli* and monocytes producing fibrogenic factors which may well determine scar formation.

Dr. *P. Ransley*: In half of our pigs, there was no sign of renal parenchymal involvement after 1 week. All animals showed parenchymal involvement after 2 weeks.

Dr. *R. White*: I want to speak to this question of the role of UTI in VUR. I have no doubt whatever from the experimental evidence that in the human being the pressure from posterior urethral valve obstruction, if it is severe and has existed for 6 months by the time the baby is born, there has been ample time for sterile IRR to occur and set up a scarring process. And I think that immature nephrons may respond to that pressure in a slightly different way than fully mature ones and so produce what we call 'dysplasia'.

Dr. *Bailey* asked earlier what was the history of these patients who turn up in chronic renal failure with bilateral VUR and no evidence of UTI. I think it is very easy to obtain a positive diagnosis of UTI but difficult to be sure that there has been no UTI previously. I can quote an example, a child that came into my care at the age of about 3 or 4 in terminal renal failure and shortly died of gross bilateral VUR. At the time we were keen on screening populations for UTI and the parents asked for their 2 other children to be screened. 1 of them had UTI, and a scarred kidney with VUR. We have observed many, many times that children who are without VUR will have recurrent UTIs. Once they reach puberty the latter cease. So your young adult in this situation may well have had UTIs as a child and got over them. I think one has to take this into account. It also seems to me that in the clinical situation, there is overwhelming evidence that UTI plays a part in the whole of this matter primary VUR.

Contr. Nephrol., vol. 39, pp. 376–377 (Karger, Basel 1984)

Closing Remarks

Priscilla Kincaid-Smith

I have a few closing remarks to make. I would like to thank the Kroc Foundation very much indeed for their generosity in allowing us this meeting in such a delightful place and looking after us so well. *John Hodson* has also asked me to make some remarks about the content of the meeting and I have been making voluminous notes, from which I've got some points I think are worth making.

In the experimental field the controversy about sterile reflux causing scarring, is now resolved. Dr. *Hodson* of course has always believed in it. Dr. *Ransley* and his group have now also demonstrated sterile scars. Another thing in the experimental field that has been re-emphasized at this meeting, is the importance of high pressures.

The Tamm-Horsfall protein (THP) story is still, in my mind, a little unclear, and we might have to wait 3 or 4 years before we sort out exactly what is the significance of THP and its antibodies. I personally still have doubts that it plays a major role in the pathogenesis of scarring.

I think one of the most important experiences described at this meeting was the benign course in the follow-up study of asymptomatic bacteriuric schoolgirls reported by Dr. *Verrier Jones*. It is all very well to say that patients run a benign course if on antibiotics for the rest of their lives (or even throughout childhood). It is a very different matter to be able to say that they also have a benign course when they are reporting only at 3-monthly intervals and then being treated only when symptomatic. This provides a much more realistic and economic way of managing these girls. I really don't consider that satisfactory conservative management should include urine tests and antibiotics on a regular basis. The major argument in favour of surgery is that it may obviate the need for regular visits of this type but its final answer as an alternative treatment has *not* yet been clarified fully. On the other side of the coin is the small population of adults that both Dr. *Bailey* and myself have identified who get worse even when their disease is apparently strictly unilateral. Which, in my opinion, may point to the fact there are many more people with reflux nephropathy (RN) than can be diagnosed on radiographic evidence. Perhaps the most important thing that has emerged on the clinical side is the great advance in radionuclide tests which will help both in the diagnosis and follow-up of our patients, and also provide another means of individual renal function tests.

Other exciting developments are the reports on controlled trials of surgery versus conservative management that are in progress. The Birmingham study is well on the way. It includes a large number of patients, and I think we can look forward to hearing really meaningful answers from it quite soon. Dr. *Bailey* has told us more today of the progress of the well-known group of infants originally described from Christchurch, New Zealand.

Finally, I just want to try to extrapolate from what we now know as to the overall incidence of RN in the population as a whole. I still consider that only a small proportion progress to end-stage disease. A calculation 4 years ago suggested that only 1 in 5,000 cases with RN progress to end-stage renal failure. Working on the basis of the published numbers per million of the population with this diagnosis who pass into end-stage renal failure, and the bacteriuric screening studies in girls and women (and I know of no studies in men to indicate how common vesico-ureteral reflux is among the male population) it seems to me that the chance of progression to end-stage renal disease is closer to 1 in 1,000 for any patient with reflux nephropathy.

It is obvious that the age at which diagnosis must be made is infancy. I still believe that perhaps the best hope so far for a screening test in infancy may lie in the THP field. I'm afraid I don't know what, but that's the impression I got from the meeting.

Appendix

Contr. Nephrol., vol. 39, pp. 378–382 (Karger, Basel 1984)

Evaluation of Home Monitoring for Bacteriuria in Children

George T. Klauber[a], *Edwin M. Meares, Jr.*[b]

[a]Tufts New England School of Medicine and Department of Pediatric Urology, New England Medical Center, Boston; Charles M. Whitney Fellow Professor of Urology Chairman, [b]Division of Urology, Tufts University School of Medicine and Department or Urology, New England Medical Center Hospital, Boston, Mass., USA

Introduction

There is considerable need for a simple and reliable method of detecting urinary tract infection (UTI) in children. Those with recurrent UTI may be at risk of developing pyelonephritis and kidney damage, especially when there are associated structural abnormalities [1]. Careful surveillance, especially of infants, is therefore mandatory. Home screening for UTI in infants has been successfully used [2, 3]. A culturing program for children with recurrent UTI using a roll-tube device was reported by *Fennell* et al. [4]. Home culturing has the advantage of availability of a first morning urine specimen and avoids the problems associated with delay of transporting samples to the laboratory.

This report covers our experience with a home urine culture kit in a study to evaluate the efficacy of such a program.

Subjects

75 consecutive children in whom data suitable for analysis was obtained were included in this study between July 1981 and March 31, 1982. Their ages ranged from 2 months to 14 years. Indications for home urine cultures were clean intermittent catheterization (CIC) in 34, vesicoureteral reflux (VUR) in 23, recurrent UTIs in 17, and neuropathic bladder (NB) in 3 (3 children on CIC also had VUR).

Table I. Results of home and office cultures for UTI showing false positive rate

	Positive	Negative	Kits used
Home	272[1]	1,846	2,118
Office	125	426	551
Total			2,680

Positives duplicated by laboratory	False-positives
229[2]	(5)[3]

[1] 98 home cultures negative upon repeat 87 pairs of positive HUCKs.
[2] Includes 125 positive office cultures and 174 positive home cultures and excludes home cultures negative on repeat.
[3] Appearance totally unlike kit colony density chart (4 yeast and 1 fungus).

Materials and Methods

Urine was collected in a U-bag urine collector in infants and a clean dixie cup in older children [1]. Cultures were plated on a 'Uri-quick' home urine culture kit (HUCK). The kit consists of a hinged clear plastic box containing cystine-lactose, electrolyte-free medium plus a special inoculating swab. The swab dispenses the same amount of urine as a standard 0.01-ml loop. Parents were trained in the use of the HUCKS without any problems. The HUCKS were incubated at room temperature for 24 h after which time *Escherichia coli* and *Klebsiella* changed the medium color to yellow, and *Proteus* to blue. Colony counts can be obtained by comparing HUCK to a colony-density chart supplied with the kit.

2,118 HUCKS were used in the home. A second series of 551 HUCKS were evaluated in the office. 272 positive home cultures and all the office cultures were duplicated in the laboratory.

Protocol for the home urine culture study was as follows: (1) An early morning urine specimen was cultured on Sunday and only the HUCK retained. (2) 24 h later the HUCK was read. Negatives were discarded. Positives were treated as follows: (a) Color change and colony count were recorded and the HUCK preserved in a refrigerator. (b) A repeat urine specimen was obtained in a sterile container, the Uri-quick culture was repeated and the container saved in a refrigerator. (c) 24 h later the Uri-quick was read and, if positive, a second sterile specimen obtained and both sterile specimens and Uri-quicks were transported on ice to our laboratory. If negative, the Uri-quick was discarded and repeated 24 h later until either two negative cultures on successive days or two positive cultures on successive days were obtained. The entire cycle was repeated on a weekly basis.

Table II. Results of home and office cultures for UTI showing false negative rate

Office cultures	Negative		False-negative
551	416		8 + (2)
False-negative cultures	>50,000		Numbers
Staph. epidermidis	100,000	bacteria/ml	2
Enterococcus	100,000	bacteria/ml	4
Enterococcus	80,000	bacteria/ml	1
Enterococcus	50,000	bacteria/ml	1
False-negative cultures	<50,000		
Enterococcus	40,000	bacteria/ml	1
Enterococcus	10–30,000	bacteria/ml	1

No other false-negatives with as many as 10,000 bacteria/ml.

Results

2,118 HUCKS were used by parents. 272 were positive. Of these positives, 98 were negative upon repeat culture. Thus, 87 pairs of positive HUCKS were transported to our laboratory (table I).

551 office cultures were duplicated using Uri-quicks and laboratory techniques. There were 426 negative HUCKS and 125 positives.

299 positive HUCKS were duplicated by the laboratory and 5 false-positives were obtained. Appearance of the false-positives were totally unlike true-positives. 4 were due to yeast and 1 to fungus and neither demonstrated the discrete scattered colonies of the true-positives (table I).

False-negatives were obtained in 8 of 416 negative office Uri-quicks. False-negatives were defined as missing a colony count in excess of 50,000 in duplicated laboratory culture. *Enterococcus* was responsible in 6 cases and *Staphylococcus epidermis* in the remaining 2. 2 additional false-negative cultures with colony counts of less than 50,000 *Enterococcus* were also noted but not considered significant. No other false-negatives with as many as 10,000 bacteria/ml were obtained (table II).

Organisms identified in 299 positive HUCKS are listed in table III; *E. coli* being responsible for 40%.

The use of antibiotics is listed in table IV. 22 children remained on antibiotic prophylaxis throughout the study. 39 remained off antibiotics and 14 children were initially off them but were later changed. 6 children on CIC received 1–3 courses of antibiotics for 7 days. A number of other children had transient UTI which subsided spontaneously and did not require antibiotic therapy.

Table III. Organisms identified in 200 positive HUCKs

E. coli	120
Enterococcus	59
Pseudomonas	38
Proteus sp.	25
Klebsiella	25
Acinetobacter	16
Citrobacter	12
Staph. saprophyticus	11
Staph. epidermidis	4
Serratia	3
Flavobacter	2
	315[1]

[1] Multiple organisms in some cultures.

Table IV. Use of antibiotic in study population

	ALL	CIC	VUR	RUTI
Remain off antibiotic	39	21[1]	5	7
Initially off but changed	14	7	1	6
Prophylaxis throughout	22	6	17	4
Totals	75	34	23	17

ALL = 75; RUTI = recurrent urinary tract infection.
[1] Includes children with transient bacteriuria, and 6 children who received 1–3 courses of antibiotics for 7 days.

Conclusions

HUCKS were found to be a reliable and simple method for UTI surveillance and screening. HUCKS are an inexpensive and convenient alternative to laboratory urine cultures, also an inexpensive alternative to antibacterial prophylaxis for some children. They provide a useful method of studying the natural history of UTI, especially in children on CIC whether on and off antibiotics.

Urine cultures can be used for subculturing and sensitivity testing. Such sensitivities are obtainable within 48 h of original plating; a similar length of time to conventional urine culture sensitivity testing. This is a decided advantage over chemical tests for the detection of bacteriuria.

As little as a few drops of urine suffices for an accurate Uri-quick culture. This is an advantage over dip slides which require a greater volume of urine.

References

1 Smellie, J.M.; Normand, I.C.S.: Experience of follow-up of children with urinary tract infection; in O'Grady, Brumfitt, Urinary tract infections. Proc. 1st National Symp., pp. 123–138 (Oxford University Press, London 1968).

2 Randolph, M.F.; Woods, S.E.; Hodson, C.J.; Klauber, G.T.: Home screening for the detection of urinary tract infections in children. Am. J. Dis. Child. *133*: 713–717 (1979).

3 Randolph, M.F.; Hodson, C.J.; Woods, S.E.; Redys, J.J.; Cope, J.B.: Home screening for urinary tract infections in children. Am. J. Dis. Child. *135*: 122–125 (1981).

4 Fennell, R.S.; Austin, S.; Walker, R.D.; Garin, E.H:, Pryor, N.D.; Sorgen, C.D.; Richard, G.A.: Home culturing program for children with recurrent bacteriuria. Am. J. Dis. Child. *130*: 501–503 (1976).

George T. Klauber, MD, Chief of Pediatric Urology, New England Medical Center, Boston, MA 02111 (USA)

Subject Index